A Nurse's Survival Guide to Critical Care
First Updated Edition

T0200569

At Elsevier, we understand the importance of providing up-to-date and relevant content. For this reason, we are continuously working on updated editions and new titles for the Series. Please visit our website to find out the latest news and the upcoming publications: https://www.uk.elsevierhealth.com/

A Nurse's Survival Guide to Critical Care

First Updated Edition

Sharon Edwards EdD SFHEA NTF MSc DipN(Lon) PGCEA RN
Senior Lecturer, Faculty of Society and Health,
Buckinghamshire New University, Uxbridge, UK

Joyce Williams RN BSc (Hons) MSc PGCert FHEA
Senior Lecturer, Faculty of Society and Health,
Buckinghamshire New University, Uxbridge, UK

ELSEVIER

Edinburgh London New York Oxford Philadelphia St Louis Sydney 2019

ISBN: 978-0-7020-7654-1

Printed in Poland
Last digit is the print number: 9   8   7   6   5   4   3   2   1

Content Strategist: Serena Castelnovo/Poppy Garraway
Content Development Specialist: Kirsty Guest
Project Manager: Anne Collett
Design: Amy Buxton

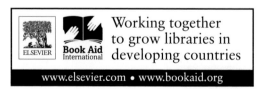

Working together
to grow libraries in
developing countries

www.elsevier.com • www.bookaid.org

Contents

Section 2
Patient Assessment and Investigations 95

Section 4
Common Conditions/Reasons for Admission

Preface

The aim of this book is to provide an insight into the critical care arena and highlight the important physiological, psychological and social areas, alongside ensuring safety in practice and emphasising legal issues and ethical and moral dilemmas that health care practitioners may face on a daily basis. This book does not profess to be the sole textbook of choice within critical care but to act in a supportive and informative way to the novice critical care practitioner and provoke further reading and use of current reading literature within the speciality.

The book, written by experts in the field as practitioners and educators, will help bridge the theory-practice gap by underpinning current knowledge and ensuring that an understanding is gained before starting your critical care placement or embarking on a career in critical care. In view of the fact that critical care is now opening up to all disciplines, the book is aimed not only at student and qualified nurses but also at student and qualified midwives, operating department practitioners, paramedics, physiotherapists, medical students and occupational therapists. The objective is that, as multi-disciplinary team members in the decision-making process within critical care, these professionals will engage in developing a better insight into the working environment. Cue question boxes have been inserted throughout the book so that discussion and thought processes may be stimulated and promote the inquisitive side of the health care professional.

For most people, the critical care environment will seem daunting and complex, embedded in sophisticated language and high technology, but for those of us who have spent a number of years in critical care, it is a homely, friendly and supportive place. We aim to put this across in our book and help open the doors to a wonderful and extraordinary speciality and in turn empower you to spend a number of years uncovering, understanding and enjoying this specialist area. Our focus is on the patient and not the technology; we aim to put across that the critical care practitioner looks after the patient and uses the technology to assist this important role, rather than vice versa.

Sharon Edwards
Joyce Williams
Buckinghamshire, 2019

Section 1

General principles of critical care

Section Outline

1.1 INTRODUCTION TO CRITICAL CARE NURSING

For some, critical care areas may be a daunting prospect, and there are many issues that you may want to know prior to going to critical care. You may also have many concerns that you would like to discuss prior to going there. This book will attempt to answer some of the questions you may have.

A critical care area is a specially staffed and equipped ward, dedicated to the management of patients with life-threatening illness, injuries, or complications. Some critical care areas are also designated for the prevention of complications or the reduction of their severity.

Remember that — even though you may not know it — there are skills you already have that you can use in critical care. Think of a skill that you have undertaken in clinical practice, and the knowledge you have gained as a student, and maybe now as a qualified member of staff. These will all equip you and prepare you for your critical care experience.

Critical Care Layout

Due to the very nature of critical care, the requirements of the department may vary from hospital to hospital. Factors such as whether the environment is purely intensive care based, coronary care or a high-dependency unit will play an important role in the overall layout. Storage space, sluices, laboratory facilities, equipment room, staff restroom, changing rooms, offices and family facilities should all be catered for within this specialist environment.

However, it is most important that the department is kept clean, tidy, safe and compliant with current building regulations. Each bed space should have adequate electricity supply, emergency supply in the event of power failure, medical gases, suction and hand washing facilities. The critical care environment should also have adequate daylight, with an external view if possible. This plays an important role in orientation, psychological and mental status for the critical care patient. Adequate communication systems, for example, telephones, computers and X-ray facilities, should be available to aid and support patient care.

The size of the critical care unit will be dependent on the needs and specialities available at that hospital. Some hospitals will mix specialities such as coronary care and high dependency, and other hospitals will keep them quite separate. In mixed critical care environments, it is fair to say that those patients who require ventilation should be separated from those who require coronary and high-dependency care. Often this is not possible but should be achieved where it is possible.

Communicating with Patients in Critical Care

Communicating with the critical care patient is essential but difficult due to the often one-way direction of the interaction. However, both verbal and/or non-verbal communication is used whether the patient is conscious or unconscious. Communication is a vital psychological activity of daily living, which is as important maintain as physical support.

Patients often express dissatisfaction with communication during their hospital stay, which relates to the quality and amount of information received and to insufficient, confusing and contradictory information being given by different health care professionals. By giving active communication, health care professionals can speed up recovery and reduce the number of complications and the need for more pain relief or sedation.

In critical care, the development of verbal skills, the giving of information and the additional use of listening skills are insufficient on their own. The bedside nurse needs to increase proficiency at monitoring and interpreting non-verbal cues from critically ill patients who are unable to communicate verbally, which may be due to their physical condition, such as breathlessness, intubation or pain.

Effective Communication

The communication pathway between patient and health care professional is probably the most important factor in minimizing patient anxiety in critical care; therefore, it is important that patients are spoken to regardless of their conscious state. Patients may be at risk of developing serious complications in critical care (see Section 5.1), and a risk assessment may need to be undertaken to identify the communication barriers (Table 1.1). Reassurance and explanations are two major components in alleviating anxiety; furthermore,

TABLE 1.1 Communication barriers within critical care.

Potential problem	
Distortion of message delivery	• Noise • Poor/bright lights • Vibration • Temperature
Distractions	• Other surrounding activities • Competing messages
Patient issues	
Psychological	• Perception altered by drug therapy and/or underlying pathology • Motivation and interest in message • Attitude/values/beliefs • Emotions/mood • Intelligence • Self-image

Physical	• Conscious level
	• Sensory deficits
	  • Hearing
	  • Sight
	  • Movement
	  • Sensation
	  • Speech
	• Constraints to movement
	• Pain

Social	• Language • Culture/lifestyle • Isolation

communication is not just about telling the patient what has happened and what is about to happen, but more about understanding the patient's fears and promoting assurance and comfort.

Methods of supportive or alternative communication:

• Mouthing
• Writing
• Facial expression
• Gesture
• Pointing
• Communication charts
• Computer-assisted aids

The Nursing Hand-Over

At the beginning of each shift, in most critical care units, a general nursing hand-over takes place whereby all staff from the previous and next shift are present. At the end of this general hand-over, a nurse will be allocated to a particular patient for that shift. At the patient's bedside, the current nurse will give a detailed hand-over to the nurse taking over about their care, treatment, drug therapy, next of kin and so on, the purpose being to ensure that information relevant to that patient's care is provided and thus minimize any disruption in patient care and uphold continuity of care. Typically, during this process, the bedside nurse uses a universally used structure that reiterates the care plan format, thus incorporating the patient's bedside observations, nursing, drug and medical charts.

At the initial phase of each hand-over, the nurse begins by giving a basic overview of the following list:

- Patient's age
- Past medical history
- Reason for admission
- Length of stay in critical care
- Major events that have occurred during admission
- Physical, psychological and social status

The checklist in Table 1.2 uses a systems approach to a routine hand-over that critical care nurses may be able to follow at the bedside. It is important to note that whichever care plan or additional structure is used, as a health care professional, you must familiarize yourself with, understand and implement your care accordingly.

Care Planning for Critical Care Patients

Within critical care, a daily nursing care plan is produced. Khandelwal et al. (2015) identified that advanced care planning in intensive care unit (ICU) can reduce length of stay in critical care. Thus, care planning is an important part of care in the critical care environment. Care planning should involve a systematic patient assessment, which is carried out at the beginning of the day shift or on patient admission; goals of care and a report is then written at the end of the shift regarding whether the aims and objectives have been met. The night staff will then re-evaluate the patient's planned care and write a report at the end of their shift. The structure and choice of care plan may vary depending on the critical care area in which you are based. This might include follow the structure of a nursing model, standardized care plans, electronic health care records. It is important to note that whichever care plan is used, as a health care professional, you must familiarize, understand and implement your care accordingly.

TABLE 1.2 Bedside hand-over information.

System	Information
Respiratory	• How is the patient's airway managed? • What size is the tracheal tube (COETT)? What is its cuff pressure? What is the length of the COETT at the lip? • What size is the tracheostomy tube? What is its cuff pressure? Is it fenestrated or non-fenestrated? How often is the inner tube being cleaned/replaced? • What mode of ventilation is the patient receiving? What is their FiO_2, respiratory rate? • If they are mechanically ventilated, what are the settings, e.g., minute volumes, PEEP, tidal volumes, pressure support? • What are the patient's arterial blood gas results? Are they stable? • What is the patient's air entry like? • Is the patient receiving any respiratory therapy, e.g., nebulizers? If so, type and how often? Reason for therapy? • Is the patient having chest physiotherapy? When did they last have any treatment? • Is the patient coughing spontaneously? Is it a strong cough? • Give details of the type of sputum being produced. Is it easy to suction? • Are there any chest drains present? Are they draining, swinging or bubbling? Is there any suction attached? Length of time in situ? Details of insertion? Are there any plans to remove them? • When was the patient's last chest X-ray? What were its findings? • What changes in treatment have been made during your shift that could affect the patient's respiratory system? • Have they been reviewed and by whom?
Cardiovascular	• What is the patient's heart rate and rhythm? Is it controlled with drug therapy? • Is the patient's heart being paced? If so, how? • Is the patient receiving anticoagulation therapy? If so, what was their last coagulation screen? • What is the patient's electrolyte balance? Have they or do they need supplementing? • Is the patient's blood pressure stable? What are the mean arterial blood pressure (MAP) ranges? Is their blood pressure being supported with any form of vasoactive drugs? Are they receiving any colloid fluids? What was their last full blood count results? • What is the patient's central venous pressure? Has any treatment been prescribed to increase or decrease the pressure? • What is the patient's body temperature? What mode of measurement was used? Are any steps being taken to actively control their temperature? • What changes in treatment have been made during your shift that could affect the patient's cardiovascular system? • Have they been reviewed and by whom?

Continued

TABLE 1.2 Bedside hand-over information.—cont'd

System	Information
Pain and sedation	• Is the patient complaining of pain? If they cannot communicate verbally, are there any symptoms that indicate that they might be experiencing pain, e.g., agitation? • Is the patient receiving analgesia? If so, does it appear to be effective? • Are there any other methods being used to alleviate pain and discomfort, e.g., repositioning, communication? • Is the patient receiving a sedative or muscle relaxant? If so, how is it being delivered? • What is the patient's sedation score? Is this score acceptable? • What changes have been made to the patient's pain and sedation treatments during your shift? • Have they been reviewed and by whom?
Neurological	• Are the patient's pupils equal and reacting to light? • Are they opening their eyes spontaneously? If not, what stimulation is required? • What form of motor response are they manifesting? Is this normal? • What form of verbal response are they manifesting? Is this normal? • Is any specialist care required to support the patient's neurology, e.g., positioning, drug/ventilation therapy? • What changes in treatment have been made during your shift that could affect the patient's neurological system? • Have they been reviewed and by whom?
Hydration and nutrition	• What type of fluids is the patient receiving? • What is their fluid balance? • What is their target fluid balance parameter? • What action is being taken if there is a discrepancy in their actual and target fluid balance? • What are the patient's blood results, e.g., albumin, protein? • What is the state of the patient's oral mucosa and skin elasticity? • What mode of nutritional intake is being used? Is the patient taking diet or fluids orally? • Are they being fed enterally? If so, are they absorbing their feed? • Are they receiving prokinetics? • What is their BMI? Has this changed and why? • What is the patient's blood sugar? Is it raised? If so, what treatment is being advised/given to the patient? • What changes in treatment have been made during your shift that could affect the patient's hydration and/or nutritional status? • Have they been reviewed and by whom?

TABLE 1.2 Bedside hand-over information.—cont'd

System	Information

Renal	• What is the patient's hourly urine output? Is there an indwelling urinary catheter?
	• What is the quality of the patient's urine?
	• Is the patient receiving any diuretic therapy? If so, how, i.e., boluses or infusion?
	• What is the patient's renal function? Has this improved or deteriorated?
	• Are they receiving a form of renal replacement therapy? If so:
	  • What type of renal replacement therapy is the patient receiving?
	  • Where is their vascular access?
	  • What fluid exchange are they receiving?
	  • What are the settings of the machine?
	  • What anticoagulation therapy are they receiving?
	  • What type of replacement fluid is being used?
	  • How much potassium do the replacement fluid bags contain?
	• What changes in treatment have been made during your shift that could affect the patient's renal function?
	• Have they been reviewed and by whom?

Gastrointestinal	• Is the patient's abdomen distended? If so, what is its size and shape? Has this changed from previous shift? • Does the patient have any bowel sounds? • When did the patient last have their bowels open? • Does the patient need, or are they receiving, a bowel management regimen? • Have they had any recent abdominal intervention, e.g., surgery? • Are there any drains present? Is there any drainage? If so, what? • What changes in treatment have been made during your shift that could affect the patient's gastrointestinal system? • Have they been reviewed and by whom?
Hygiene and skin integrity	• What is the overall condition of the patient's skin integrity? • How often is the patient being turned? Does the patient's overall condition tolerate being manually turned? • Is the patient nursed against a pressure-relieving mattress? If so, is it still an appropriate treatment? • What personal hygiene regimen is being used for the patient? • What condition are the patient's eyes? Are they receiving any specific eye care regimen? • What is the condition of the patient's mouth? What is their score on the Oral Assessment scale? Does this correspond to their mouth care regimen?

Continued

TABLE 1.2 Bedside hand-over information.—cont'd

System	Information
	• Have any referrals been made to specialist practitioners related to hygiene or skin care, e.g., tissue viability nurse, chiropodist? • Are there any wounds? If so, what is their overall condition? • What IV access does the patient have? • What is the condition of the patient's IV access sites? • How long have the lines been in situ? • When do they need to be resited? • When were they last redressed? • What changes in treatment have been made during your shift that could affect the patient's hygiene and/or skin management? • Have they been reviewed and by whom?
Psychological, social and cultural	• If the patient is conscious, what is their psychological state? • If the patient is unconscious, what was their psychological state? • Are there any factors that may be influencing their general wellbeing? • Does the patient have any next-of-kin? If so, what are their contact details? • When did they last visit/phone? • What information has been given to them? • Are there any specific circumstances about visiting or information-giving? • Are there any difficulties in their relationship with each other or the patient? • What degree of support are they giving to the patient? • What is the patient's social situation? • Does the patient have any specific cultural or religious needs? If so, what has been done to ensure that they have been met? • What has changed during your shift that could affect the patient's psychological, social and cultural status? • Have they been reviewed and by whom?
Medications and infusions	• What drug therapy is the patient receiving? • When are they next due? • Are there any problems with the prescription? • Have any drugs been withheld? If so, why? • Do any infusions/infusion lines need changing in the near future?
Microbiology	• What is the patient's infection status? • Are there any results from microbiology? • Does the patient require barrier nursing? • What changes in treatment have been made during your shift that could affect the patient's infection status? • Have they been reviewed and by whom?

COETT, cuffed oral endotracheal tube; *PEEP*, positive end-expiratory pressure.

Care Bundles

The use of care bundles in critical care is currently being promoted. Care bundles are a group of evidence-based care interventions that when implemented together can result in improved quality of care (Lavallee et al., 2017) and outcomes (Bogert et al., 2015). The individual interventions within each bundle are all supported by a well-established evidence base. Care bundles are a direct way of improving the delivery of clinical care (Gao et al., 2005). The theory is that when several evidence-based interventions are grouped together in a single protocol, it will improve patient outcomes, reduce unnecessary morbidity, reduce length of stay and thus increase critical care capacity. It is based on measuring the actual provision of therapeutic interventions according to standards, informed by evidence set by clinicians. At the same time, it reduces unwarranted variation in clinical care and ensures that patients across the country with the same clinical condition are consistently managed. Examples of two care bundles are given in Table 1.3. Additional critical care bundles will be explored as the intervention arises throughout this book.

Care bundles are proposed to be easy to develop, implement and audit, providing practitioners with a practical method of implementing evidence-based practice.

The steps to a care bundle are as follows:

- Agreement by clinical staff to reduce morbidity and mortality
- Select a small number of elements to be measured, scan available evidence
- Agree local guidelines for therapeutic interventions
- Use simple methods to measure and give feedback
- Facilitate creative discussion to develop ways for improving the elements of care

It is recommended that care bundles be monitored through hospital clinical audit. Feedback of data from some critical care units in England has shown effects on service outcome related to throughput and cost. The best results for

TABLE 1.3 Examples of two care bundles.

Elements of a ventilator care bundle	Elements of a tracheostomy care bundle

• DVT prophylaxis
• Peptic ulcer prophylaxis
• Prevention of ventilator-associated pneumonia by elevation of the head of the bed
• Managing sedation effectively
  • Oral care with chlorhexidine
  • Subglottic aspiration
	• Humidification
	• Tube patency/inner tube care
	• Suctioning
	• Safety equipment availability
	• Cuff pressure
	• Tracheostomy dressing/tapes

care bundles have been collectively and consistently incorporated into the daily routine of critical care.

Integrated Care Pathways

Integrated care pathways are structured multidisciplinary guides to good practice, placed in an appropriate timeframe, which detail anticipated steps in the care of patients with common clinical conditions such as asthma and diabetes. Medical algorithms or decision tree approaches may be added to incorporate treatments, for example, if a patient has condition or symptom A, B or C, then intervention X is preferred.

The Multidisciplinary Team

Medical Staff

- This may involve a clinical director of critical care areas within the hospital, or the responsibility of critical care may be split up into medical or surgical directorates.
- Management of the critical care environment may also involve the use of specialist intensive care practitioners, which is generally preferred.
- Some critical care areas are staffed by specialists from other disciplines, such as anaesthesia or medicine, who often have clinical commitments elsewhere.
- Generally responsible for patient treatment and management.

Physician's Associate

- Is a new role who is under the supervision of doctors in charge of running the critical care area
- May have some responsibilities in patient care and management

Physiotherapist

- Assist with patient's respiratory function
- Preserve existing motor skills, restore mobility, and consider the functioning of all limbs whether strong or weak
- Work towards reducing stiffness, contractions and spasticity
- Re-educate motor function, coordination and balance

Occupational Therapist

- Restore patient's ability to perform activities of daily living − relearn practical skills if necessary
- Evaluate patient's perceptual and cognitive functions

- Adapt objects that improve daily living activities
- Assess the need for modifications to the home

Speech and Language Therapist

- Assess patient's swallowing and gag ability
- Provide specialized speech therapy, communication advice and aids to assist speech, if required

Dietician

- Advise on nutritional and fluid requirements — whether it should be liquid, thickened or pureed food
- Advise regarding enteral or parenteral feeding requirements and regimen

Social Worker

- May discuss long-term or short-term care options with patient and family
- Support families and patients by assisting with social issues
- Arrange benefits
- Provide assessment for home adjustments and/or the need for home adjustments

Other Staff

- Secretarial support may be required specifically for critical care areas
- Porters may be involved in transporting specimens, patients or equipment during the day and night to and from the critical care area
- Local chaplains, priests or relevant officials from all religions when there is a need for their services
- A designated-ward clinical pharmacist is invaluable but may not be available in all critical care areas
- Technicians, to service, repair and develop equipment

Working as a Team

Working as a team is essential if care is to be carried out efficiently in critical care. The team consists of not only those working in the multidisciplinary team (MDT) but also many other personnel from both within and outside the critical care setting. These may include:

- The police
- Security
- Specialist hospitals
- Laboratories, for example, technicians, laboratory staff

- Support staff, for example, phlebotomists, electrocardiogram (ECG) technicians
- Theatres
- Specialist nurses, for example, diabetic, wound care, resuscitation, pain
- Other wards/departments, for example, pharmacy, X-ray
- Relatives and friends
- Patients
- Ambulance personnel

Liaison and effective communication inside and outside the critical care team is essential to ensure optimum patient care.

The role of the critical care practitioner are as follows:

- Provides one-to-one care
- Undertakes and assists with evidence-based care
- Gatekeeper of psychological/physiological care
- Care of relatives and significant others
- Record vital signs/documentation of care
- Combines patient information to determine if the patient is deteriorating, improving or suffering from a complication following drug therapy, interventions or investigations
- Care for intravenous (IV) and other invasive lines, for example, arterial or central venous pressure (CVP) lines
- Key role in the understanding of and safe practice in the administration and management of drugs
- Ability to prioritize care
- Intuitive knowledge
- Ability to provide individualized/holistic care
- Works within the MDT:
  - Medical and surgical teams
  - Physiotherapist
  - Occupational therapist
  - Social worker
  - Pharmacist
  - Radiologist
  - Medical technicians
- Works in other departments, for example, theatres
- Takes part in ethical and moral decision-making
- Is open to changing practices and innovations
- Has awareness of personal and professional development
- Encourages and supports others to develop themselves and enrol on study days and courses
- Supports and educates less-qualified colleagues, for example, as a mentor for student nurses gaining clinical experience in critical care as part of their training or as a preceptor for newly qualified nurses

- Plays a major role in communicating with others
- Key role in team building, which involves working together to benefit patient care

Areas Open for Consideration as to the Role of the Critical Care Practitioner

- Limitations:
  - Environment − where we work, no natural light, confined space, television, teaching room.
  - Management styles − dogmatic, authoritarian, laissez-faire − influences on practice.
  - Resources available − confined to monitoring equipment, dressings and drugs available.
  - Medical practices − generally doctors have the final say; nurses need to express their views so that they are effective advocates for their critical care patients.
  - Advances in technology − often these impinge on our practice as patients are often critically ill but need to understand and appreciate that these technologies cannot and do not save all patients.
  - Knowledge of nurses − confines practices to level of knowledge/education.
  - Government legislation.
- Multiskilling:
  - Increased autonomy − professionalism of critical care practitioners.
  - Expansion of the critical care practitioner's role, for example, taking of bloods; cost-effectiveness versus caring for critically ill patients.
- The legal implications in practice, for example, litigation of extended role.
- The scope of professional practice − the rules governing health care professionals.
- It is important to remember and be aware of the outside influences that often govern how we practise and how we would like to practise.

Computer Technology in Critical Care

The application of computer technology within a critical care setting can be seen as important, widespread and diverse. Its application to patient care within this highly technological environment is the key to its success and therefore requires a fundamental insight and understanding of its use by health care practitioners.

The critical care area is a complex environment with rapidly changing patients, personnel, policies and procedures. Continuing specialist care of this highly technologically demanding environment requires an enormous amount of data collection, analysis, interpretation, report writing and auditing, with much of this information undergoing repeated transcription. Therefore, it is apparent that one of the vital reasons for computerizing the critical care environment is to minimize duplication of data entry and allow the health care professional to focus upon the critically ill patient. Computer technology within a critical care setting is capable of:

- Detecting variations in physiological parameters
- Calculating critical care scoring systems
- Identifying important aspects of care or service
- Identifying indicators
- Establishing thresholds for these indicators
- Monitoring and reporting the important aspects of care by collecting and organizing the data for each indicator
- Evaluating care when limits are reached to identify problems or opportunities for improvement of care
- Taking action to resolve identified problems
- Assessing the action and documenting improvement
- Communicating the relevant information in report form
- Processing correlations in a short period of time and storing results
- Telemedicine uses the world of Internet where physicians can diagnose patients remotely via video or send photographs/X-rays for quick diagnosis

More recently there has been the potential to implement more complex systems:

- Clinical decision support systems
- Automated dispensing devices
- Medication systems and procedures
- Computer physician order entry
- Health care information systems
- Electronic medical records

Yet, adopting these technologies is costly to implement and maintain, and there are potential problems with patient privacy. It is also worth noting that these technologies are reliant on user input to ensure patient data are accurate and complete.

However, these technologies may be seen to reduce Health Care Practitioner (HCP) time in documentation, ordering of medication and risk to patients but can create new problems such as 'alert fatigue' as often technology has an override system, which can be easy putting into question the safety of such system. This might include silencing alarms if they begin to irritate the nurse working with the new technology. There is also a danger of the possibility of professional's overreliance on the technology and the danger of putting too much trust in the ability of systems to provide clinical decision support rather than their own judgement.

1.2 HEALTH AND SAFETY

Violence, Bullying and Harassment

Violence

Violence orientated towards staff members is any incident in which a health professional experiences abuse, threat, fear or the application of force arising out of the course of their work, whether or not they are on duty. Violence may take the form of aggression, abuse, threat or attack (Ferns, 2006). The management of violence is necessary when the person

- shows a predisposition to violence,
- makes a physical attack on another person or object and
- becomes disturbed to the extent that his/her behaviour is considered a threat to his/her own safety and the safety of others.

The following principles underlie the management of violent persons.

1. Prevention of violent incidents is the foremost principle; this may not always be possible with regard to patients if physiological causes are the reason for the violence:
   a. Brain tumours
   b. Endocrine imbalance
   c. Hyperthyroidism
   d. Hyperglycaemia
   e. Convulsive disorders
   f. HIV encephalopathy
   g. Dementia
   h. Neurological impairment
   i. Alcohol/substance abuse
   j. Pain
   k. Side effects of medication
   Violence and unnecessary restraint can be averted if a physiological reason can be identified and reversed promptly.
2. Restraint for violet persons:
   a. Is always therapeutic, never corrective, and the best method where a one-to-one violent confrontation arises is to use a breakaway technique. Should not risk physical injury or be minimized; any restraint should be appropriate to the actual danger or resistance shown by the person.
3. In all situations of violence, the locally agreed policy/procedure for the nursing management/care of violent persons should be adhered to. The aspects of policy for violence should include
   a. Environmental and organizational factors
   b. Anticipation and prevention of violence
   c. Action following an incident

When restraint is necessary, the risk of physical injury should be minimized; any restraints should be appropriate to the actual danger or resistance shown by the person.

Workplace Bullying and Harassment

The issue of bullying in the workplace is extremely prevalent yet remains under-researched in literature (Edwards and O'Connell, 2007). Although bullying appears to be categorized under the classification of violence, numerous studies do appear to adopt it as an individual issue. Bullying is a form of violence. Without a doubt, bullying exists in all areas of society, from toddlers to the very aged. It is not specific to gender, race, age or profession. Bullying takes many forms and can be subtle, indirect, direct or completely explicit. Regardless of its format, the consequences of bullying behaviour can be detrimental to the critical care nurse's psychological and physiological well-being. Unfortunately, bullying is rife in the health care sector, especially in the nursing profession.

The impact of bullying on the victim can have an enormous range of consequences, including psychological and physical effects impacting on his/ her personal and professional life. Individual responses include victims giving up their job to avoid the perpetrators; experiencing psychological stress, moodiness and recurring nightmares; re-experiencing the trauma, to name but a few.

Dealing with bullying can be varied:

- Confronting the perpetrator can be successful
- Seeking support from friends and family
- Seeking support from a counsellor
- Writing down incidences by keeping a record of times, dates and incidents

As professionals, it is important to support colleagues if situations occur and follow the processes in place is to discourage a workplace bullying culture.

Legislation, Policies and Guidelines

All employees of the National Health Service (NHS), including critical care nurses, should not have to experience any form of violence, aggression or bullying behaviour. There are various national and governmental policies, guidelines and legislation from 1974 to the present to protect them from such horrifying ordeals. The Government has developed guidelines (ACAS, 2014) directed at employees and employer's responsibilities for preventing bullying and harassment in the workplace. There are also resources available for employers in order for them to effectively prevent and reduce the incidence of bullying and harassment.

Procedures for dealing with aggressive patients, withholding treatment, developing local policies, development of counselling services for victims, dealing with complaints, methods of staff training and education against violence, how to record and monitor harassment, and relevant legislation are all outlined in detail in the Zero Tolerance for workplace violence and website. Employers and employees of all Trusts should have access to this information, and members of the public should be made aware that any form of aggressive behaviour would not be tolerated.

Although in theory with all of the published guidelines available, there should be a reduction in violence, bullying and harassment in practice. However, violence and bullying against staff still occur. Reasons why these policies are not working need to be further explored. Perhaps, NHS staff are not aware of their existence or employers are choosing not to implement them in their Trusts. Regardless, the issue of violence and aggression against health care professionals until it is dealt with appropriately may not be reduced.

In order for a change in the working environment to occur, various actions must occur. Primarily, critical care staff must accept that there is a need to alter practice and have a shared vision of a healthier working climate:

- The ethic of caring between each other − critical care staff will function more profitably in a happy, team-working environment.
- Education and training − greatest method for overcoming change is through education. The need for education and training on how to manage and deal with abusive/violent patients and bullying is essential.
- Provide policies, protocols and guidelines of workplace violence that exist within the hospital, including management of intra-staff bullying and abuse.

Infection Control

Patients who are admitted to the critical care environment are immunologically vulnerable and invariably have a reduced immune response. This may be due to the individual patient's general condition, their inability to take nutrition or fasting practices in hospital. It might be due to prescribed treatments or drug therapies. Therefore, the health care professional must be vigilant in relation to infection control practices as a patient's immune system can be severely reduced putting the patient at risk of obtaining a hospital-acquired infection (HAI). Listed below are a number of conditions and situations that make patients susceptible to infection while in critical care.

Non-Steroidal Anti-Inflammatory Drugs

These drugs are prescribed to relieve pain. They work by reducing the release of prostaglandin during the inflammatory response. Prostaglandin has a number of roles in the body; it

- sends messages to the brain and pain may be felt;
- stimulates the inflammatory response and leads to swelling and pressure on localized nerve endings, resulting in pain;
- stimulates the clotting cascade, so any interference with its release can induce bleeding from the nose, vagina or wounds, etc. and
- controls renal blood flow, and if prostaglandin is reduced, then glomerular filtration rate (GFR) is reduced, leading to sodium and water retention, reduced kidney function. Consequently, non-steroidal anti-inflammatory drugs (NSAIDs) should not be prescribed for patients with renal dysfunction.

This information serves to help critical care practitioners understand the particular information as to side effects and restrictions and considerations when taking this group of drugs. NSAIDs are acid and increase the acidity of the stomach and can lead to the formation of ulcers, and strict adherence to administering these drugs with food at meal times is essential (Galbraith et al., 2007). In addition, it is essential that patients taking NSAIDs should not take other protein-bound anticoagulants, such as aspirin, as NSAIDs displace high-protein-bound drugs from protein sites, causing more free anticoagulants. It should also be noted that these drugs reduce the inflammatory response and, as such, healing may also be delayed.

Broad-Spectrum Antibiotics

Broad-spectrum antibiotic therapy may be prescribed pending culture, and sensitivity results in critical care. However, the use of these is not without consequences:

- Broad-spectrum antibiotics not only destroy the invading bacteria but also devastate the normal intestinal flora present in the mucous membranes.
- Broad-spectrum antibiotics destroy resident flora living in the mouth and vagina, allowing pathogens (commonly *Candida albicans*, which causes thrush) to colonize, leading to fungal infections.
- Overuse of broad-spectrum antibiotics can lead to the emergence of resistant microorganisms.

Antibiotic prescribers need to consider the future treatment of infection and have a duty to patients, as there is a reduction in the discovery of new age antibiotics reducing available therapeutic options.

Antacids

Antacids are drugs that neutralize acidity of the stomach, which can give rise to an increase in the production of bacterial growth in the stomach and small and large intestines, leading to diarrhoea.

The Administration of Chemotherapy and Radiotherapy

Chemotherapy

- The administration of chemotherapy can depress the bone marrow, leaving it less able to produce sufficient amounts of red blood cells (RBCs), white blood cells and platelets. The reduction in white blood cells (neutrophils and monocytes, which mature into macrophages) leaves the body more susceptible to infection.
- The administration of chemotherapy can lead to an increased risk of patients becoming neutropenic, which can lead to an increased risk of sepsis.

Radiotherapy

- Radiation can cause irritation of the skin, leading to breakdown allowing bacteria to enter the body.
- With some types of radiation therapy, the effect on the immune system can be similar to chemotherapy.

Steroids

Corticosteroids are anti-inflammatory and reduce the production of chemicals that cause inflammation:

- Steroid hormones are synthesized by the adrenal cortex, and cortisol is the naturally occurring steroid in the body.
  Corticosteroids are steroid hormones either produced by the body or are manmade.
- The suppression of the immune processes by corticosteroids can result in an increased susceptibility to infection and impair wound healing (Galbraith et al., 2007).
- Inflammation is part of innate immunity, and a critical care patient may be exposed to bacteria, which would not normally breach the innate immune defences.

A Reduced Nutritional Intake

Nutritional intake (e.g., glucose, fats, protein, vitamins and minerals) is required to produce the cells and molecules of innate immunity, as most phagocytes, complement factors, acute phase proteins, clotting factors and mediators are made from proteins, vitamins, minerals, carbohydrates and fats (see Section 2). During and following exposure to bacteria, the cells and molecules of immunity may become depleted; if nutrients are not available, new molecules and cells cannot be produced, reducing the body's innate and acquired immune defences against infection. With continued fasting practices often observed on the wards, the mechanisms of inflammation cannot be switched off due to a reduction in anti-inflammatory molecules and, in this event, can lead to serious complications, such as adult respiratory distress syndrome (ARDS), systemic inflammatory response syndrome (SIRS) and multiple system organ failure (MSOF).

The nutritional requirements for wound healing (see Section 2) include an adequate protein intake. Proteins supply the amino acids necessary for repair and regeneration of tissues and produce many of the proteins involved in the immune responses. Fibrous tissue is protein based, and hence, scar tissue will have poorer tensile strength in those who are protein depleted. Vitamin A is necessary for re-epithelialization, and vitamin C is required for collagen synthesis and capillary integrity. Zinc deficiency is thought to be associated with delayed wound healing. Zinc supplements have been shown to promote venous ulcer healing in those who were zinc depleted.

Nutrition affects the body's ability to fight infection, and a patient admitted to hospital may have suppressed nutrition before admission or obtain poor nutritional support while in hospital (Richards and Edwards, 2018). In addition, there are hospital practices, which exacerbate bad nutrition and hence the patient's immune response:

- Preoperative patients only need to be fasted between 4 and 6 h, less in some surgeries.
- Postoperative feeding should be initiated immediately; leaving fasting until the return of bowel sounds is traditional, ritualistic and unnecessary.
- The prescription of 5% dextrose solution to maintain nutrition only promotes malnutrition as 1 L of 5% dextrose solution contains 170 kcal.

There are a number of assessment tools available to determine state of nutrition (see later).

Changes Associated with Ageing

There are many body processes that deteriorate due to age, including the innate immune system; the elderly are at greater risk of developing complications due to:

- Increased risk of infection — fibroblast activity decreases with age, and the elderly are especially vulnerable to infection as they
  - have a reduced innate immune system and
  - do not take an adequate diet.

- Reduced healing processes:
  - Collagen fibres in the skin decrease in number, and the skin becomes wrinkled and loses its elasticity.
  - There is a loss of some subcutaneous fat.
  - The skin becomes thinner in areas not exposed to sunlight and less resistant to trauma.
  - Bruising may result from quite minor injuries.
  - Mitosis occurring in the basal layer of the epidermis is slowed, delaying wound healing.
- Reduced ability to maintain body temperature:
  - Temperature regulation is affected due to an impaired ability to sense changes in the ambient temperature and impaired hypothalamic mechanisms. Decreased metabolic processes, together with problems with mobility and exercise compound the problem.
  - Sweat gland production decreases since the number of glands diminishes.

Types of Infections

Organisms that cause infection are made up of cells. A cell consists of a nucleus, which contains the genetic information unique to that cell (often referred to as DNA; a code that, when translated, creates the specific proteins and enzymes necessary to build and operate the cell; a cytoplasm enclosed in a semi-permeable membrane; and, in some instances, an outer cell wall.

Cells are placed into groups according to their structure, but generally two distinct types of cell can be identified:

- Eukaryotic (differentiated and undifferentiated) − include the cells of plants, animals, protozoa, fungi and algae, which are made up of many differentiated cells.
- Prokaryotic (unicellular) − less complex and only form single-celled organisms; these include all bacteria and viruses.

Bacteria

- Bacteria are made up of carbohydrates and amino acids in the form of peptidoglycans, which determine the gram-staining properties of bacterial cells, which provide a provisional identification of a microorganism, especially if the infection is potentially life-threatening, so appropriate antibiotic therapy can be started immediately:
  - Gram-negative cell walls stain pink under a microscope, as they only have a thin layer of peptidoglycans and include. meningitis, chlamydia, Helicobacter and Pseudomonas; and gram-positive cell walls stain a crystal violet colour due to the thick layer of peptidoglycans and include *Staphylococcus aureus*, clostridium perfringens and group A streptococcus

- The majority of antibiotics work by interfering with the synthesis of peptidoglycans.
- Many bacteria (e.g., *Escherichia coli*, *Pseudomonas* spp.) are motile, capable of rapid movement generated by long threadlike flagella that extend from the cell surface and can survive in water. Non-mobile bacteria tend to survive in dry environments.
- Some bacteria (*Clostridium* and *Bacillus* spp.) have the ability to produce spores, cells enclosed in a resistant casing that is difficult to destroy by heat or chemicals. Spores are formed when the bacterium is exposed to adverse environmental conditions, for example, no food, high/low temperature or a reduction in oxygen. When conditions improve, the spores germinate, and the cell starts to multiply. In this way, spore-forming bacteria can survive for very long periods.
- Bacteria require different forms of energy for growth and replication such as aerobic, anaerobic or facultative.

A combination of all these can be used to help identify the organism.

Bacterial Growth and Replication

Bacteria grow in a variety of environments. The nutrients they need vary widely, but they contain complex molecular systems that can use a wide variety of substances as energy sources. They can synthesize all their required organic and inorganic molecules from simple starting substances such as water, carbon dioxide, nitrogen, phosphorus, sulphur and oxygen (Table 1.4).

Awareness of microorganisms leads critical care nurses to

- Appreciate the importance of drying equipment and surface areas thoroughly;
- Appreciate which bacteria are more likely to be found in a wet or damp environment;
- Appreciate which bacteria form spores and are able to survive without food and
- Prevent the multiplication of bacteria by removing potential sources of nutrients, for example, urine, blood, skin scales.

Health care professionals, hospital workers and relatives can all help to reduce the risk of transmission of HAI in critically ill patients, who may have reduced immune defences, by removing the bacteria's energy source.

Identification of Bacteria

- Microscopy — looking at bacteria under a microscope identifies their shape: round (cocci); oblong (bacilli or rods).
- Culture — bacteria are grown in special media to identify the organism; incubation at around body temperature encourages the bacteria to grow rapidly.

TABLE 1.4 The substances required for bacterial growth and replication.

Energy source	Substances
Organic carbon	The sun
Carbon	Glucose, carbon dioxide
Nitrogen	Found in cells, e.g., proteins, ammonia or nitrates, e.g., urine, atmospheric nitrogen
Inorganic ions	Sodium, potassium, magnesium, sulphate, phosphate
Environmental factors	
Water	Gram-negative bacteria die in the absence of water, a useful infection control measure; others are more resistant to drying out, e.g., staphylococci, or are able to form spores (*Clostridium*) and can survive for months in dust particles, recommencing multiplication when a supply of water is resumed
Oxygen	A wound with a good oxygen supply is unlikely to support anaerobic bacteria; in contrast, a pressure sore with a poor blood supply is unlikely to support aerobic bacteria
Temperature	Many bacteria die in high temperatures, and as such represents a systemic response
pH (acid or alkaline)	Determined by the presence of hydrogen ions, most bacteria prefer neutrality (7.35–7.45), but some microorganisms can grow in acid or alkaline environments
Concentration of solution	Some microorganisms can stand various concentrations of salt, e.g., very strong or dilute solutions, therefore to kill all germs in a salt bath is impossible as such enormous quantities are necessary to achieve a final concentration and as such is of no actual value

Courtesy: Edwards SL (2005) Innate defences (Chapter 6.1), In: Montegue, S, Watson, S, Herbert RA. Physiology for Nursing Practice, Edinburgh: Elsevier.

Oxygen-free incubation cabinets are required if the pathogen, for example, from infected pressure ulcers, is likely to be anaerobic.

- The appearance of colonies — bacteria grow in distinct groups or colonies and the size, colour and shape of these differ markedly between species.

Viruses

Viruses are not cells; they are simple pieces of nucleic acid made from either DNA or RNA (ribonucleic acid), protected by a protein coat and sometimes enclosed in an envelope made from lipids. Viruses are very small and can only replicate inside living cells.

- A virus enters the nucleus of a host cell, where it instructs the cell's own mechanisms to copy the nucleic acid and use it to make viral proteins.
- The new virus made by the host cell is released, generally destroying the host cell in the process.
- Most viruses are fragile and cannot survive outside a living cell for long, but some can survive in the environment or on hands for some time prior to transmission to a new host.
- Viruses are fairly resistant to some disinfectants, and outbreaks of viral gastrointestinal or respiratory infections can therefore occur both in the community and hospital.

Identification of Viruses

- Virus culture — viruses cannot be grown like bacteria and need to be grown in tissue or cell culture.
- Serological tests — infection by a virus may stimulate the release by the body of distinct antibodies into the blood. Detection of such antibodies is the basis of serological testing.
- Serum antibodies — different types of antibody appear in the blood during the course of an infection. These can indicate whether the person has had the infection in the past or is recovering from it.

Fungi

These are plant-like organisms often described as moulds or yeasts depending on how they grow. Often, a species can grow as both yeast and a mould depending on the availability of oxygen and nutrients. Yeast cells, for example, *Candida albicans*, are larger than bacterial cells but can still only be seen with the aid of a microscope and have a characteristic microscopic appearance.

Infection Control Practices

It is important to remember that, while in hospital, patients may have a reduced innate response to an invasion of the body by bacteria and/or viruses; therefore, infection control practices are imperative (Wilson, 2012; Table 1.5). Continuous audit is essential to ensure every effort is being taken to prevent the spread and multiplication of microbes.

Moving and Handling

Patients in critical care will require moving and handling. Moving and handling is part of working and caring for patients at the bedside. It is important that the practice of moving and handling is undertaken safely, and

TABLE 1.5 Infection control practices.

Type	Reasons	Practice
The use of a single room	This is generally used to protect staff and other patients in the ward area (isolation) or to simply protect the patient due to immunosuppression (protective isolation).	Protective clothing is not generally required – visitors do not go from patient to patient, are not in contact with other patients, and do not handle infectious material. Hand-washing before and after the visitor leaves the room is all that is necessary.
Hand-washing	Hand contamination is responsible for a large proportion of cross-infection, and hand-washing is the most important method of preventing the spread of infection (Wilson, 2012).	Thorough hand-washing before attending a patient ensures the majority of microorganisms acquired transiently from other patients are removed. An awareness of microorganisms demonstrates the importance of thoroughly washing and drying hands.
Protective clothing	The transmission of microorganisms on staff clothing is possible, but unlikely. It is more likely to arise on the front. Uniforms contaminated with body fluids increase the microbial load; plastic aprons provide adequate protection as they are impermeable.	Plastic aprons over cloth gowns if there is a risk of spillage. Disposable gloves for any activity – discard after use and wash hands. When no contact occurs with other patients, infection is unlikely to spread when the nurse leaves the room.
Masks and eye protection	Recommended for infections that are spread by respiratory droplets. They do not work when wet, as damp masks do not filter microorganisms effectively. Efficiency diminishes when worn for long periods. Easily contaminated by the hands during repositioning or removal, and as such are unreliable against airborne infections (Wilson, 2006), especially viral.	Not necessary for most procedures. They are important to protect health care workers and should be worn for any activity where there is a risk of body fluid splashing into the face.

Continued

TABLE 1.5 Infection control practices.—cont'd

Type	Reasons	Practice
Waste material	If contaminated with blood or body fluids, it should be discarded in a yellow waste bag, in the patient's room. The outer surface of waste bags does not become significantly contaminated, thus there is no reason to enclose the waste in a second bag.	All body fluids should be safely discarded directly into a bedpan washer or macerator.
Equipment	Beds, curtains, bedclothes, toys, bedpans, sphygmomanometers. The majority of microorganisms are not able to survive in the absence of moisture, warmth and nutrients; thus, as long as the equipment and other surface areas are kept clean and dry, the potential for the multiplication of bacteria will be removed.	Certain microorganisms can form spores that are able to survive when food is scarce; hot water or special chemicals may be required for cleaning.

the correct hospital policy or procedure is undertaken. Any manual handling operation must meet two objectives:

1. The handler needs to employ minimal effort.
2. The patient must experience minimal discomfort.

These objectives can be achieved, and the risk of injury reduced by undertaking a comprehensive assessment of the task's requirements. Poor technique when handling patients can result in injury to the mover(s) and the patient, accidents leading to injury to both mover(s) and patient and discomfort and a lack of dignity for the patient being moved. Risk assessment must be undertaken when manual handling cannot be avoided, and there is a risk of injury.

When moving and handling people, there is a risk of causing harm, a risk assessment needs to be undertaken as to the possible severity of that harm.

People handling risk assessment is the likelihood of a particular situation causing harm, taking into account the possible severity of that harm. People handling risk assessment should include the following and use the acronym TILEE:

- Task — the job to be undertaken, for example, sit the patient up in the bed, walk the patient to the toilet, bed bath a patient, etc.
- Individual — the nurse and includes the skills/experience of the person(s) who is going to be involved and takes into consideration the height of nurses involved in the task.
- Load — the patient is the load; involves ascertaining details of the patient's weight and abilities:
  - Ask the patient to raise their legs while sitting.
  - What does the patient understand by simple commands?
  - Why is the patient in hospital?
  - Do they require analgesia before moving?
  - Are there any drains, catheters, cardiac monitoring, and trailing flexes?
- Environment — consider the area surrounding the patient, what are the constraints, consider safety and trailing flexes.
- Equipment — what is the most appropriate equipment to use, have the staff been trained in using it, what safety checks need to be carried out before using the equipment?

Moving and handling procedure in critical care needs to do a risk assessment prior to the moving and handling event. This must be documented, which is part of the professional duty of care. It is important to remember that safe moving and handling impacts on all nursing activities, for example, making a bed, wound dressings, taking a patient's blood pressure and stocking shelves.

When suitable equipment such as hoists, small handling aids and electronic profiling beds are provided, these should be used, well maintained, serviced, in good working order and placed close at hand.

Training and education in the use of manual handling equipment and practices should be an ongoing process with yearly updates for all staff. The aim is to have fewer nurses injured and to increase comfort and safety for patients. Factors that contribute to safer handling are as follows:

- Trained, fit staff
- Adequate supervision
- Ergonomic assessments
- Planned maintenance
- Repair and replacement of equipment
- Control of purchasing
- Suitable and sufficient handling aids
- Influencing attitudes of patients and relatives

- Reporting and investigation of incidents
- Competent agency staff
- Sufficient staff.

Many patients may be able to move themselves or assist nurses while being moved and should be encouraged to help in ways compatible with their capabilities or health status.

The principles of safer manual handling for critical care nurses are as follows:

- Assess unavoidable handling tasks and update assessment regularly.
- Channel the effort through your legs to protect your back.
- Move your feet in turn, not your body. Turn feet successively in the direction of movement (rather than twist at the waist).
- Bend your knees when appropriate but avoid over bending.
- Keep close to the load (when safe to do so).
- Maintain the natural curves of your spine and avoid twisting.
- Wear a uniform that allows unrestricted movement at shoulders, waist and hip, with non-slip shoes that provide support.
- Try to vary your tasks (so that different muscle groups are used in turn).
- Relax and move smoothly; avoid sudden movements.
- Remember to look after yourself with enough rest, suitable exercise and a healthy diet.
- If in doubt, seek advice. **Do not risk it.**

Safeguarding Adults in Critical Care

Nurses have a responsibility to safeguard the patients in their care and if appropriate undertake training (Ochieng and Ward, 2018). Safeguarding is ensuring that adults are safe and free from abuse and neglect while in critical care. Critical care patients often suffer from sensory and mental impairment and so are more dependent on others. During this time, relatives and loved ones need to be assured they are safeguarded from the risk of abuse or neglect. These might include

- Poor professional practice
  - Poor care standards
  - Lack of positive responses to complex needs
  - Rigid routines
  - Inadequate staffing and insufficient knowledge base within the service
- Unacceptable treatments
  - Withholding food and drink
  - Seclusion
  - Unnecessary and unauthorized use of restraint
  - Inappropriate/overuse of medication

In addition, it is the responsibility of staff to alert others to any concerns about or suspected abuse of an adult prior to admission. This includes working together to identify those who might be at risk from or suspected of abuse or neglect. There are a number of areas that constitute abuse (RCN, 2015):

- Domestic violence
- Sexual abuse
- Psychological abuse
- Financial or material abuse
- Modern slavery
- Discriminatory abuse
- Organizational abuse
- Neglect and acts of omission
- Self-neglect

There are also patterns of abuse:

- Serial — a person seeks out/grooms a vulnerable individual
- Long-term — domestic violence
- Opportunistic — theft as money or valuables are lying around
- Situational — due to pressure of work
- Neglect — due to stress outside of work, for example, debt, alcohol or mental health problems.

Summary

All nurses must respond if there are any concerns about safeguarding:

- Be aware of what constitutes abuse/engage in training
- Recognize any signs of abuse
- Share any safeguarding concerns
- Report/document any concerns
- Refer to other agencies
- Share relevant information with other agencies/teams
- Participate in investigations
- Reflect on the incidences and learn from them

1.3 EMERGENCIES AND LIFE-THREATENING CONDITIONS

Critical Care Outreach/Acute Life-Threatening Events Recognition and Treatment

The majority of hospital trusts provide critical care education for ward-based staff. Different forms of outreach services have evolved depending on the local priorities and resources. The acute life-threatening events recognition and treatment (ALERT) course generally provides this education for ward nurses and junior doctors (Smith et al., 2002). The whole basis of the programme is to improve ward nurses' knowledge of vital signs and identification of patients at risk in an attempt to reduce the number of patients requiring admission to critical care.

In the event of a patient's worsening condition, a ward nurse will alert the critical care outreach team before contacting the doctor. Critical care outreach teams are nursing led and organized from the local ICU/intensive therapy units. They act as a link between the ICU and ward areas. The role of the outreach nurse, once they have been made aware of a patient's deteriorating condition, varies from respiratory intervention such as administration of oxygen to instigation of noninvasive ventilation and fluid challenges to patients who are hypotensive and oliguric.

While working in critical care areas as part of their clinical experience, undergraduate student nurses in their second or third year of training are encouraged to attend the ALERT sessions or accompany an outreach team within the hospital. Currently, there are a number of other courses that HCP can undertake to facilitate their development in identifying a deteriorating patient and instigate the necessary interventions:

• Awareness why anticipating and responding is essential.

Bedside Emergency Assessment Course for Healthcare Staff

National Early Warning Scoring

Patients when critically ill often have abnormal physiological values present; most commonly observed prior to further deterioration are changes in six physiological parameters. Combining these with basic observations of the airway, breathing, circulation, disability and examination (ABCDE), measure of fluid balance and neurological status forms the basis of this simple system of early detection:

• A + B − Respiration rate (per minute)
• A + B − Oxygen saturation (%):
  • SpO_2 scale 1 used if target range is within normal limits
  • SpO_2 scale 2 used if target range is 88%−92%, for example, in hypercapnic respiratory failure
  • Air or oxygen?
• C − Blood pressure (BP), mm Hg, score uses systolic BP only
• C − Pulse beats/minute
• D − Level of consciousness or confusion
• E − Temperature in degree Celsius

Deviations from the normal score points a total are calculated. There are four trigger points that determine a clinical response (RCP, 2017):

- A low National Early Warning Scoring (NEWS; 1–4) should prompt assessment by a registered nurse
- A single (red score; 3 in a single parameter) is unusual but should prompt urgent review by a clinician
- A medium NEWS (5–6) is a key trigger and should prompt an urgent review by a clinician or acute team nurse
- A high NEWS (7 or more) is a key trigger and should prompt emergency assessment by a clinician/critical care outreach team

These levels should alert the nurse to deterioration in the patient's condition and those that require additional clinical assessment (Table 1.1). These parameters form the basis of the NEWS scoring system. It is used to aid early detection of patients' deteriorating conditions on acute general or surgical wards. The NEWS is a simple scoring system to be used at ward level utilizing routine observations taken by nursing staff. Nurses are identifying those patients at risk of deterioration and then scored according to their physiological parameters.

ABCDE Initial Assessment for the Critically Ill Patient

When a patient's condition is deteriorating, it is important to consider the A–E initial assessment (Table 1.6) in conjunction with the NEWS guidelines given above:

Airway

- Is it clear (if the patient can speak it is likely the airway is open); obstructed or protected; can the patient speak in full sentences.
- Use the look, listen and feel approach to determine air entry.
- Is there any noise heard during breathing such as snoring (partial obstruction by the tongue); gurgling, which indicates secretions, vomit or blood is in the upper airway; inspiratory stridor, which is an indication of an obstruction above the larynx.

Breathing

- Look for chest movement, listen for air entry and feel if the chest is moving
- Is the patient distressed or using their accessory muscles?
- Is the respiratory rate high or low (12–15 normal), include pattern and depth of breathing?
- Colour – is the patient cyanosed?
- What is the oxygen saturation?
- Is the patient using their accessory muscles?

TABLE 1.6 Underlying principles of the ABCDE approach to CPR.

Airway	Breathing	Circulation	Disability	Exposure
Difficulty in talking	Look at accessory	Perfusion	Glasgow coma scale	Remove clothes for
Difficulty in breathing	muscles	Pulse rate – radial and femoral	Optimize ABC	examination
Distress, choking	Cyanosis	Blood pressure falling	Treat cause:	Look for injuries,
Shortness of breath	Respiratory rate	Organ perfusion	Naloxone for opioid	bleeding, rashes etc.
Treatment is to head tilt; suction	Listen to breathing	Bleeding, fluid, urine output	toxicity	Avoid heat loss
may be needed, intubation, oxygen	Feel expiration	Treatment: airway, breathing,	Blood glucose if,	Maintain dignity
therapy; patient condition should	Treatment: airway,	monitoring, IV access, take bloods	3 mmol/L give	
guide direction.	oxygen, treat	Call for help, treat cause, fluid	glucose	
	underlying cause,	challenge	Check drug chart	
	support if	Acute cardiac		
	inadequate.	syndrome – unstable angina/MI		
		Oxygen, aspirin 300 mg orally,		
		GTN spray or tablet, morphine		

CPR, cardiopulmonary resuscitation; IV, intravenous; MI, myocardial infarction; GTN, Glyceryl trinitrate.

- Are the chest and abdomen moving in the same direction?
- Is there an expiratory wheeze (collapse during expiration)?
- Listen to the patient's chest, are there any rattling noises (indicating secretions)
- Bronchial breathing, is it absent or reduced? (may indicate a pneumothorax, a medical emergency), or pleural effusion
- Is air entry equal on both sides?

Circulation

- Is the patient pale or cyanosed (may indicate peripheral vein collapse and may be difficult to cannulate) or haemorrhage?
- What is the patient's urine output?
- What is the BP, it may be normal because compensatory homeostatic mechanisms increase peripheral resistance in response to reduced cardiac output (CO), so it is not a good indicator of shock (see later), more significant is pulse pressure which is the difference between systolic and diastolic BP and should be between 35 and 45 mm Hg. If increased suggestive of arterial vasoconstriction and reduced indicative of vasodilatation and sepsis.
- What is the heart rate (HR); is the pulse bounding (sepsis) or weak (reduced CO)?
- Check the capillary refill time should be less than 2 s.

Disability

- Check A = if patient spontaneously alert, V = responding to verbal stimulus, P = responding to painful stimuli, U = unresponsive.
- Check Blood Glucose level
- Pupil reactions to light (bilateral pinpoint drug overdose, opiates, brain stem involvement, stroke). Unilateral dilated unresponsive to light (brain stem death, cancer, lesion, cerebral oedema)
- Glasgow Coma Scale (GCS) if time.

Exposure

- Get a full medical history from the patient, relatives or friends
- Undertake a thorough head to toe physical examination after correction of any compromise to ABCD is secured
- Temperature if not taken elsewhere − hypothermia from theatre
- Blood results − electrolytes, U&Es, K^+, Na, Hb
- Fluids − fluid balance chart, input and output, increase in weight
- Gastrointestinal Tract (GIT) − abdomen, surgery, drains, blood loss, wound infection, bowel habits sounds

- Haematology — clotting, haemoglobin (Hb), white blood count (WBC)
  - Lines — source of sepsis, IV, drains, catheters, etc.
- Medication — prescribed drugs given, nephrotoxic drugs given, monitored digoxin/vancomycin, drug interactions, allergies

Provide appropriate interventions A—E then return to NEWS to recognize any further deterioration and review if score improves or deteriorates.

Emergencies

Shock

This is a condition whereby the cardiovascular system fails to perfuse body tissues adequately with oxygen and nutrients (Edwards, 2005). This brings about a widespread disruption of cellular metabolism. This results in functional disturbances at organ/tissue level. The causes of shock are generally any factor, which affects blood volume, BP, or cardiac function.

BP can be used as a basis for defining shock, which is explained in two forms (Table 1.7):

1. Hypotensive shock — further subdivided into:
   a. Low cardiac output shock characterized clinically by cold skin
   b. High cardiac output shock characterized by warm skin
2. Normotensive or hypertensive shock — BP is compensated.

Another classification is recognized by type and aetiology:

1. Distributive: septic, neurogenic, anaphylactic, drug and toxin-induced shock
2. Cardiogenic: cardiomyopathy, arrhythmic, mechanical
3. Hypovolaemic: haemorrhagic, non-haemorrhagic
4. Obstructive: pulmonary or vascular

These forms or classifications of shock may be helpful for accident and emergency staff to use as they are based on parameters that are relatively quick and easy to measure, and the classification is broader in terms of aetiology suitable for this particular area of nursing. A more traditional classification is by categorizing shock according to the primary defect that produced it. With this system, there are five forms of shock: anaphylactic, septic, neurogenic, cardiogenic and hypovolaemic.

Anaphylactic Shock

Anaphylaxis occurs when a sensitized person is exposed to an antigen to which he or she is allergic. The antigen enters the body and combines with immunoglobulin E antibodies on the surface of the mast cells and basophils (Edwards, 2001). Anaphylaxis is a systemic immediate hypersensitivity

TABLE 1.7 Classification of shock according to blood pressure response.

Type of shock	Initial presentation	Result	Treatment
Hypotensive shock	Cold skin: low cardiac output and high peripheral resistance	Low CVP (caused by large loss of circulating volume)	Responds well to IV fluid replacement
		High CVP (caused by cardiac failure)	Responds poorly to IV fluids; may respond to vasodilators, which decrease cardiac work
	Warm skin: high cardiac output	Vasodilatation (caused by gram-negative or gram-positive sepsis)	Treatment difficult due to the development of arteriovenous shunts
		Vasodilatation (caused by spinal anaesthesia or drugs)	Responds well to vasopressor drugs and fluid administration
Normotensive/ hypertensive shock	Blood pressure maintained in spite of shock being present	Baroreceptor reflex: the normal physiological compensatory mechanism	Administration of vasopressor drugs Pheochromocytoma: responds to alpha sympathetic blocking drugs

CVP, central venous pressure; *IV*, intravenous.

reaction that mediated an inflammatory immunological release of mediators with potentially life-threatening consequences. Mast cells and basophils are primarily found in the lungs, small intestines, skin and connective tissue. An antigen−antibody reaction occurs, which induces the release of histamine and prostaglandins into the blood. This causes:

- Selective vasodilatation (systemic circulation and the heart) and vasoconstriction (pulmonary bed, hepatic and other large veins) and
- Increased capillary permeability (causing movement of circulating fluids into the interstitial space, thus causing a relative hypovolaemia)

This in turn leads to:

- A reduced CO and low arterial pressure and
- A fall in cellular perfusion − metabolic demands are not met, resulting in acidosis, coagulopathies and capillary pooling and stimulation of the inflammatory/immune response (IIR)

The implications of this for the patient are as follows:

- Bronchospasm − cough, dyspnoea, chest tightness, wheezing, high respiratory rate
- Oedema formation in the glottis and pharynx − hoarseness, dysphagia, airway obstruction, sudden death, inspiratory stridor leading to cyanosis
- Oedema in the lungs and subcutaneous tissue
- Changes in cardiac function, for example, reduced contractility and dysrhythmias (Fig. 1.1) − hypotension, tachycardia, oliguria

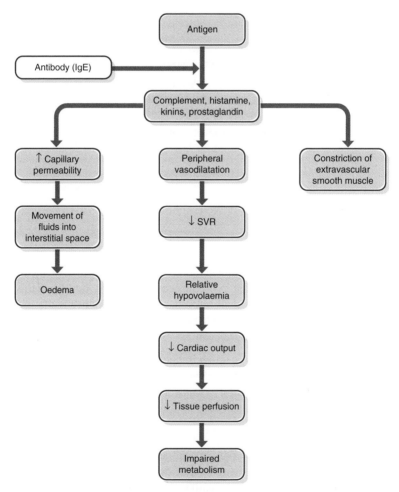

FIGURE 1.1 Anaphylactic shock. SVR 5 systemic vascular resistance.

Immediate Interventions for Anaphylactic Shock Reaction
Adrenaline.

- Adrenaline works on adrenergic receptors in the body of which there are both alpha and beta types.
- Alpha-receptors action reverses vasodilation and capillary leak. This reduces mucosal and cutaneous oedema, as well as shock. Improves BP and coronary artery perfusion. Decreases antio-oedema and urticaria.
- Beta 1 adrenergic stimulation has positive inotropic and chronotropic effects on cardiac activity. Beta 2 receptor action dilates the airway smooth muscle. Inhibits further mediator release.
- The administration should be intramuscular to all patients with anaphylactic shock or definite breathing difficulty. Adult dose is 500 µg (0.5 mg), which is equivalent to 0.5 mL of 1 in 1000 solution. Nearly always effective if given early. A second dose may be given in 5–10 min if there is no improvement.

Hydrocortisone.

- Hydrocortisone (as sodium succinate) 200 mg can be administered intramuscularly or by slow IV injection, after severe attacks to help avert further release of mediators.
- Particularly important in those with asthma who are at increased risk of fatal anaphylaxis if they have been treated with steroids previously.
- Steroids such as hydrocortisone are definitely valuable, as they probably act earlier than thought and their action persists after the adrenaline has worn off. They block the manufacture of prostaglandin and leukotrienes, which are also important mediators.

The triggers for an anaphylactic shock are as follows:

- Peanuts, nuts, fish, shellfish.
- Medications such as antibiotics, aspirin, IV contrast used in some imaging tests.
- Other causative agents: NSAIDs, anaesthetics, muscle relaxants, latex and radiocontrast media.
- Stings from bees, wasps, hornets and ants.

Anaphylaxis is often unpredictable, and so the critical care nurse needs to focus on how she/he can decrease risks. Strategies:

- Ensure that a detailed patient history and full physical examination is done.
- Consider the route of the medicine and the rate of the medicine and/or fluid.
- Identify patients with known causes of anaphylaxis.

TABLE 1.8 Microorganisms associated with septic shock.

Type of bacteria	Microorganisms	Occurrence
Gram-negative	Escherichia coli Klebsiella Enterobacter Pseudomonas aeruginosa Serratia Proteus Bacteroides fragilis (anaerobe)	50% of all cases
Gram-positive	Staphylococcus aureus Streptococcus pneumoniae Alpha-haemolytic streptococci	10% of all cases
Fungi	Candida	2% of all cases

- Sound knowledge of the medicine, as some cross-react and also are contraindicated if there is a known history of anaphylaxis.
- The greater the number of years since the last administration of the offending agent, the less the chance of a recurrence.

Septic Shock

This is caused by an overwhelming infection in the blood and may be the result of a suppressed immune system, a massive burn injury or anything else that can introduce an infecting organism into a compromised victim.

- The most common organism is a gram-negative enteric bacillus, such as *Escherichia coli, Pseudomonas,* or gram-positive *Staphylococcus aureus* (Table 1.8).
- These organisms enter the vascular system and release endotoxins, which cause an interstitial fluid leak, increased vascular permeability and vasodilatation, leading to shock.

The result of septic shock is tachycardia and a high CO (Fig. 1.2). In this state, the patient may feel warm, have a high temperature, a low circulating volume owing to venous pooling, increased capillary permeability and third-space fluid shift. CO is maintained at a normal/high level by the increasing tachycardia, but if volume loss is not corrected, hypovolaemia will persist, CO will decrease, and the skin will become cool. As in all other types of shock, the primary problem is tissue hypoperfusion; consequently, nutrients and oxygen fail to be delivered to cells.

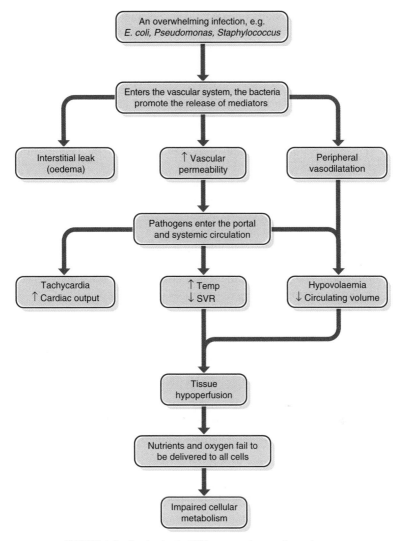

FIGURE 1.2   Septic shock. SVR = systemic vascular resistance.

The results of septic shock are as follows:

- Tachycardia.
- High CO − maintained at a normal/high level by the increasing tachycardia.
- The patient feels warm and has a high temperature.
- A low circulating volume owing to venous pooling, increased capillary permeability and third space fluid shift.

If volume loss is not corrected, hypovolaemia will persist, CO will decrease, and the skin will become cool. As in all other types of shock, the primary problem is tissue hypoperfusion; consequently, nutrients and oxygen fail to be delivered to cells. Sepsis can be treated with antibiotics.

Treatment guidelines have been produced to improve survival from sepsis:

- The sepsis 6 standardized by the inclusion of three ins and three outs, which need to be completed within the first hour following the recognition of sepsis:
    - Three ins are administration of oxygen therapy, IV fluid administration, IV antibiotics
    - Three outs are blood measure of lactate, blood cultures and urine output
- Quick sepsis organ failure assessment is used to determine the extent of a person's organ function or rate of failure:
    - Heart failure − fluid balance chart positive balance, increase in weight, changes in vital signs, coughing up frothy sputum
    - Renal failure − changes in blood results increase in urea and creatinine, reduced haemoglobin; fluid balance chart reduced urine output, positive balance, increase in weight; urinalysis contains protein
    - Liver failure − changes in liver function tests, urinalysis contains bilirubin, jaundice
    - Respiratory failure − changes in respiratory rate, pattern and depth, oxygen saturation, arterial blood gases (ABGs)
    - Neurological abnormalities − confusion, disorientation, changes in Glasgow coma scale
- Sepsis survival campaign is around interventions that may need to be included in addition to the sepsis 6:
    - Consideration of the family/initiate palliative care
    - Blood analysis
    - Intubation/ventilation
    - Continuous monitoring of blood glucose levels
    - Prevention of stress ulcers, deep vein thrombosis/pulmonary embolism (PE) and pressure ulcers
    - Renal replacement therapy
    - Sedation/analgesia
    - Nutrition such as enteral feeding

These standardized treatment guidelines are mainly for medical practitioners, but there is no reason why nurses cannot consider these areas in the management and care of their patients with sepsis.

Systemic Inflammatory Response Syndrome

SIRS is a type of shock that presents with all the signs of sepsis/septic shock due to a nonspecific insult, such as ischemia, pancreatitis, with no evidence of an infectious origin. This is often referred to as SIRS. This is when inflammatory mediators have entered the bloodstream and lead to widespread systemic inflammation.

SIRS criteria are as follows:

Body temperature <36 or >38°C
HR >90 bpm
Respiratory rate >20 per minute or $PaCO_2$ <4.3 kPa
WBC <4 × 10^9/L, >12 × 10^9/L

When two or more of these criteria are present without evidence of infection, a patient may be diagnosed with SIRS. It is important to consider SIRS when all the signs of sepsis/septic shock are present without any history of infection. Thus, all the signs of sepsis/septic shock might be ignored, as the patient does not have an infective focus.

Neurogenic Shock

Neurogenic shock causes changes to smooth muscle in the walls of the circulatory vessels due to inappropriate nervous system action, which leads to an imbalance between parasympathetic and sympathetic stimulation. There is a loss of sympathetic tone, causing widespread peripheral vasodilatation and a severe reduction in BP and hypotension (Fig. 1.3). The hypotension often observed in neurogenic shock can give the appearance of hypovolaemia or hypovolaemic shock. There is reduced vascular tone leading to a decrease in systemic vascular resistance (SVR), inadequate CO, reduced tissue perfusion and impaired cellular metabolism.

The following are the causes of neurogenic shock:

- Brain stem injury at the level of the medulla
- An injury to the spinal cord
- Spinal anaesthesia

Neurogenic shock may mask signs and symptoms of other types of shock. If neurogenic shock is present, there should be a heightened suspicion for an undetected source of haemorrhage.

Cardiogenic Shock

Cardiogenic shock is a severe circulatory failure due to a primary defect in the pumping activity of the heart. The circulatory collapse becomes so profound

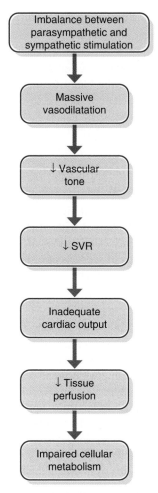

FIGURE 1.3 Neurogenic shock. SVR 5 systemic vascular resistance.

that myocardial contractility is decreased, and the body is unable adequately to compensate as CO drops.

- This occurs when the heart, due to impaired myocardial performance, cannot produce an adequate CO to sustain the metabolic requirements of body tissues.
- Myocardial infarction (MI) is the most common cause of cardiogenic shock, as the area infarcted becomes dysfunctional, and, depending on the size of the infarction, stroke volume and CO may decrease with a concurrent increase in left ventricular end-diastolic pressure (Edwards, 2002).

Compensatory mechanisms are stimulated by the decrease in BP, and catecholamines are released. This causes an increase in HR, contractility, BP and SVR to maintain arterial pressure.

The compensatory mechanisms improve blood flow for a time, but more oxygen is required by the already ischaemic cardiac muscle to pump blood into the constricted systemic circulation, consequently increasing cardiac workload. The heart becomes more ischaemic, and cardiac failure worsens. The result is to jeopardize potentially viable tissue and worsen left ventricular function. As CO continues to decline, BP and tissue perfusion decrease, which results in cardiogenic shock and ends with the patient's death (Fig. 1.4). Arrhythmias or pulmonary oedema often complicate cardiogenic shock.

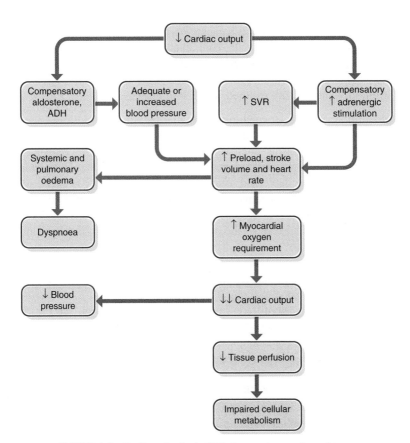

FIGURE 1.4 Cardiogenic shock. SVR 5 systemic vascular resistance.

Hypovolaemic Shock

- This is the most common type of shock.
- It is the state that results from hypovolaemia, and shock occurs due to a decrease in the circulating fluid volume so large that the body's metabolic needs cannot be met.
- The decline in blood volume produced by continued bleeding, plasma loss, bleeding disorders, water or fluid shifts, dehydration or high temperature (Richards and Edwards, 2014) decreases venous return and CO.
- The decrease in intravascular volume primarily affects tissue perfusion.

The degree of shock depends on the amount of blood/circulating volume lost:

- 15% of total blood volume can be lost without causing any serious symptoms
- Above 15%, homeostatic mechanisms start to ensure major organs receive blood, with a weak pulse, pale, cool, clammy skin
- Between 30% and 40%, BP begins to drop
- Above 40%, organs will begin to fail, and urine output may cease
- If blood volume is not restored, death will ensue

In addition, the rate at which blood/circulating volume is lost, the age and general physical condition of the patient and the patient's ability to activate compensatory mechanisms contribute to severity. Numerous compensatory mechanisms to increase venous tone are activated when the circulating volume and venous return are decreased. As a result, venous capacity is decreased to match the smaller blood volume, and adequate transport of oxygen and nutrients is maintained.

If the fluid loss exceeds the ability of homeostatic mechanisms to compensate for the loss, the CVP, diastolic filling pressure, stroke volume, and systemic arterial BP will fall. As the severity of shock increases, blood is pooled in the capillary and venous beds, with further impairment of the effective vascular volume available for oxygen transport and tissue perfusion (Fig. 1.5). To identify the different types of shock in a patient, see Fig. 1.6.

Patients in shock will not uncommonly have components of more than one of the forms of shock. For example, patients in cardiogenic shock may also be hypovolaemic due to loss of fluid into the tissues as a result of high venous pressures or increased capillary permeability. Hypovolaemia is also frequently a complication of septic shock, and in late stages of hypovolaemic shock, patients usually have some degree of cardiac failure and vasomotor collapse complicating their shock picture.

Fluid replacement therapy (FRT) needs to be administered using crystalloids that contain sodium in the range of 130–154 mmol/L, with a bolus dose of 500 mL over <15 min (NICE, 2017).

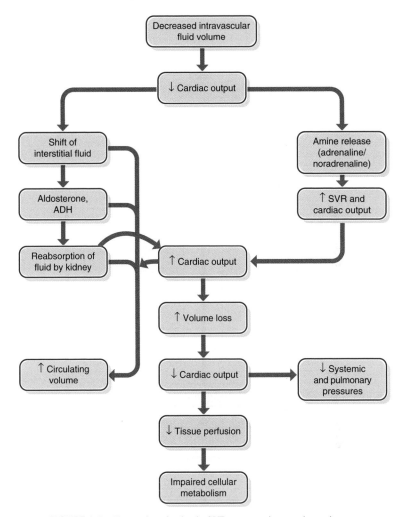

FIGURE 1.5 Hypovolaemic shock. SVR = systemic vascular resistance.

The Stages of Shock

In shock, irrespective of the initial cause, the end result is always the same, that is, the tissues fail to receive oxygen and nutrients and to rid themselves of waste products. It is inadequate tissue and cell perfusion, which causes widespread disruption to cellular metabolism (Fig. 1.6).

Shock is a very complex syndrome, as the problem concerns not only the amount of blood volume but also delivery in terms of blood flow to organs and cells of the body. There are a number of variables that affect the course of shock, such as the age and the general state of health of the person before the shock insult (see later).

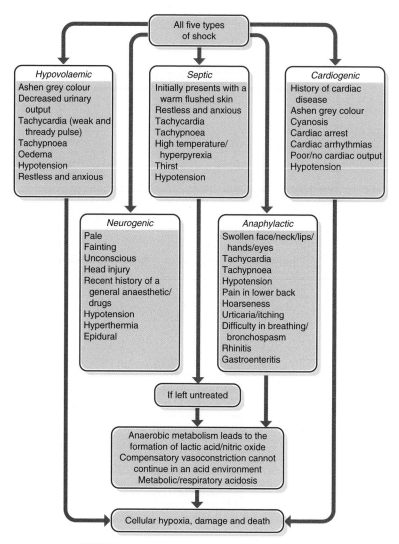

FIGURE 1.6   Signs and symptoms of all types of shock.

It is the responsibility of the nurse that the development of shock must be prevented. This includes early interpretation of observational and measurable data to recognize its early development. For easy understanding and recognition of shock, it can be divided into three stages: compensated, progressive or uncompensated and irreversible. These stages are not distinct and should be regarded as a continuum.

There has been debate recently regarding whether there are three or four stages of shock, with the addition of an initial stage included in some literature. The initial stage of shock is mentioned, but evidence to its relevance to nursing practice is debatable.

Stage 0 — The Initial Stage

Some new literature on shock proposes an initial stage of shock whereby cellular metabolism switches from aerobic to anaerobic and produces lactic acid (Garretson and Malberti, 2007). However, this stage can be asymptomatic, does not show visual clinical signs, and as a result, some disregard the existence of the initial stage (Richards and Edwards, 2014). Some of the literature that describes an initial stage of shock includes processes that are more likely to be clinically evident during the progressive stage of shock, for example, anaerobic metabolism and an increased production of lactic acid. There is limited evidence that this stage has clinical significance, as the compensatory stage of shock will be recognized almost immediately before any signs of the initial stage can be determined.

Stage 1 — Compensated Shock

The compensatory stage of shock begins as the body's homeostatic attempt to maintain cardiovascular dynamics and stabilize the circulation in the face of whatever defect is causing the shock. The compensatory mechanisms involved are as follows:

Sympathetic Nervous System

- Sympathetic nervous system — initiated by the decrease in arterial pressure that stimulates baroreceptors.
- Responds to any decrease in arterial BP, whether it is due to haemorrhage, peripheral blood pooling or a decrease in myocardial contractility.
- A decrease in circulation causes the pressure exerted by the blood in the artery (BP) to reduce.
- The increase in resistance caused by baroreceptor control is not uniform throughout the body's organ systems. Some systems are given preference as to the amount of blood flow they will receive, varying the distribution of CO, with some organs being well perfused and others being hypoperfused.
- This decreases the rate of firing of both the carotid sinus and the aortic arch baroreceptors and supplies sensory information to the cardiovascular centre in the medulla of the brain, which regulates BP. This regulating reflex increases:
  - Sympathetic nervous system (SNS) discharge, which will increase HR
  - Myocardial contractility and peripheral resistance by vasoconstriction of blood vessels
  - Total peripheral vascular resistance
  - Arterial BP
  - Myocardial afterload

Release of Noradrenaline and Adrenaline

- This difference in distribution of CO is due to the distribution of alpha (to gut, skin) and beta (heart, lungs) adrenergic receptors in the body (Table 1.9).

TABLE 1.9 Adrenergic receptors.

Neurotransmitter	Receptor type	Major locations	Effects of binding
Adrenaline (released by adrenal medulla)	Beta$_1$	Myocardium, sphincters of the GIT, renal arterioles.	Increased heart rate and strength; stimulates renin release by kidney; lipolysis in adipose tissue leading to increased blood glucose level; decreased digestion and GIT motility.
	Beta$_2$	Smooth muscles of the bronchioles, skeletal muscles, blood vessels supplying the brain, heart, kidneys, mast cells, the uterus, and liver cells.	Bronchodilation; increased skeletal muscle excitability; vasodilation of blood vessels in the brain, heart, kidneys and skeletal muscle; decreased bile secretion and increased glycogenolysis; stabilization of the membrane of the mast cell.
Noradrenaline	Alpha$_1$	Blood vessels; smooth muscle of the GIT, all sympathetic target organs except heart.	Constricts blood vessels; decreases GIT motility, slows digestion, decreases bile secretion, increases glycogenolysis.
	Alpha$_2$	Presynaptically and found on all adrenergic nerve terminals.	When adrenergic stimulation is excessive and leads to build-up, the stimulation of these receptors results in inhibition even though the stimulation persists.

- These receptors respond to catecholamines (adrenaline and noradrenaline) liberated from postganglionic sympathetic nerve endings and the adrenal medulla.
- Stimulation of the adrenal glands occurs early in shock, mainly due to stress, and activates the SNS, which causes a release of catecholamines (noradrenaline and adrenaline).
- Circulating concentrations of adrenaline during shock can increase within 5−60 min of injury.

- Adrenaline increases arteriolar resistance, which helps to support perfusion pressure in the face of a relatively low CO.
- Noradrenaline leads to vasoconstriction of certain organs and tissues, which will be hypoperfused (GIT, skin, skeletal muscles) and may cause problems when and if the shock continues. The vasoconstriction of the GIT due to the effect of noradrenaline can be the major contributor to the production of lactic acid early in shock.
- In addition, adrenaline:
  - increases circulating glucose concentrations by inhibiting insulin secretion, consequently raising blood glucose level;
  - stimulates pancreatic glucagon release and gluconeogenesis and
  - stimulates beta receptors in the heart, increasing myocardial contractility (inotropic effect) and HR (chronotropic effect), which improves CO and increases BP.

The vasoconstriction of the GIT and a reduction in blood supply, due to the action of noradrenaline, can lead to gut cells reverting to anaerobic metabolism and an early rise in lactic acid production.

Renal Autoregulation

- The kidneys play a complex role in restoring extracellular fluid volume and increasing systemic BP.
- This system is stimulated principally when there is a decrease in BP.
- This elaborate set of interlinked processes involves the renin–angiotensin–aldosterone system (RAAS).
- A decrease in kidney perfusion activates the renin–angiotensin–aldosterone mechanism.
- Renin is released by the kidneys, and angiotensinogen is catalytically combined to renin to produce angiotensin I and travels to the lungs.
- Once in the lungs, angiotensin I is converted to angiotensin II by the angiotensin-converting enzyme.
- Angiotensin II has three primary actions:
  - It can enhance the effect of noradrenaline and directly cause vasoconstriction of the peripheral vasculature, which will directly increase the BP by increasing the SVR to maintain BP in the face of a worsening shocked state.
  - Antidiuretic hormone (ADH) will stimulate the reabsorption of water in the renal tubules increasing circulating volume.

- Aldosterone causes increased sodium and a net movement of water reabsorption in the renal tubules resulting in a further increase in intravascular circulating volume, resulting in increased venous return to the heart, CO, and BP, thus providing a longer term compensation for shock. This leads to a reduction of urine output often observed in the early stages of shock.

Arterial Chemoreceptors

There are two types of chemoreceptors — central and peripheral, which transmit impulses to the medulla in the brain, which regulates BP.

Central chemoreceptors:

- Sensitive to a reduction in carbon dioxide, hydrogen ions and pH in blood.
- An increase in carbon dioxide causes vasodilatation and a decrease in BP.
- A decrease in carbon dioxide or pH causes vasoconstriction and a reflexive increase in BP.

Peripheral chemoreceptors

- Sensitive to changes in oxygen concentration of the blood.
- A decrease in arterial oxygen concentration causes vasoconstriction and a reflexive increase in BP.
- Smooth muscle layers in blood vessels carry out these BP changes.
- If hypoxia occurs due to shock, then patients are at risk of having an increased BP, and heart conditions or varicose veins can compound this, which can further increase their resistance and thus BP.
- Osmoreceptors
  - Osmoreceptors are highly specialized hypothalamic neurons, which continually monitor the solute concentration (and thus water concentration) of the blood.
  - If concentrations of sodium (the major cation in extracellular fluid) are increased, as in the case when there is a loss of extracellular water, osmoreceptors in the hypothalamus are stimulated.
  - When solutes threaten to become too concentrated, as in conditions that cause an increased sodium concentration (excessive sweating, inadequate fluid intake, burns), the osmoreceptors transmit excitatory impulses to the hypothalamic neurons and release ADH.
    - Once in blood, ADH targets kidney tubules and inhibits or prevents urine formation — the tubule cells respond by increasing water absorption at the renal collecting duct and returning it to the circulation.
    - As a result, less urine is produced, and blood volume increases, improving venous return to the heart, CO, and BP.
    - Urinary output will decrease, and the sense of thirst will be aroused.

Capillary Dynamics

- When compensatory mechanisms cease to respond to stimulus, BP will start to drop, leading to a change in capillary hydrostatic pressure (HP) compared to colloidal oncotic pressure (COP) in the capillaries and interstitial fluid. In this instance, fluid will be drawn from the interstitial fluid (ISF) spaces to bring up BP. In a well-hydrated patient, this can maintain BP lengthening the compensatory stage of shock.

Elderly patients are not usually well hydrated, and Interstitial Fluid (ISF) content, as a consequence, is reduced; thus, this group of patients will deteriorate much quicker when in a state of shock.

Generally, the clinical picture of a patient in the compensatory stage of shock is:

- Tachycardia, narrowing pulse pressure, increase in temperature and blood glucose level due to the effect of catecholamines;
- Pale skin colour, cool to cold skin due to the redistribution of blood away from the skin and clammy due to the activation of sweat glands by the SNS;
- Decrease in urine output due to selective vasoconstriction of the renal bed and the actions of ADH and aldosterone;
- Absent bowel sounds due to the reduced GIT motility from the action of noradrenaline;
- An increase in BP and rate and depth of respiration;
- Mental state alterations ranging from restlessness to coma and
- Complaining of thirst.

These protective mechanisms, observed in the compensatory stage of shock can maintain circulation and BP. These mechanisms will eventually cease to function, and circulatory failure will ensue. If the metabolic acidosis, circulatory failure or volume is not corrected or treatment instigated, progressive shock will occur in a short space of time.

Stage 2 – Progressive or Uncompensated Shock

Once shock has developed, the course it takes is complex. Certainly, the prognosis in some forms of shock – particularly hypovolaemic shock – is excellent if treated in the early compensatory stage. Once shock has progressed into this stage, the outcome is no longer as predictable. As shock progresses, there are deleterious changes:

Oxygen Supply and Demand

- An imbalance between oxygen supply and tissue demand is fundamental to the nature of shock. The demand for oxygen by the cells outweighs supply.

- Oxygen supply and demand are maintained in balance as long as oxygen is supplied to the body and carbon dioxide is eliminated through ventilation, perfusion, diffusion and cell metabolism.
- Under normal circumstances, whole body oxygen consumption (VO_2) is maintained over a wide range of oxygen delivery (DO_2) by varying oxygen extraction. For example, as VO_2 increases so does DO_2. When VO_2/DO_2 increases and DO_2 falls below a critical level, this gives rise to an oxygen debt, and hypoxia occurs.
- The events following shock place increased demands on these processes, and when overwhelmed, the victim of shock is at risk of pulmonary complications, leading to a supply–demand deficit and hypoxia.

Cellular Energy Production

- Nutrients, such as glucose and fatty acids, as well as oxygen, enter the cell across the cell membrane.
- Shock results in an inadequate flow of nutrients and oxygen to the cell.
- This causes a reduction in adenosine triphosphate (ATP) concentrations in the mitochondria of the cell, which fall within 15 min following hypoxia. Mitochondrial activity is diminished due to a lack of oxygen for glycolysis leading to anaerobic metabolism. The end product of anaerobic metabolism by the cell is lactic acid, which rapidly builds up in the blood, leading to a reduction in the energy available for cell work and eventually lowers the pH.
- This gives rise to a decrease in the energy available for cell work, consequently leading to metabolic acidosis, and tissue and organ dysfunction.
- Poor blood flow also impairs the normal removal of carbon dioxide, which is converted to carbonic acid, further lowering blood pH.
- Lactic acidosis also reduces myocardial contractility, and arteriolar responsiveness to further adrenaline and noradrenaline release, potentiating vasomotor collapse, stimulates the intravascular clotting mechanism.
- Acidosis has the beneficial effect of shifting the oxyhaemoglobin dissociation curve to the right, thereby facilitating the release of oxygen from Hb.
- Eventually, a large number of inflammatory mediators are released from damaged cells into the circulation, resulting in progressive vasodilatation, myocardial depression, increased capillary permeability and eventually intravascular coagulation.
- These substances include histamine, serotonin, kinins, lysosomal enzymes, and endogenous mediators.
- If cellular acidosis becomes extreme, cellular dysfunction becomes intemperate, and if permitted to continue, may finally become irreversible.

Cellular Membrane Disruption

- If cellular acidosis due to hypoxia becomes extreme, the hypoxic cell swells, becomes distorted and finally ruptures (Fig. 1.7).
- The shortage of ATP changes the normal ionic gradients across the cell membrane, with a rapid efflux of potassium from the cell, and movement of sodium and chloride into the cell.
- An increased sodium in the interior of cells results in water also entering the cell, driven by osmotic forces, causing cellular swelling and distortion, which may interfere with organelle function and lead to disintegration of the mitochondrial matrix.

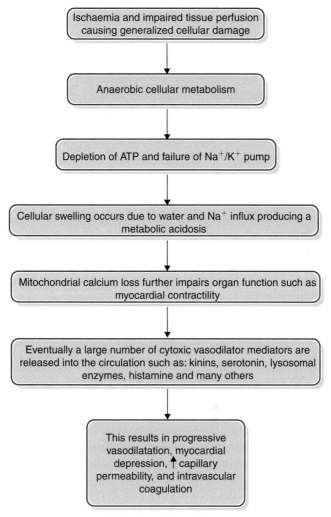

FIGURE 1.7   Cellular changes common to all forms of shock.

- This is why just delivering to patients with shock an adequate or higher oxygen concentration than normal does not always lead to prevention or recovery from cellular hypoxia, and aerobic respiration is not always fully restored.

The Role of Calcium

- The influx of calcium into the cell during shock is dysfunctional also because of a lack of ATP.
- Intracellular calcium is an important signalling system responsible for the activation of phospholipases and proteases, and its derangement results in membrane disruption.
- As a result, calcium accumulates in the mitochondria, causing structural derangement of the organelles, and may be the hallmark of irreversible cellular injury and eventually cell death.

The Role of Lysosomes Within the Cell

- Lysosomes are important cell structures, which are affected during shock.
- Contain enzymes, which function as a system for the breakdown of cell waste
- The lysosomal membrane is ordinarily quite stable, but it becomes fragile when the cell is injured or deprived of oxygen.
- Lysosomal membrane instability is made worse by the lack of ATP, and the cell starts to use its own structural phospholipids as a nutrient source.
- Eventually, the lysosomal membrane becomes more permeable and may rupture, allowing the release of lysosomal enzymes, resulting in self-digestion of the cell.
- The use of steroids in shock is thought to help stabilize the lysosomal membrane and prevent lysosomal-enzyme damage to the cell.

Cellular Fluid Shifts

- Any type of shock will automatically trigger an inflammatory response (see Section 4).
- The normal body response will be to send nutrients, fluids, white blood cells and clotting factors to the damaged site to repair tissue, prevent infection and, if necessary, stem blood loss.
- Capillaries vasodilate and become more permeable to allow these factors to reach the site of injury, leading to localized swelling and lymphatic blockage.
- The increased permeability causes movements of fluids, allowing water, electrolytes and other particles (such as albumin) into the interstitial spaces, and are known as a third-space fluid shift.
- When a third-space fluid shift occurs, a patient can appear paradoxically 'dry' or hypovolaemic as fluid has moved into the intravascular spaces yet may still have the same excess amount of body water.

- The vasodilatation is caused by the release of cell mediators (e.g., histamine, kinins, complement) from the damaged endothelium and causes a reduction in BP and peripheral vascular resistance and an increase in HR, further compounding the appearance of a hypovolaemic state.

Coagulation Defects

- Early in shock, changes in blood coagulation can be seen. Hypercoagulability occurs as a result of the stimulation of the IIR.
- Systemic changes in coagulation also occur as a result of the effects of catecholamines, lysosomal enzymes and acidosis.
- Platelet aggregation is increased in response to stress. This process of hypercoagulability may at first be compensatory if the cause of the shock is haemorrhage, but later it can produce drastic problems.
- The combination of hypercoagulation and stagnation of the blood in the capillaries may be responsible for microemboli developing during or following shock.
- These microemboli enhance tissue ischaemia and the progression of shock by decreasing the already poor blood flow through the capillaries to the tissues, damaging organs and leading to multiple organ failure.
- Late in shock, a state of hypocoagulability may develop owing to loss of clotting factors through:
  - Haemorrhage,
  - Replacement of lost volume — crystalloid/non-crystalloid solutions causing haemodilution and
  - The blood being deficient in clotting factors and a decrease in the production of clotting factors.

The progressive stage of shock is predominantly marked by continuing hypoperfusion, cellular changes and hypoxia, leading to a reduction in BP and deteriorating organ function. How far the deterioration in organ function goes will vary from person to person, but organ function will largely determine the course and outcome. However, some organs bear the brunt of the body's effort to compensate for a decrease in systemic pressure, and as a result, these organs will suffer damage, and dysfunction will appear early in the shock syndrome. The point at which organ dysfunction becomes irreversible is not clear. The major organs affected are the kidneys, liver, GIT, heart, lungs and brain (Table 1.10).

Stage 3 — Refractory (Irreversible) Shock

- This is the final stage of shock and is where severe cellular and organ dysfunction leads to general decline and death.
- In this stage, it may be possible to return arterial pressure to normal for a short while, but tissue and organ deterioration continue, and no amount of therapy will reverse the process.

TABLE 1.10 Effects of shock on specific organs.

Organ	Effect	Result
Kidneys — the most important and apparent organ affected early in shock	Renal blood flow is reduced early. As the total renal blood flow falls, the GFR is reduced, and the kidney will release renin. The GFR is preserved for a time, but oliguria nevertheless occurs, due to ADH and aldosterone secretion.	When there is a reduction in oxygen and energy, the reabsorptive functions for sodium and water are lost, and the renal tubules undergo necrosis. Acute tubular necrosis of the kidney commonly occurs in shock, and if severe may lead to acute renal failure, contributing to late deaths following resuscitation.
Liver — a highly complex organ having multiple functions	It is sensitive to ischaemia; both hepatic arterial and portal venous blood flow are reduced in shock. Early in shock, the liver releases large amounts of glucose as the result of adrenaline-induced glycogenolysis and gluconeogenesis.	In uncompensated shock, all liver functions are depleted, including bile and cholesterol formation, protein synthesis, gluconeogenesis, lactate metabolism, detoxification and glycogen storage, and the phagocytic activity of the Kupffer cells is depressed.
The GIT	The GIT suffers an early reduction of oxygen in shock, due to ADH, angiotensin II and catecholamines. There is, however, a threshold whereby the reduction in blood flow affects food/gut motility and absorption, and produces lactate in large amounts. The gut is the major source of lactic acidosis in haemorrhagic shock.	In shock, the gut mucosa barrier loses its integrity and is permeable to bacterial and endotoxins from the intestinal lumen, resulting in damage/necrosis of the intestinal wall by digestive enzymes. This may then allow pathogens to enter the portal and systemic circulation, causing infection and multiple organ failure.
Lungs — necessary for ventilation and perfusion for oxygenation and removing waste gases	In shock, the reduced pulmonary blood flow results in an imbalance between oxygen supply and tissue demands. These are compensated for by hyperventilation due to chemoreceptor stimulation, and thus, arterial partial pressure of oxygen is well maintained.	Ventilation and/or perfusion and gas exchange are poor or do not take place, resulting in progressive atelectasis ARDS, respiratory muscle fatigue from respiratory muscle hypoperfusion, and respiratory failure.

TABLE 1.10 Effects of shock on specific organs.—cont'd

Organ	Effect	Result
Heart — early deaths are associated with unsupportable reductions in cardiac function	The heart muscle relies on the delivery of oxygen and nutrients to its cells via the coronary arteries and has a very high oxygen requirement. Thus, a major reduction in cardiac blood flow quickly renders the heart muscle ischaemic.	Blood flow during shock is relatively preserved due to homeostatic compensation. Myocardial dysfunction occurs if there is a reduction in coronary blood flow exceeding the limits of compensatory mechanisms. Eventually, the heart ceases to function adequately as a pump, causing a decrease in cardiac output. Failure of the circulatory pump intensifies the deficient oxygen delivery throughout the remainder of the body, as well as to the heart itself.
Brain — most susceptible to hypoxic injury because it depends on glucose and oxygen to function	Although protected by the homeostatic vasoconstriction and by its own autoregulation, if the systolic blood pressure falls below 60 mm Hg, the capacity for autoregulation is exceeded.	Mental state abnormalities are associated with poor outcome, as respiratory alkalosis, hypoxaemia and electrolyte disturbances start to appear. If blood flow continues to deteriorate, autoregulation can no longer maintain normal cerebral metabolism. Unconsciousness and irreversible brain damage rapidly occur.

ADH, antidiuretic hormone; *ARDS*, adult respiratory distress syndrome; *GFR*, glomerular filtration rate.

- So much tissue damage and necrosis have occurred, so many mediators and toxins have been released into the systemic circulation, and acidosis is so profound that even a return of normal CO and arterial pressure will not reverse the downward progression.

At this point, there is an almost total depletion of ATP stores, which are very difficult to restore once they are gone. There is usually vasomotor failure due to central nervous system (CNS) ischaemia. The vasomotor centres become so depressed that no sympathetic activity occurs. The vascular bed is generally dilated owing to the CNS depression, acidosis, and toxins. Deterioration will continue, and death will ensue.

Other Considerations

There are a number of variables that affect the course of shock, such as the age of the person, their general state of health before the shock insult, hypothermia and pain.

Age

- The elderly injured patient requires special attention in relation to shock, as they have:
  - Slowed blood circulation
  - Structural and functional changes in the skin
  - An overall decrease in heat-producing conservation activities
  - Decrease in shivering response (delayed onset and decreased effectiveness)
  - Slowed metabolic rate
  - Sedentary lifestyle
  - Decreased vasoconstrictor response
  - Diminished or absent sweating
  - Desynchronization of circadian rhythm
  - Undernutrition
  - A decreased perception of heat and cold
- Therefore, they are at more risk of developing late-stage shock following injury than a younger person.
- They are more likely to be suffering from dehydration, and if prolonged, this can severely enhance hypovolaemic shock.
- Dehydration itself is a critical state; added to any other form of shock, it can precipitate and progress very early to multiple organ failure.

General State of Health

- A patient suffering any medical condition is in danger of the effects of shock appearing early due to the inability of the body to initiate homeostatic autoregulation mechanisms.
- Hypertension can affect the circulation by damaging the walls of the systemic blood vessels.
- A prolonged high pressure within these vessels stimulates the vessels to thicken and strengthen to withstand the stress.
- The thickening gradually becomes sufficient to narrow the blood vessels' lumina, reducing the patient's ability to compensate during shock states.
- Heart failure reduces the supply of nutrients to body tissues and causes circulatory stasis, pulmonary congestion and increased stress on the body. This is a serious condition, which, in situations that cause shock, can enhance the physiological processes and influence the patient's recovery. Arteriosclerosis and atherosclerosis frequently affect the peripheral

arteries, which influences the survival of the body's extremities, most commonly the lower extremities, during shock.

- It is imperative to take the patient's general state of health into account, as shock in these patients is more likely to occur due to the patient being more susceptible to low flow states, microemboli and loss of limb.
- Pain (see p. 264)
  - The goals of trauma teams have expanded to include controlling pain, which can increase an already taxed energy requirement.
  - The presence of pain can interfere with obtaining accurate and reliable measurements, which can lead to false, inaccurate readings (e.g., increase in BP, heart and respiratory rate) and, as such, delay the detection of shock.
  - Pain needs to be identified early, and nurses should provide tools to help patients assess and communicate their pain.
- Hypothermia
  - A high majority of shock patients may suffer from hypothermia, which is a result of prolonged exposure to cold environments (surgical procedures, trauma).
  - Hypothermia is characterized by a marked cooling of core temperature below 35°C.
  - A temperature of below 35°C is below the hypothalamic set point and results in attempts to conserve and generate body heat.
  - Vasoconstriction occurs, and muscle tone increases, providing an increase in heat production and a decrease in heat loss, thus maintaining body temperature at normal.
  - In extreme cold, these mechanisms can no longer produce enough heat to maintain normal temperature, and hypothermia ensues.
  - Hypothermia affects virtually all metabolic processes in the body, and these effects can delay the diagnosis of shock.

Cardiopulmonary Resuscitation

Basic Life Support

The instigation of resuscitation in the event of a cardiac arrest occurring in critical care is to save lives.

The Sequence of Basic Life Support

First, ensure you are safe, check the environment for spillages or wires, check the victim's response by gently shaking their shoulders and ask loudly 'Can you hear me' or 'Are you alright'. If there is no response, call for help. Assess the airway, breathing and circulation before initiating active interventions:

- A − Airway maintenance: open the airway and ensure it is secure, insert a Guedel's airway if available

- B — Breathing, look, listen and feel for normal breathing for no more than 10 s, if available, maintain breathing using bag and mask
- C — Circulation, start chest compressions

The ABCDE approach when determining a cardiac arrest is slightly different to that of assessing a deteriorating patient.

In a hospital situation, call the resuscitation team; if outside, dial 999.

The purpose of basic life support is to maintain adequate ventilation and circulation until help arrives. Airway, breathing and circulation is always the priority order. The sequence of action is as follows:

1. Ensure the safety of yourself and the patient.
2. Check responsiveness of the patient. Ask 'are you alright?', give a verbal command and gently shake the shoulders.
3. If the patient responds by answering or moving, leave in position (if safe), assess condition and get help. If she/he does not respond, shout for help and then open the airway by tilting the head and lifting the chin.
4. Keeping the airway open, look, listen and feel for breathing for up to 10 s before deciding that breathing is absent.
5. If the patient is breathing, turn into the recovery position, check for continued breathing, get help. If she/he is not breathing, turn him/her on to his/her back and remove any visible obstruction from the mouth.
6. Assess casualty for signs of circulation.
7. If no signs of circulation, start compressions at the centre of the sternum mid nipple line; depress 1.5—2 in or 4—5 cm at a rate of 100 times per minute.
8. Combine compressions and rescue breathing at a ratio of 30:2.
9. Continue resuscitation until the casualty shows signs of life and/or help arrives.

Intermediate Cardiopulmonary Resuscitation (CPR)

- Many calls in practice are periarrests, which have implications for survival and soon will take over from cardiac arrest calls.
- The chain of survival includes four key interrelated steps to optimize survival:
  - Early recognition and call for help as most cardiac arrests are predictable:
    - A drop in BP and reduced oxygen saturation.
    - When these signs occur, a precardiac arrest call can be given.

TABLE 1.11 Respiratory and cardiac reasons for cardiac arrest.

Airway problems	Cardiac problems	
	Primary	Secondary
Central nervous system	Coronary syndrome	Asphyxia
Blood	Dysrhythmia	Hypoxaemia
Vomit	Increased blood pressure	Blood loss
Foreign body	Heart disease	Hypothermia
Trauma	Valve disease	Septic shock
Infection	Drugs	
Inflammation	Hereditary	
Laryngospasm	Electrolytes	
Bronchospasm	Acid–base changes	
Inhalation/burns	Electrocution	
Drugs (suppression)		
Pain (breathing inadequately)		
Pneumothorax/haemothorax		
Chronic obstructive pulmonary disease		
Pulmonary embolism		
Adult respiratory distress syndrome		

- If these are not picked up, the patient could go on to a cardiac arrest.
- The areas of BP, heart and respiratory rate and oxygen saturation need to be tracked to determine changes in physiology to incorporate early warning systems.
- Early CPR – the reasons for patients' cardiac arrest are listed in Table 1.11:
  - Treat life-threatening problem
  - Reassessment
  - Assess effects of treatment
  - Call for help early – concentrate on this
  - Personal safety
  - Patient responsiveness
  - Vital signs (breathing deteriorates first and so changes first)
- Early defibrillation
- Early advanced life support and standardized postresuscitation care

Adult tidal volume is 500 mL, and dead space (air not involved in gaseous exchange) is up to 250 mL. Ventilation using bag and mask should reflect this, and breaths given (adult) need to be greater than 250 mL to be effective.

During CPR, consider potential reversible causes (4Hs and 4Ts)

- The 4Hs:
  - Hypoxia
  - Hypothermia
  - Hypo/hypokalaemia
  - Hypovolaemia
- The 4Ts:
  - Tamponade
  - Tension pneumothorax
  - Toxins
  - Thrombosis

Then continue with:

- Check electrode position
- Airway/oxygen
- IV access (variable rates of absorption from sites, e.g., radial, CVP)
- Give uninterrupted compressions
- Follow the CPR algorithm

Advanced Life Support

The Resuscitation Council (UK) recommends guidelines and protocols to manage shockable rhythms, such as VT and VF, and non-shockable rhythms, such as asystole and pulseless electrical activity. The protocol stresses early defibrillation and advanced care. Advanced life support involves:

- Following the guidelines set out by the resuscitation council (UK).
- Giving 1 mg adrenaline and sequences of 2:15 compressions/ventilation.
- Advanced airway care (intubation) after the first DC shock; once achieved, ventilation can proceed.
- Gaining venous access.
- Intubation — Advanced airway management using endotracheal intubation, oesophageal tracheal airways or are types of supraglottic airways that keep the patient's airway open during anaesthesia or unconsciousness. There is a range of these type of airways available:
  - Laryngeal mask airway (LMA)
  - iGel supraglottic airway
  - Extraglottic airway device
  - Oesophageal tracheal combitube

Fluid Overload

An increase in circulating volume can occur for many reasons:

- Past Medical History (PMH) of MI
- Circulation problems prior to admission, for example, heart failure and peripheral vascular disease
- Kidney problems, for example, renal failure
- Cirrhosis of the liver
- Following IV FRT given after surgery or shock:
  - Too much salt
  - Sluggish arterial and venous circulation caused by a stagnant flow of blood through the circulation due to continued bed rest or immobility

Prior to problems being observed (cyanosis and pale skin) or measured (BP and CVP) in the patient's condition, these processes activate compensatory mechanisms to maintain homeostasis, for example, atrial natriuretic peptide (ANP). ANP is released by the atria of the heart and exerts a potent diuretic effect, thus off-loading excess water and salt to protect the body against fluid overload.

Factors that Can Precipitate Fluid Overload

There are many specific conditions, which can precipitate fluid overload, by:

- Reducing the body's ability to maintain homeostasis in the event of an increase in circulating volume;
- Stimulating control mechanisms that accelerate the symptoms of fluid overload, for example, the RAAS and
- Causing the flow of blood to become turbulent, increasing SVR and BP.

All these conditions may hasten fluid overload during or following an IV infusion. The most common of these are hypertension, heart failure and peripheral vascular disease.

In all cases of fluid overload, there is an increase in circulatory volume. When the body is functioning normally, it is almost impossible to produce an excess of total body water. However, this can occur during IV treatment with either a crystalloid (normal saline, Hartmann's solution, 5% dextrose) or colloid (blood, gelofusine, albumin solutions, haematocele).

Blood Transfusion In this situation, blood velocity reduces, and blood flow becomes slow, leading to pooling of blood in the peripheries, lungs, liver, kidneys and possibly the brain. The heart can no longer pump the increasing amount of volume around the circulation. As the signs of heart failure increase and the kidneys become swamped with fluid and start to receive a lower blood supply, renal failure ensues. The complications of pulmonary oedema, cardiac failure, renal failure, ascites, cerebral oedema and peripheral oedema can be very serious if not treated quickly.

In the majority of cases when a blood transfusion is being administered, a diuretic is generally given with each or every alternate unit. This is even more important in patients who have problems with maintaining an adequate circulation.

Salt/Water Overload A fluid overload can occur with both crystalloid and colloid similar to those observed when giving whole blood:
Crystalloid Fluid. — The effects can be an overload of both salt and water (isotonic volume excess) or just salt (hypertonic volume excess) or a dilutional low sodium (hypotonic volume excesses).

Hypotonic volume excesses can lead to a dilutional hyponatraemia, whereby all blood contents are reduced. This is a life-threatening state, and if a patient has had a significant amount of FRT, blood results need to be monitored for any signs of reducing values.

Colloid Fluid. — The effect is an increase in COP drawing water/fluid from the ICF space into the circulation leading to a fluid overload.

Colloid fluid should be used sparingly. If the cause of fluid overload is due to the overuse of colloids, the excess fluid cannot be easily removed by diuretics, as protein does not appear in urine and cannot be offloaded by the kidney.

Obstetric and Gynaecological Emergencies

Pregnant women can be admitted to critical care either while pregnant or following delivery. Ventilating a pregnant woman is complex due to the physiological changes that occur during pregnancy, which can lead to many additional complications, some of which are life-threatening to mother and baby. The physiological changes of pregnancy can mask some of the standard measurements/observations used to monitor or diagnose these conditions.

The Physiological Changes of Pregnancy

Physiological alterations occur gradually, beginning in early pregnancy and continuing throughout gestation. The body makes physiological adaptations during pregnancy to maintain maternal homeostasis to meet the demands of foetal growth. Virtually all organ systems are affected.

Cardiovascular Changes

Maternal blood volume increases markedly. The increase in total volume for a single pregnancy is between 1000 and 1500 mL, more in multiple gestations. Blood volume rises by 30%−50%, and CO increases 20%−40% and may be decreased up to 30% in the supine position. This fluid overload of pregnancy ensures adequate perfusion for foetal and maternal needs and is a protective mechanism for the blood loss that occurs with delivery but imposes a 40% increase in maternal cardiac workload. Healthy expectant mothers adjust to the cardiovascular changes.

There is an elevation of oestrogens and progesterone during pregnancy; this:

- Increases plasma renin;
- Increases aldosterone levels, promoting sodium and water retention;
- The increase in progesterone level:
  - decreases SVR
  - produces vasodilatation of the peripheral vessels
- Increases HR by 10−15 bpm by the 14th week of pregnancy and
- Mean arterial BP decreases very little.

Respiratory Changes

Observed during pregnancy are necessary. The foetus must obtain oxygen and eliminate carbon dioxide through the mother. Maternal oxygen requirements increase in response to the growth and metabolism in the mother's body. The changes in tidal volume begin in the first trimester and progressively increase.

The diaphragm elevates about 4 cm, causing a decrease in the length of the lungs. To compensate, the lower rib cage flares. The minute ventilation increases by 50% by term because of the increase in respiratory rate by 15% and the tidal volume by 30%−40%. Combination of these decreases the arterial carbon dioxide tension ($PaCO_2$). The reduction in carbon dioxide is stimulated by progesterone, which increases levels of carbonic anhydrase in RBCs, facilitating carbon dioxide transfer. This results in an increase in ventilation and decrease in arterial partial pressure of carbon dioxide. The pH is not altered from the non-pregnant level of about 7.35−7.45; the fall in arterial partial pressure of carbon dioxide is matched by a fall in plasma bicarbonate. The kidneys and the renal excretion of bicarbonate maintain normal acid−base balance.

Oxygen consumption is greater, because of:

- The increase in circulating Hb.
- The increase in total oxygen-carrying capacity.
- There is an increase in the demand for oxygen and an increase in oxygen uptake by the cells of all organs, as well as the foetus.

This can result in a reduction in arterial partial pressure of oxygen. The functional residual capacity and residual volume of the lung are decreased.

Respiratory changes during pregnancy accelerate hypoxic tissue damage if the pulmonary system suffers insult.

Renal Changes

These changes occur in pregnancy, and these are dilatation of the renal parenchyma (especially the right), renal pelvis and ureters. The mother's kidneys must handle the increased metabolic and circulatory requirements of pregnancy. Pregnancy requires an increase in water to supply the foetus, placenta, amniotic fluid, and expanded maternal blood volume. At least 6.5 L of extra water is retained during a normal pregnancy. Fluid retention is due to increases in:

- Adreno-corticosteroids
- Tubular reabsorption
- Retention of sodium
- Circulatory stasis in the lower extremities

As a result:

- Urine output increases
- Specific gravity decreases
- Glucose and small amount of leukocytes may be present in the urine secondary to increased GFR

The abrupt increase in metabolism of albumin in early pregnancy, total protein and colloid osmotic pressure decreases during pregnancy. Sodium reabsorption by the kidneys is heightened during pregnancy to meet foetal needs and maintain the expanded maternal blood volume. Urine pooling is likely, resulting in a risk of urinary tract infection. The growing uterus displaces the bladder superiorly and anteriorly.

Immunological Changes

The developing foetus within the uterus is considered an allograft (a graft between two individuals of the same species but of different genotype). There are consequent changes in the body's defence mechanisms, which result in immune suppression. During pregnancy, maternal IgG is decreased due to placental transport. IgM and IgA levels do not change significantly, but complement activity increases.

Cellular immune response is decreased, resulting in high susceptibility to viral and bacterial infections. A contributing factor may be the physiological changes pregnancy induces in the structure and function of various systems.

Haematological Changes

These are reflected in the increase in the plasma volume and increase in erythrocyte volume, resulting in a physiological anaemia of pregnancy.

This anaemia is most apparent from the seventh month. An increase in clotting factors and fibrinogen may result in hypercoagulation and thrombus formation in women with decreased mobility. Therefore, both Hb and haematocrit values are lower during pregnancy. However, during pregnancy, the production of RBC increases to deliver more oxygen to cope with the increasing demand required by the organs of the body and the developing foetus, but the overall erythrocyte count will decrease because of physiological haemodilution.

Effects on Monitoring

The physiological changes in pregnancy affect the monitoring a pregnant woman requires while in critical care.

HR and BP. The maternal HR increases by 15–20 bpm, and mean arterial BP decreases by 10–15 mm Hg. As pregnancy progresses, mild tachycardia and a low BP indicate normal changes, rather than shock. An elevated BP may indicate pre-eclampsia and is never normal during pregnancy.

The ECG. As pregnancy progresses, the heart becomes displaced upward and to the left. This results in a slight anterior rotation; therefore, a left axis deviation may be noted in V_1 and V_2 in lead III of a 12-lead ECG. Flattened or inverted T waves also may be noted in lead III. Small Q waves may also be identified. These are considered to be normal findings related to anatomic changes of pregnancy and are not necessarily caused by an MI.

Skin Temperature. It can be a useful guide to determining the severity of hypovolaemia. During hypovolaemia, circulation to the major organs is maintained, leading to:

- Cool extremities
- An increase in BP
- Improved circulation to the body's major organs

A pregnant woman in shock may present with warm, dry skin rather than cool, clammy skin, due to circulating progesterone.

Ventilation Changes

Oxygen requirements during pregnancy can be 10%–20% above the non-pregnant state. Supplemental high-flow oxygen is always given to the injured pregnant patient. Since the pregnant patient may lose 15%–35% of blood volume before showing signs of shock fluid, replacement and oxygen are essential. The changes in tidal volume, respiratory rate and minute volume should be monitored in the event that a pregnant woman requires intubation. The result is an overall hyperventilation of the pregnant patient. This will lead to a chronic respiratory alkalosis, compensated by the excretion of bicarbonate to maintain normality during pregnancy.

Pulse Oximetry

Oxygen consumption and demand are greater during pregnancy, resulting in a reduction in oxygen saturation. This is combined with a decrease in functional residual capacity and seriously reduces the ability of the pregnant patient to compensate for any respiratory compromise. This process reduces oxygen reserves available. Consequently, during pregnancy, oxygen saturation may drop very quickly in response to the cessation of oxygen or hand ventilation.

Colloid Oncotic Pressure

Colloid oncotic pressure (COP) is the pressure exerted by proteins in the plasma to draw fluid into the vascular system. In a balanced physiological state, the COP would prevent excess fluid being reabsorbed from the blood circulation by the lymphatic system. During pregnancy, this state of physiological balance changes. The COP decreases because of the haemodilutional effect of pregnancy exerted on plasma albumin.

Administering IV fluids to pregnant women can further dilute plasma colloid concentration. This may result in an increase in BP and a reduction in COP and increase the risk of generalized pulmonary oedema. Colloid solutions must also be administered with caution as they can serve to increase circulating volume and BP within the vasculature. If there is capillary or vascular damage, proteins will leak across the membrane, giving rise to the appearance of a reduced circulating volume and a low BP.

Urine Output

During pregnancy, urine output might be expected to reduce due to the effect of aldosterone and vasopressin to maintain the expanded maternal blood volume.

Trauma Injury During Pregnancy

Anatomical and physiological changes during the gestational period predispose pregnant women to accidental injury; as the pregnancy progresses, alterations in balance and gait increase the likelihood of falls. The enlarging abdomen becomes more susceptible to injury from blunt and penetrating trauma. The most common causes of trauma are as follows:

- Motor vehicle accidents
- Falls, industrial accidents
- Burns
- Firearm injuries
- Direct assaults to the abdomen caused by violence or battering

The effects of trauma on pregnancy depend on:

- Length of gestation
- Type and severity of the trauma
- Degree of disruption of uterine and foetal physiology

Severe Pre-Eclampsia

This is also known as pregnancy-induced hypertension (PIH). No one has identified the aetiology. Investigations have identified:

- Calcium
- Antithrombotic agents
- Angiotensin II
- Prostaglandins
- Hereditary factors

  PIH is associated with

- Hypertension
- Proteinuria
- Oedema from vascular endothelial damage.

  The damaged endothelium results in plasma leakage out of blood vessels. COP decreases, and protein enters the extravascular space. A woman with PIH is at risk of hypovolaemia, alteration in tissue perfusion and cellular oxygenation.

Disseminated Intravascular Coagulation

Disseminated intravascular coagulation (DIC) is an acquired coagulopathy, which never occurs as a primary disorder but arises as an intermediary mechanism of disease in numerous underlying conditions:

- Pre-eclampsia in normal pregnancy
- Haemodilution, which is common because of the increased plasma volume leading to a lower-than-normal haematocrit
- Plasma leakage from the blood vessels, which results in an increase in haematocrit activating the intrinsic pathway

  DIC involves all aspects of coagulation. DIC occurs due to overstimulation of normal haemostasis; the patient simultaneously develops microvascular thrombi and haemorrhage.

Pulmonary Oedema

Pulmonary oedema during pregnancy comprises of an excessive accumulation of fluid in the interstitial spaces, alveoli, or cells within the lungs. This inhibits adequate diffusion of carbon dioxide and oxygen. It can develop for a number of reasons in pregnant women:

- Due to the physiological changes of the cardiopulmonary system
- From drug therapy such as tocolytic agents to prevent preterm labour
- Due to severe pre-eclampsia

Haemolysis, Elevated Liver Enzyme, Low Platelet Count Syndrome

Haemolysis, elevated liver enzyme, low platelet count syndrome may accompany severe pre-eclampsia. It is associated with significant perinatal mortality and morbidity. Liver enzymes become elevated as hepatic endothelial damage eventually leads to ischaemia and decreased liver function.

Rupture of the Gravid Uterus

This is an uncommon but serious obstetric emergency. It presents a lethal threat to both foetus and mother. Such a rupture usually involves a previous uterine scar from caesarean section or myomectomy. Occasionally, it occurs spontaneously or following blunt trauma.

Myocardial Infarction

MI during pregnancy is a rare event. Some 5% of individuals younger than 40 years are now experiencing MI, usually accepted as the childbearing years for women. With the trend toward delaying pregnancy and factors such as stress and hypercholesterolaemia, MI during pregnancy is expected to increase. MI is thought to occur because of:

- The dynamic alterations in the cardiovascular system during pregnancy
- The additional stressors, which may precipitate myocardial ischaemia or infarction in susceptible women
- Systemic hypertension
- Hypervolaemia/fluid overload
- Alterations in cardiovascular anatomy, which may also affect coronary artery perfusion

Pulmonary Embolism

This is a major cause of maternal morbidity and mortality during pregnancy. Anatomical, physiological and biochemical changes seen during pregnancy and the postpartum period predispose to thrombus formation. Relaxation of the venous system and compression of the inferior vena cava encourage venous pooling in the lower extremities. Venous stasis and hypercoagulability lead to the development of DVT formation with the potential for development of a PE.

Amniotic Fluid Embolism

Amniotic fluid embolism (AFE) is the cause of 5%–10% of maternal deaths; between 25% and 50% of patients with suspected or proven AFE die within the first hour. Overall mortality is as high as 86%. Amniotic fluid is thought to enter the maternal circulation due to placental abruption. Amniotic fluid contains:

- Prostaglandins
- Leukotrienes
- Foetal debris

The AFE causes:

- Complement activation
- Pulmonary vasoconstriction
- Blockage of pulmonary capillaries with resultant damage and release of further mediators

Clinical presentation:

- Severe dyspnoea, cyanosis
- Sudden cardiovascular collapse
- Coma or convulsions during labour
- May occur earlier during pregnancy, during delivery, or in early puerperium

It is difficult to diagnose and has many differential diagnoses.

Blood Loss

These generally relate to bleeding and blood loss. The result is generally shock, leading to a reduction in supply of oxygen and nutrients to tissues. Inadequate tissue and cell perfusion cause widespread disruption to cellular metabolism and organ and tissue dysfunction. This can lead to stimulation of the inflammatory response and widespread swelling and further fluid loss.

The physiological changes that occur during pregnancy can lead to obstetric emergencies that can put the mother and baby at risk. It is imperative to instigate early interventions to prevent shock and severe loss of fluid and mother and baby mortality.

Chest Drain Insertion

Chest drains are used in many different clinical settings; however, all personnel involved in the insertion of a chest drain should be adequately trained. The use of premedication, unless contraindicated, is required to reduce patient anxiety and stress levels, as the procedure can be distressing to the patient.

Indications:

- Pneumothorax − trauma, CVP insertion
- Tension pneumothorax after initial needle relief
- Persistent or recurrent pneumothorax after simple aspiration
- Large secondary spontaneous pneumothorax in patients over 50 years
- Malignant pleural effusion
- Empyema
- Pleural effusion
- Traumatic haemopneumothorax
- Postoperative, for example, cardiothoracic or thoracic surgery

Risks Associated with Chest Drain Insertion:

- There is a risk of haemorrhage; therefore, where possible, any coagulopathy or platelet deficit should be corrected prior to chest drain insertion. For elective chest drain insertion, anticoagulants should be stopped and time allowed for their effects to resolve.
- The differential diagnosis between a pneumothorax and bullous disease requires careful radiological assessment so as to give the appropriate

treatment. Similarly, it is important to differentiate between the presence of collapse and a pleural effusion when the chest X-ray shows a unilateral 'whiteout'.
- Lung tissue densely adherent to the chest wall throughout the hemithorax is an absolute contraindication to chest drain insertion.

Consent

If the patient is unconscious, the best interest rule takes effect. If this is not the case, then prior to commencing a chest tube insertion, the procedure should be explained fully to the patient and consent recorded in accordance with national guidelines.

The Patient's Position

- The preferred position for drain insertion is with the patient on the bed, slightly rotated on their side, with their arm on the insertion side placed behind their head to expose the axillary area.
- An alternative is for the patient to sit upright leaning over an adjacent table with a pillow or in the lateral decubitus position.

Insertion

- All the equipment required should be made available before commencing the procedure.
- The usual sterile gloves and gown, skin antiseptic solution, sterile drapes, gauze swabs, syringes and needles are necessary.
- Additional equipment for this procedure are:
  - Local anaesthetic – lidocaine or cream can be placed on the site prior to insertion
  - Scalpel
  - Suture material
  - Instrument for blunt dissection, for example, Fraser Kelly
- Aseptic technique should be employed during tube insertion.
- Confirming drain site insertion – if fluid or free air cannot be aspirated with a needle at the time of local anaesthesia, then a chest tube should not be inserted without further imaging guidance.
- Imaging should be used to select the appropriate site for chest tube placement.
- Position of chest tubes:
  - The most common is in the mid-axillary line. This minimizes any risk to underlying structures, for example, internal mammary artery, and avoids damage to muscle and breast tissue resulting in unsightly scarring.

- A more posterior position may be chosen. It is not the preferred site as it is more uncomfortable for the patient to lie on after insertion coupled with a risk of the tube kinking.
- For apical pneumothorax, the second intercostal space in the mid-clavicular line is sometimes chosen but is not recommended routinely as it may be uncomfortable for the patient and may leave an unsightly scar.
- Drain size — small-bore drains are recommended as they are more comfortable, but there is no evidence that either size is therapeutically superior. Large-bore drains are used for drainage of an acute haemothorax to monitor further blood loss and for their dual role of thoracic cavity drainage and assessment of continuing blood loss.
- Substantial force should not be used on insertion of the chest drain as this risks sudden chest penetration and damage to essential intrathoracic structures. This can be avoided either by the use of a Seldinger technique or by blunt dissection through the chest wall, into the pleural space, before tube insertion.
- Incision — equal or similar to the diameter of the tube being inserted. Once the local anaesthetic has taken effect, an incision is made just above and parallel to a rib.
- Blunt dissection of the subcutaneous tissue and muscle into the pleural cavity is universal and essential to prevent damage to essential intrathoracic structures.
- Position of tube tip — aimed apically for a pneumothorax or basally for fluid drainage. However, any tube position can be effective at draining air or fluid, and an effectively functioning drain should not be repositioned solely because of its poor radiographic position.
- Securing the drain — large-bore chest drain incisions should be closed by a suture appropriate for a linear incision.
  - 'Purse string' sutures must not be used.
  - Two sutures are usually inserted, the first to assist later closure of the wound after drain removal, and the second, a stay suture, to secure the drain.
  - Large amounts of tape (sleek) and padding to dress the site are unnecessary, and concerns have been expressed that they may restrict chest wall movement or increase moisture collection.
  - A transparent dressing allows the wound site to be inspected regularly by nursing staff for leakage or infection.

Management of the Chest Drainage System

- Chest X-ray must be available after the drain is inserted to ensure that the lung has reinflated.

- Fluoroscopy, ultrasound and computed tomography (CT) scanning can all be used as adjunctive guides to the site of tube placement.
- The use of ultrasonography-guided insertion is particularly helpful for empyema and effusions, as the diaphragm can be localized and the presence of loculations and pleural thickening defined.
- If an imaging technique is used to indicate the site for drain insertion, but the procedure is not carried out at the time of imaging, the position of the patient at the time must be clearly documented to aid accurate insertion when the patient returns to the ward.
- It is recommended that ultrasound is used if the effusion is very small or initial blind aspiration fails.
- Prophylactic antibiotics should also be administered in trauma cases.
- Furthermore, as a chest drain may potentially be in place for a number of days, aseptic technique is essential to avoid wound site infection or secondary empyema.
- A chest drain should never be clamped as the presence of a tension pneumothorax can never be ascertained in every case.

Closed System Drainage

- All chest tubes should be connected to a single flow drainage system, for example, underwater seal bottle or flutter valve.
- The tube is placed under water at a depth of approximately 3 cm with a side vent, which allows escape of air, or it may be connected to a suction pump. This enables the operator to see the air bubble out as the lung re-expands in the case of pneumothorax or fluid evacuation rate in empyemas, pleural effusions or haemothorax.
- The continuation of bubbling suggests a continued visceral pleural air leak, although it may also occur in patients on suction when the drain is partly out of the thorax, and one of the tube holes is open to the air.
- The respiratory swing in the fluid in the chest tube is useful for assessing tube patency and confirms the position of the tube in the pleural cavity.
- The use of a Heimlich flutter valve system allows earlier mobilization and the potential for earlier discharge of patients with chest drains.

Disadvantages of the Underwater Seal 'Closed System' Drainage

- Obligatory inpatient management
- Difficulty of patient mobilization
- Risk of knocking over the bottle

Suction

When chest drain suction is required, a high-volume/low-pressure system should be used. Appropriately trained staff must nurse the patient. The use of high-volume/low-pressure suction pumps has been advocated in cases of non-resolving pneumothorax or following chemical pleurodesis. If suction is required, this may be performed via the underwater seal at a level of $10-20$ cm H_2O.

A high-volume pump, for example, Vernon—Thompson, may be required to cope with a large leak. The use of a low-volume pump, for example, Roberts pump, is inappropriate in cases of rapid flow as it is unable to cope with the demand, thereby effecting a situation similar to clamping and risking formation of a tension pneumothorax. A wall suction adapter may also be effective, although chest drains must not be connected directly to the high negative pressure available from wall suction.

Removal of the Chest Tubes

If a chest tube for pneumothorax is clamped, this should only be with a view to removing the chest drain following X-ray to ensure that the lung has remained expanded. However, there is no evidence to suggest that clamping a chest drain prior to its removal increases success or prevents recurrence of a pneumothorax and it may be hazardous. It is therefore generally discouraged. Clamping a chest drain in the presence of a continuing air leak may lead to the potentially fatal complication of tension pneumothorax. In the event that a patient with a clamped drain becomes breathless or develops subcutaneous emphysema, the drain must be immediately unclamped and medical advice sought. The patient should be managed in a specialist ward with experienced nursing staff, and the patient should not leave the ward environment.

The tube should be removed either while the patient performs a Valsalva manoeuvre or during expiration with a brisk firm movement while the nurse ties the closure suture. The drain should not be removed until bubbling has ceased, and a chest X-ray demonstrates lung reinflation.

Patients Requiring Assisted Ventilation

During the chest tube insertion, a patient on a high-pressure ventilator (especially with positive-end expiratory pressure [PEEP]) should be disconnected from the ventilator at the time of insertion.

Documentation

- The presence and use of an appropriate chest drain observation chart should be maintained.
- The frequency of chest drain complications should also be recorded.
- The use of analgesia and a patient pain assessment scoring system should be used to monitor its effectiveness.
- The duration of chest tube placement and its drainage should also be recorded, noting colour and consistency.

Status Asthmaticus

Asthma is the most common chronic disease of childhood, affecting 5%−10% of children and resulting in approximately 400,000 hospitalizations annually. Episodes are associated with obstruction that occurs in predominantly small-to-medium airways and that reverses partially or completely, either spontaneously or with treatment. Not all patients who present with wheezing have asthma; some may have one of a variety of other causes of obstructed airways:

- Bronchiolitis
- Pneumonia − viral, bacterial, atypical
- Congenital abnormalities, for example, vocal cord paralysis, tracheal or bronchial stenosis, gastro-oesophageal reflux, vascular ring
- Enlarged lymph nodes from infection or tumour
- Foreign bodies in trachea, bronchus or oesophagus
- Cystic fibrosis
- *Aspergillus*
- Anaphylaxis
- Toxic fume exposure

Status asthmaticus is an acute exacerbation of asthma that does not respond adequately to initial treatment with bronchodilators, aminophylline or theophylline and steroids. The condition becomes progressively worse. The asthma may have been left untreated. With a delay in medical treatment, particularly treatment with systemic steroids, patients have a greater chance of dying.

Typically, patients present with the condition a few days after:

- Onset of a viral respiratory illness
- Exposure to a potent allergen or irritant
- Exercise in a cold environment.

It can also vary from acute to chronic phase with:

- Associated bronchospasm
- Airway inflammation
- Mucus plugging
- Carbon dioxide retention
- Hypoxaemia
- Pulsus paradoxus
- Respiratory failure
- Lung hyperinflation
- Ventilation/perfusion (V/Q) mismatch
- Increased dead-space ventilation

The primary mechanical event in status asthmaticus is a progressive increase in airflow resistance. Mucus plugging and mucosal oedema or inflammation is the major cause for the delayed recovery in status asthmaticus. The combination of hypoxia, hypercapnia and acidosis, along with the mechanical effects of increased lung volumes, may result in cardiovascular depression or cardiovascular arrest.

Patient Assessment

- Evaluation should centre on the 'ABC':
  - Airway: can the patient maintain own airway?
  - Breathing: what is the degree of air exchange? Is the patient hypoxic?
  - Circulation: how is their perfusion?
- History-taking and a more detailed examination
  - Is there any previous history of wheezing?
  - If the patient is a known asthmatic, what are their regular medications?
  - Are they compliant with asthma current asthma medication?
  - Time of the last bronchodilator?
  - Previous hospitalizations, were they intubated?
  - When was their last course of steroids?
  - When did this exacerbation begin?
  - Are there any precipitating factors?
  - General medical history, including any medications.
  - Use the clinical asthma score
    - The higher the score, the more serious the asthma attack
- Monitor vital signs
  - Temperature: fever may indicate upper respiratory tract infection, pneumonia or other source of infection
  - Check pulse, respiratory rate and BP.
- Respiratory assessment (see p. 130)
  - Check breath sounds and undertake chest examination, order chest X-ray.
  - Is there symmetry of breath sounds? If there is asymmetry, this may be due to mucus plugging and atelectasis.
  - Increased wheezing unilaterally and addition of stridor may indicate the presence of a foreign body.
  - Significantly decreased breath sounds unilaterally may indicate pneumonia or a pneumothorax.
  - The use of accessory respiratory muscles may correlate with the severity of airway obstruction. Wheezing is a less sensitive indicator of the degree of obstruction present.
  - Feel for the presence of crepitus in the neck or chest wall, signifying air leak and significant obstruction.
- Cardiac examination
  - HR and BP
  - Normal heart tones
  - Signs of a murmur or evidence of preexisting heart disease

- Neurological examination
  - Alert, conscious, verbal or unconscious
  - Confusion suggests significant hypercapnia or hypoxaemia and necessitates immediate action

Investigations

- Pulmonary function tests.
- Chest X-ray − this should be obtained in any patient with severe status asthmaticus in order to:
  - Define extent of the condition;
  - Ascertain whether there is any evidence of extra-alveolar air and
  - Differentiate other disease entities.
- ECG − this may show right axis deviation, 'p' pulmonale, and a right ventricular strain pattern, as the pulmonary vascular resistance is elevated in the presence of hyperinflation, hypercarbia or hypoxaemia.
- ABGs − these are not always indicated during an asthma exacerbation.
- ABGs are indicated if:
  - You cannot determine the severity of the exacerbation.
  - You believe the patient's respiratory function is worsening.

Serial ABGs may be necessary to evaluate progression of disease if you feel the patient is difficult to evaluate clinically.

Treatment

- Oxygen delivery
- Continuous monitoring
- Frequent assessment of work of breathing and breath sounds
- An arterial line may be indicated if the attack is severe; this will allow for frequent ABGs and BP monitoring
- Standard drug therapy includes steroids, beta-agonists, for example, bronchodilators, and possibly IV beta-antagonists. Additional therapy might include aminophylline or theophylline, noninvasive ventilation or ventilation
- Additional therapies may include magnesium, ketamine, antibiotics, diuretics

Intubation and Mechanical Ventilation

- There are no widely agreed upon guidelines for when asthmatics require intubation; it can be difficult and dangerous for the asthmatic, so it is avoided if at all possible.
- The difficulty arises as to whether it is or is not possible.
- Indications for intubation are:
  - Apnoea or failure to breathe, for example, fatigue
  - Diminished level of consciousness with inability to protect the airway

- Severe hypoxia and/or hypercapnia despite supplemental O_2
- Cardiovascular collapse
- Complications of ventilation
  - Pneumothorax or lung/lobar collapse
  - Cardiovascular compromise or collapse
  - Aspiration during intubation
  - Worsening bronchospasm making it difficult to ventilate because of high pressures
  - Mucus plugging
- Concerns related to ventilatory weaning
  - Presence of bronchospasm as the patient awakes
  - Increased coughing due to presence of endotracheal tube
  - Consider extubation with background sedative
  - High FiO_2 requirement upon extubation

General Management Issues

- Fluids and electrolyte balance – maintain hydration with IV fluids.
- Prophylactic gastrointestinal protection – asthmatics are usually on relatively large doses of steroids. It may be appropriate to treat them with an H_2 blocker drug to prevent ulcer formation.
- Antibiotics – antibiotics are to be used if a bacterial pneumonia, sinusitis or other bacterial infection is the cause of the patient's asthma exacerbation.
- Chest physiotherapy – controversial; if used, evaluate patient before and after treatments; known to create more wheezing immediately but may be necessary if there is considerable atelectasis or mucus plugging.
- Hyperventilation should be avoided
- Assessment of air trapping
  - Measure intrinsic PEEP
  - Absence of pause between expiratory and inspiratory sounds
  - Timing of audible expiratory wheeze following ventilatory disconnection
  - Increasing $PaCO_2$

Diabetic Emergencies

Hypoglycaemia

- Occurs when blood glucose falls below 3.5 mmol/L.
- Does not occur in diabetes that is diet-controlled but may occur in type II diabetics on oral hypoglycaemics such as tolbutamide or gliclazide; more common in patients receiving insulin.
- Commonest cause of diabetic coma.

Causes:

- Too much insulin (accidental or deliberate)
- Missed or delayed meal or snack
- Excessive exercise with no reduction in insulin
- Alcohol inhibits gluconeogenesis and binges may precipitate hypoglycaemia

Clinical features:

- Pallor
- Trembling
- Sweating
- Feeling 'lightheaded'
- Blurred vision
- Tachycardia
- Increasing confusion – sometimes aggression
- Incoherent speech

Hypoglycaemia can occur very rapidly and if a critical care nurse notices a change in behaviour in a patient with diabetes and he or she becomes irritable or lethargic, seek help immediately. Glucose or glycogen may be administered.

Diabetic Ketoacidosis

- This occurs when there is insufficient insulin in the body; the cells cannot utilize glucose, and it accumulates in the blood.
- Deterioration is generally slow, and the patient may have been feeling unwell for months.
- A hyperglycaemia is present; ketones can be smelt on the breath, and ketones and glucose are present in the urine in increased amounts.
- The condition produces a severe metabolic acidosis due to the over-production of ketones; nausea and vomiting and a reduced potassium level may occur leading to electrolyte imbalance.
- Dehydration will occur due to loss of excessive water; this lowers BP, and a rapid and thready pulse occurs.
- Respiration becomes deep and rapid in an attempt to excrete excess metabolic acids.
- Drowsiness and coma will occur if treatment is not instigated and indicate severe metabolic derangement.

Causes:

- Untreated diabetes – undiagnosed condition.
- Illness – as patient does not feel like eating, they omit their insulin.
- Vomiting and a total omission of insulin.

It is important that insulin is never totally suspended when a patient is ill.
Treatment:

- Assessment of conscious level.
- Suction machine in case of vomiting.
- Monitoring of vital signs.
- IV infusion of fluids to replace loss of water (normal saline); potassium may need to be added.
- Monitoring of blood glucose level.
- Monitoring of ABGs.
- Cardiac monitoring.
- Insulin therapy titrated to the blood glucose measurement.
- Once blood glucose has fallen to 11 mmol/L, IV fluid may be replaced with a dextrose solution.

Status Epilepticus

This refers to a life-threatening condition in which the brain is in a persistent state of seizure. There are many variations of the definition, but it can safely be defined as one continuous or recurrent seizure without regaining consciousness between seizures for more than 30 min. Status epilepticus among epileptics is often associated with poor compliance, alcohol withdrawal and metabolic disturbances. If the status epilepticus is a primary presentation, it is normally associated with a brain tumour or abscess.

Although there is no consensus over a classification system for status epilepticus, classification is necessary for appropriate management of the condition because effective management depends on the type of status epilepticus. In general, the various systems characterize status epilepticus according to whether the seizures arise from a localized region of the cortex or from both hemispheres of the brain.

The other major categorization hinges on the clinical observation of overt convulsions: therefore, status epilepticus may be convulsive or non-convulsive in nature. The rate of mortality from status epilepticus among elderly adults is high. The primary determinants of mortality in persons with status epilepticus are duration of seizures, age at onset and aetiology. Patients with anoxia and stroke have a very high mortality rate that is independent of other variables. Patients with status epilepticus occurring in the setting of alcohol withdrawal or low levels of antiepileptic drugs have a relatively low mortality rate.

Pathophysiology

Generalized convulsive status epilepticus is associated with serious systemic physiological changes resulting from the metabolic demands of repetitive seizures. Many of these systemic changes result from the profound autonomic changes that occur during status epilepticus. These include:

- Tachycardia
- Cardiac arrhythmias
- Hypertension
- Pupil dilatation
- Hyperthermia

These changes occur because of the massive catecholamine discharge associated with continuous generalized seizures. Systemic changes requiring medical intervention include:

- Hypoxia
- Hypercapnia
- Hypoglycaemia
- Metabolic acidosis
- Other electrolyte disturbances

Treatment:

- Involves the use of potent IV medications that may have serious adverse effects.
- Ascertain that the patient has tonic-clonic status epilepticus, and that prolonged or repetitive seizures have occurred.
- A single generalized seizure with complete recovery does not require treatment.
- Once the diagnosis of status epilepticus has been made, treatment should be initiated immediately. Necessary interventions include:
  - Maintaining airway and adequate oxygenation
  - Assess:
    - cardiovascular status, for example, HR/BP
    - temperature
    - the aetiology
    - laboratory results
  - Obtain ABGs
  - Obtain IV access and commence IV fluids
  - Commence appropriate drug therapy
  - Neurological assessment, for example, focal intracranial lesions; may need CT scan
  - Ascertain when medications were last taken
  - Consider other investigations, for example, electroencephalography (EEG), lumbar puncture.

Pharmacological Management (See Section 6)

Rapid treatment of status epilepticus is crucial to prevent neurological and systemic pathology. The treatment goal should always be diagnosis and termination of seizures. For an antiepileptic drug to be effective in status epilepticus, the drug must be administered intravenously to provide quick access to the brain without the risk of serious systemic and any neurological adverse effects.

Many drugs are available each with their own advantages and disadvantages. There is no ideal drug for treatment of status epilepticus; a number of considerations influence the choice.

Role of EEG in Diagnosing Status Epilepticus

- The EEG is extremely useful in the diagnosis and management of status epilepticus.
- Although overt convulsive status epilepticus is readily diagnosed, EEG can establish the diagnosis in less obvious circumstances.
- EEG can help to confirm that an episode of status epilepticus has ended, particularly when questions arise about the possibility of recurrent episodes of more subtle seizures.
- Patients with status epilepticus who fail to recover rapidly and completely should be monitored with EEG for at least 24 h after an episode to ensure that recurrent seizures are not missed.
- Monitoring also is advised if periodic discharges appear in the EEG of a patient with altered consciousness who has not had obvious seizures.
- Periodic discharges in these patients suggest the possibility of preceding status epilepticus, and careful monitoring may clarify the aetiology of the discharges and allow the detection of recurrent status epilepticus.

Trauma

Patients with severe multiple trauma require care and attention to their primary injuries. This may include surgery; dressings; IV fluids, for example, blood, crystalloid or colloid; oxygen; drugs and/or resuscitation. However, there is now a sophisticated understanding of the complex metabolic response of the human body to traumatic injury. Following trauma, the initial physiological responses that occur are neuroendocrine response; oxygen supply and demand; alterations in metabolism; IIR; and posttrauma capillary leak. These physiological responses are initiated to protect the body from cell/tissue/organ damage.

Neuroendocrine Response to Injury

One of the earliest responses to injury is neuroendocrine activation, which is intimately linked in the control of tissue function. Neuroendocrine activation occurs in response to cytokine release from the site of injury and stimulates the

SNS, hypothalamus, pituitary and adrenal glands. The nervous system generates biochemical agents that act as hormones and the endocrine system produces substances that mediate activity within the CNS.

Following an insult, activation of the neuroendocrine system stimulates the release of numerous substances into the circulation, including:

- Catecholamines (adrenaline and noradrenaline) via the SNS and adrenal cortex, causing tachycardia, increased CO and BP, rate and depth of respiration, blood flow redistribution, glycogenolysis, gluconeogenesis and lipolysis.
- Glucocorticoids via the hypothalamus releasing corticotrophin-releasing hormone, while the anterior pituitary gland secretes adrenocorticotrophic hormone. The adrenal cortex then releases cortisol, a glucocorticoid, which causes gluconeogenesis, proteolysis and lipolysis, anti-inflammatory and cell-protective effects to prevent damage from excessive activation of the metabolic response.

The effect of catecholamines occurs almost immediately, effecting change in target organs with extreme rapidity and intensity. HR can double in 3–5 s, CO can increase fourfold, and selective vasoconstriction and vasodilatation occur to redistribute the circulating volume to vital organs (heart, brain).

The neuroendocrine response in injury protects the body from the effects of injury. However, it causes:

- An increase in oxygen consumption and myocardial work.
- Redistribution of blood flow away from the 'non-vital' gut, which may result in translocation of bacteria and endotoxins into the circulation, resulting in septic shock.
- High catecholamine levels, which can lead to arrhythmias, causing cardiac arrest in a compromised heart.

Therefore, if this response is prolonged, it is believed to contribute to shock and MSOF.

Inflammatory/Immune Response

The wound or injury site plays a role in the systemic response as the wound produces extensive inflammation by attracting nutrients, fluids, clotting factors and large numbers of neutrophils and macrophages to the damaged site. These are activated to:

- Protect the host from invading microorganisms.
- Limit the extent of blood loss and injury.
- Promote rapid healing of involved tissues.

This activation is known as the IIR and represents a major physiological event in the body, which leads to an increased capillary permeability causing the swelling, redness, pain and oedema often observed in inflammation and stimulation of coagulation and fibrinolysis. The IIR is initiated to protect the host and promote healing and is necessary for survival, but it can lead to an uncontrolled intravascular inflammation that ultimately harms the host. This can be observed in such conditions as:

- ARDS.
- SIRS.
- DIC.
- MSOF.

Therefore, trauma requires immediate intervention as the process outlined above can lead to serious, irreversible consequences and death. The nurse's immediate role is in:

- The administration of oxygen.
- The instigation and administration of adequate nutrition.
- Maintenance of an adequate circulating volume.

For more information related to trauma see Section 4.

1.4 LIFE-THREATENING COMPLICATIONS/OUTCOMES

Patients frequently survive the initial insult as a result of aggressive treatment with fluids, blood, vasoactive drugs, resuscitation and so on. However, they are now at risk of dying days or weeks later of progressive organ failure despite expensive intensive and critical care. This occurs when the physiological protective mechanisms mentioned above become over stimulated and destructive.

This may occur due to the initial insult (mild or severe) but may be complicated by shock, infection, additional surgery or MI. If the body is continually hit by other problems, this may lead to persistent inflammation and ischaemia, leading to impaired gas exchange (ARDS), SIRS and/or DIC. These conditions may subsequently cause severe organ dysfunction 2–21 days following the initial insult, which appears unrelated or remote from the original site of injury.

Adult Respiratory Distress Syndrome

ARDS results from injury to the alveolar capillary membrane and pulmonary endothelial damage that leads to increased pulmonary capillary permeability, atelectasis and interstitial non-cardiogenic pulmonary oedema from leakage of fluid into the interstitial spaces and alveoli. It is caused by an inflammatory response involving neutrophils, macrophages and lymphocytes. It can occur in isolation, but it more often develops as a secondary insult following the initial injury. It exacerbates tissue hypoxia and activates mediators of the inflammatory response.

Destruction of the endothelial cells and leakage of protein into the alveoli reduce the action of surfactant, and gas exchange abnormalities occur. The compliance of the lung decreases substantially, and the resistance of both the airways and the lung tissue increase. Hypoxaemia occurs that does not respond to increasing amounts of inspired oxygen, as well as decreased pulmonary compliance, respiratory alkalosis, dyspnoea, tachypnoea and the appearance of diffuse, fluffy infiltrates on chest X-ray films without evidence of cardiogenic causes.

Causes of and symptoms/signs of ARDS include:

- Capillary endothelium damage − cell damage, thickened alveolar walls
- Pulmonary capillary leak − alveolar oedema − shunting, low compliance − pulmonary fibrosis
- Surfactant inactivation − low functional residual capacity − atelectasis − hypoxaemia
- Shock
- Infection − septicaemia, pneumonia
- Trauma − lung contusion, blast injuries, fat embolism, head injury, non-thoracic trauma
- Aspiration − gastric acid, near drowning
- Inhalation − smoke, corrosive gases, oxygen toxicity
- Blood − DIC, massive transfusion, postcardiac surgery
- Metabolic − renal failure, pancreatitis, liver failure
- Drug abuse − heroin, barbiturates
- Miscellaneous − high altitude, radiation, eclampsia, raised ICP

Systemic Inflammatory Response Syndrome

SIRS is characterized by persistence of the acute inflammatory response due to failure of the downregulatory mediators to overcome the excessive and persistent IIR. The IIR becomes so grossly amplified and distorted due to prolonged systemic hypoperfusion that it cannot stop. The risk factors associated with immune dysfunction are either host related or treatment related. Patients with SIRS are identified by the manifestation of the following criteria:

- Body temperature 38 or 36°C
- HR 100 bpm
- Systolic blood pressure <90 mm Hg or mean blood pressure <60 mm Hg
- Alternatively on vasoactive agents to maintain a systolic blood pressure >90 mm Hg
- Tachypnoea >20 bpm
- White cell count >4 × 10^9 or 12 × 10^9 cells/L

Overstimulation leads to immune dysfunction and widespread tissue necrosis or a series of discrete infectious or traumatic injuries. The net effect of the massive assault by these inflammatory mediators is widespread damage to the vascular endothelium, resulting in:

- Increased vascular permeability
- Vasodilatation
- A procoagulant state
- Progressive destruction of the visceral organs

The increased permeability leads to pooling of fluid in the systemic circulation; in addition, the release of coagulation factors influences the formation of microemboli that can cause ischaemic injuries to multiple target organs, particularly the lungs, liver, gastrointestinal tract and kidneys. Thus, SIRS can result in MSOF, defined as a failure of at least two distinct organs or organ systems that may be remote from the site of initial injury.

Disseminated Intravascular Coagulation

DIC is an acquired coagulopathy that never occurs as a primary disorder but arises as an intermediary mechanism of disease in numerous underlying conditions. DIC can occur due to any underlying disease states, acute or chronic. It involves all aspects of the coagulation cascade, which can lead to dysfunction in any organ system, hence the word 'disseminated'.

DIC occurs due to overstimulation of normal haemostasis due to:

- Blood transfusion reactions
- Cancer especially leukaemia
- Inflammation of the pancreas
- Sepsis
- Liver disease
- Pregnancy complications
- Surgery or anaesthesia
- Severe tissue injury, for example, burns or major trauma/head injury

These result in disseminated coagulation and excessive fibrinolysis throughout the body. The overstimulation and dissemination of blood coagulation in DIC produce a unique clinical situation whereby the patient simultaneously develops microvascular thrombi and haemorrhage:

- Microemboli block blood vessels and cut off blood supply to organs such as the liver, brain or kidneys.
- Haemorrhage or serious bleeding, even from a minor injury or without injury; this is due to a lack of clotting proteins, which have been consumed by the development of microemboli.

The symptoms are as follows:

- Bleeding from at least three different sites:
  - Blood in stool or urine
  - Neurological changes associated with bleeding in the brain
  - Bruising on the skin
  - Bleeding from wound sites, surgical sites, IV lines or catheter sites
  - Bleeding from the nose, gums, mouth
- Blood clotting:
  - Symptoms associated with organ dysfunction caused by blood clots reducing or blocking blood flow and oxygen to organs such as the liver and kidney
  - Necrosis of areas of the skin caused by blood clots
  - Coughing up blood, difficulty in breathing caused by blood clots in the lungs
  - Chest pain due to a heart attack caused by clotting in the heart
  - Headaches/confusion/memory loss associated with stroke caused by clotting in the brain

The combination of bleeding and clotting makes it distinguishable from many other conditions but makes it very difficult to treat, which involves supportive treatments:

- Plasma transfusion to replace blood clotting factors – platelets, fresh frozen plasma or cryoprecipitate
- Heparin to prevent blood clotting

Compartment Syndrome

Acute compartment syndrome is a common condition in which there is a raised pressure within a closed fascial space (Edwards, 2004). The increased pressure reduces capillary perfusion below the level necessary for tissue viability. This condition is serious. Inability of the patient to identify pain may mask its progression.

The muscles of the legs are grouped into compartments that are formed by thick layers of fairly inelastic tissue called fascia. Within the compartments are the nerves and blood vessels that supply the limbs. The legs consist of four compartments, each containing a major nerve (Table 1.12). If this condition goes unrecognized, it can have devastating consequences for a critical care patient. The delay in diagnosis can affect the patient's future quality of life.

The syndrome is fairly common following a soft tissue injury. Young men, in particular, are at risk of compartment syndrome, especially those with a clotting disorder and those taking anticoagulant therapy, where the risk of intra-compartment haemorrhage following trauma is increased.

TABLE 1.12 The four compartments of the leg and nerve supply.

	Compartments of the leg	Nerve supply
1.	Anterior	Deep peroneal
2.	Deep posterior	Tibial
3.	Lateral	Superficial peroneal
4.	Superficial posterior	Saphenous

Sites of Compartment Syndrome

- The anterior compartment is the most frequent site.
- Followed by the lateral compartment and the deep posterior compartment.
- Between the two compartments of the forearm.
- The three compartments of the thigh.
- Can occur in the abdomen, making it difficult or impossible to close following surgery.
- Can occur in an open wound if the skin laceration is not sufficient to decompress the oedema or haemorrhage.
- Observed in diabetic patients.
- Lower limbs following malignant hyperthermia.

Increase or swelling in the compartment contents may be caused by bleeding, infiltration of IV fluid, or posttraumatic or ischaemic swelling.

Causes of Compartment Syndrome

Crush injury, compression bandages or constrictive devices may decrease the compartment size of the leg or arm. Other causes include:

- Fracture (tibia—fibula fractures, usually in the middle or distal third of the leg, or supracondylar fracture of the humerus)
- Excessive exercise of a muscle group
- Surgical procedures including closure of fascial defects
- Major vascular surgery
- Bleeding disorders
- Snakebite
- Burns
- IV drug abuse
- Weightlifting
- Postischaemic swelling

The prognosis in this condition is directly dependent on the interval between the onset of the intra-compartment ischaemia and the initiation of its effective treatment.

Pathophysiology of Compartment Syndrome

The initial injury, whether traumatic, haemorrhagic, surgical or vascular or a complication of another condition, leads to localized swelling in the muscle compartments. This is due to the stimulation of the inflammatory response detailed earlier.

Further oedema forms when there is an increase in HP either at the arterial end of the capillary or at the venous end (Edwards, 2004). This will raise the pressure of blood in the capillary and cause an increase in the rate of filtration. Larger amounts of fluid will move into the interstitial space and cause the further collection of fluid in the compartments.

Elevated perfusion pressure is the physiological response to rising intra-compartmental pressure. As intra-compartmental pressure rises, autoregulatory mechanisms are overwhelmed, and a cascade of injury develops. A normal resting intramuscular pressure is 0—8 mm Hg. The pain and paraesthesia appear at a pressure of between 20 and 30 mm Hg. An ICP measure of 30 mm Hg is often used as a basis for performing a fasciotomy.

Using this method severely reduces the number of patients who undergo such surgery, with no adverse effects on those who do not. The ideal pressure threshold for performing a fasciotomy is still not known.

If the patient has a compartment pressure exceeding 30 mm Hg and has findings compatible with compartment syndrome, then prompt therapy to decrease the compartment pressure is necessary. If the compartment pressure is greater than 40 mm Hg, emergency treatment is needed. At this point, blood flow through the capillaries stops. In the absence of flow, oxygen delivery stops. This result in local tissue ischaemia, leading to intracellular oedema, which in turn further increases intra-compartmental pressure.

The interrupted supply of oxygenated blood to cells results in anaerobic metabolism and loss of ATP, and cellular membrane disruption (Edwards, 2002; Fig. 1.8). This may finally lead to irreversible cell damage, loss of limb and death. Necrotic muscle will never recover, hence the seriousness of this condition and the importance of recognizing the warning signs. The surrounding tissue suffers further damage and stimulates the release of mediators and stimulation of the IIR, developing a vicious cycle.

Myoglobinuria

When muscle tissue suffers necrosis, it releases myoglobin. Myoglobinuria is often known as rhabdomyolysis and is a life-threatening complication of severe muscle trauma. It is an excess of myoglobin, an intracellular muscle protein, which appears in the urine following major muscle trauma. Muscle damage releases the myoglobin into the circulation; it can cause visible, dark reddish-brown pigmentation of the urine.

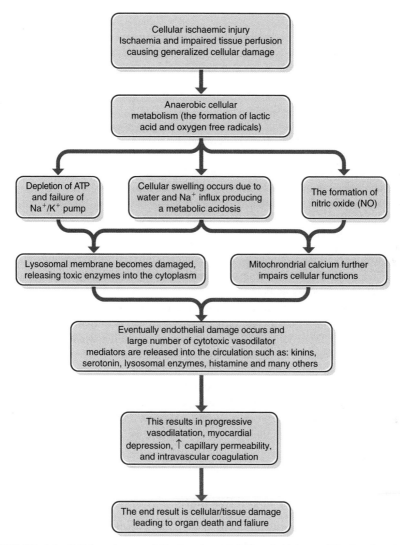

FIGURE 1.8 Cellular changes following hypoxic/ischaemic injury. ATP 5 adenosine triphosphate.

The renal threshold for myoglobin is low, approximately 0.5 mg/100 mL of urine, so that only 200 g muscle need be damaged to cause visible changes in the urine. Priorities of myoglobinuria include identifying and treating the compartment syndrome and preventing life-threatening renal failure. Myoglobinuria from muscle death may result in acidosis and renal failure as well as amputation of the involved extremity, sepsis and death. Therefore, early diagnosis of compartment syndrome is essential.

Patient Management

Although ischaemia is a major feature of compartment syndrome, only rarely will the pressures be sufficient to occlude arterial blood flow. For early recognition, more subtle skills and knowledge are required:

- Pain (out of proportion to the apparent injury): in conditions where the risk of compartment syndrome is high, a certain low level of pain/discomfort should be advocated − high doses of morphine can mask the symptoms.
- Paraesthesia may be an early complaint, but if allowed to persist may not be reversible.
- Pulselessness is not common or noted as an early sign; it appears at a much later stage and generally implies a vascular injury.
- Sensory deficit − numbness occurs because the excess pressure within a compartment hampers the activity of sensory nerves carrying messages toward the brain.

However, all these signs can only be identified in a fully conscious patient and are also present following vascular injury. A nurse has to be vigilant in clinical observation and examination.

Full recovery of compartment syndrome is probable when the treatment is started within 4−8 h of the onset of symptoms. Compartment pressure measurement (Table 1.13) should be at the top of the list when compartment syndrome is considered. If the compartment pressure is not relieved, a fasciotomy is indicated to decompress the compartment and allow reperfusion of the muscle. Fasciotomy has a high complication rate because it transforms a closed lesion into an open wound. The open wound can be allowed to heal by second intention or undergo skin closure (within 4 days), skin grafting or flap coverage. However, the combination of an open wound and necrotic muscle may contribute to the development of life-threatening infection and other complications such as acidosis, renal failure and loss of limb.

Persistent/Permanent Vegetative State

PVS is defined as 'an organic body capable of growth and development but devoid of sensation and thought'. A persistent vegetative state is a condition of wakefulness without awareness. It can be partially or totally reversible, or it can progress into a persisitent vegetative state (PVS).

- A persistent vegetative state usually present 1 month after the brain damage, but it can be irreversible.
- A PVS implies that the patient will not recover.

PVS implies a loss of forebrain function. In PVS, the brain stem remains intact, and therefore, the patient may be deeply unconscious but will retain the ability to breathe spontaneously without the aid of a ventilator. Alternatively,

TABLE 1.13 Measuring intra-compartmental pressure.

Type	Procedure	Advantages and disadvantages
Wick catheter	Uses polyglycolic acid suture wicks connected to a pressure transducer.	It is an accurate method and allows continuous measurement; other methods require repeated insertion of needles. May lead to coagulation around insertion site, and wick left in the insertion wound.
Simple needle manometry	Uses an 18-G needle and a simple mercury manometer.	The injection of saline is required into the tissues during the reading. Not as accurate as the wick method.
Infusion technique	Uses a syringe infusion pump to infuse 0.7 mL saline per day via a 19-G needle and allows continuous measurement.	The insertion of saline can increase pressure 2−4 mm Hg.
Slit catheter	Made from epidural catheter tubing; slits are used to reduce clotting problems.	Continues to use an infusion system but easier than the wick method.
Central venous pressure manometer	An 18-G needle is attached to a simple CVP manometer.	It is quick, no special equipment is needed. It suffers from some inaccuracies similar to the simple needle manometer technique.
Side-ported needle	Allows the measurement of several compartments using the same needle.	This method cannot be used for continuous monitoring.
Fibreoptic transducer	This method is very expensive and only available in specialist units.	It is easy to use, allows continuous monitoring.

CVP, central venous pressure.

the patient in PVS may appear to be awake but is unresponsive to stimulation and has a vacant look. PVS patients can survive for many years with good nursing care and adequate nutritional support.

- A vegetative state may be short-lived; the term persistent vegetative state implies that the state has continued for more than 1 month.
- PVS implies that a prediction is being made − the patient will not recover.
- Cerebral function is lost, but sleep−wake cycles are present.
- Eyes open spontaneously in response to external stimuli such as voice or touch.

- The individual maintains BP and breathing without support, and brain stem reflexes (pupillary, chewing, swallowing) are intact.
- The cardiovascular, gastrointestinal and renal functions are maintained, although the patient is doubly incontinent.
- No discrete localizing motor responses are present.
- The individual does not speak any comprehensible words or follow commands.

Locked-In Syndrome

The locked-in syndrome is caused by an insult to the ventral pons and is usually an

- Infarct
- Haemorrhage
- Trauma

The patient has characteristics such as:

- Quadriplegia.
- Preservation of consciousness, thought and the level of arousal.
- Intact cognitive functions.
- Patients retain vertical eye movement, facilitating some form of non-verbal communication.
- The individual cannot communicate either through speech or through body movement but is fully conscious.
- Patients can live for longer than 10 years despite limited recovery, but with some small improvements in physical recovery can improve quality of life and enable patients to return to live with their families.

Section 2

Patient assessment and investigations

Section Outline

2.1 IDENTIFICATION OF PATIENT NEEDS/PROBLEMS

Early Warning Scoring

Patients admitted for the ward to critical care may often be secondary to abnormal physiological values and deterioration in their clinical status. Commonly observed are deranged readings in blood pressure (BP), pulse rate and oxygen (O_2) saturation, altered cognitive function and reduced urine output (UO).

The National Early Warning Score (NEWS) or track and trigger systems have been used to aid the early recognition, timely intervention and management of the deteriorating patient in the acute setting. However, there have been concerns over the years with inconsistency with varying systems' parameters in prompting escalation of care, the limitations of the NEWS 1 scoring and the links to increased morbidity and mortality. As a result, patients who presented with critical illness when using these systems — particularly the NEWS 1 — received suboptimal care. Since then, NEWS 2 (RCP, 2017) was approved and introduced with an increased sensitivity to the signs and symptoms of the deteriorating patient to prompt timely interventions. The patient will be scored according to their physiological parameters:

- Pulse
- BP
- Respiratory rate
- UO
- Temperature
- Sedation level

Combining these scores with the patients' baseline or trend should prompt an initial intervention if the total is between 1 and 4. This should be followed by the fundamental and more comprehensive airway, breathing, circulation, disability and exposure assessment conducted by a registered nurse and appropriate clinical intervention. If appropriate, scores of 3 in a single parameter or >4 should trigger a response from the medical team, an outreach team or a medical emergency team.

Acute Physiology and Chronic Health Evaluation (APACHE) Scoring

Acute Physiology and Chronic Health Evaluation (APACHE) is a scoring system, which was designed and used for patients admitted to the critical care setting as a measure of illness severity and an indicator of in-hospital mortality. A score is applied within the first 24 hours using the worse values. An incremental score has a greater correlation to and increased risk of mortality. APACHE has now gone into its fourth version. The calculated score may also support the decision-making process in determining clinical input, resource allocation and predicting quality of care.

APACHE introduced in 1981, initially used 34 physiological variables, this was simplified by APACHE II (1985) with an acute physiological score from 12 physiological variables added to a score derived for age and chronic health. However, the scoring was made more complex based on the inclusion of diseases. APACHE III was introduced in 1991 to address some of the imperfections of the former version; this was further updated in 1998. It was then remodelled and superseded by APACHE IV in 2006 lending itself to good discrimination, refined predictor variables and detailed statistical methods. This version also broadened its applicability to both intensive care units (ICUs) and specific patient groups. The scoring includes 142 variables and is considered more sensitive in predicting hospital mortality and length of stay (Knaus et al., 1991; Venkataraman et al., 2018; Vincent and Moreno, 2010).

The physiological variables used are as follows:

- Age
- Core temperature
- Mean arterial pressure (MAP)
- Heart rate
- Respiratory rate (ventilated or self-ventilating)
- Oxygenation
  - FiO_2, 50% record AaO_2
  - FiO_2, 50% record PaO_2
- pCO_2 and pO_2
- Arterial pH
- Serum potassium
- Serum sodium

- Serum creatinine
- UO
- Urea
- Blood sugar level
- Albumin
- Bilirubin
- Haematocrit
- White cell count
- Glasgow Coma Scale (GCS)
- Chronic health condition
  - Chronic renal failure/heart disease
  - Cirrhosis
  - Hepatic failure
  - Metastatic carcinoma
  - Lymphoma
  - Leukaemia/myeloma
  - Immunosuppression
  - AIDS
- Admission information
  - Pre-ICU length of stay in days
  - Origin
  - Readmission
  - Emergency surgery
- Admission diagnosis
  - Nonoperative
  - Postoperative

The 26 variables may produce a combined score up to a maximum of 286. The APACHE II scoring system is mainly used in the United Kingdom, mainly due to its simplicity and its validation in clinical trials. However, it important to acknowledge that the APACHE score does not predict individual outcomes and may lack validation for its use with the diverse population and healthcare systems.

Simplified Acute Physiological Score (SAPS)

Simplified Acute Physiological Score (SAPS), such as APACHE scoring, can be used to establish the severity of the clinical condition and predict the risk of death in the critically ill patient. It uses weighted physiological variables to determine this prognosis. It is validated in 1984, revised in 1993, producing SAPS 2 and further refined in 2005 resulting in SAPS 3. The SAPS 3 model was devised to ensure that it was globally representative. Therefore, it acknowledges the increase of major diseases, the improvement in diagnostic technology, geographical variations of diseases and illness and therapeutic interventions in managing these caseloads. A customized equation is used to calibrate the data using statistical techniques to produce geographically representative findings. It requires the collection of 20 physiological variables, which have been divided into three main subsets. These include essential patient characteristics prior to admission, the reason for admission and the acute clinical status prior to or on admission to the ICU. This information is collated within the first 1 hour prior to or after admission to the ICU. The score ranges from 0 to 217 (Vincent and Moreno, 2010).

The following are patient information prior to admission

- Age
- Comorbidities
- Therapeutic drug requirements prior to ICU
- Intrahospital location
- Hospital length of stay before ICU

Circumstances leading to admission to the ICU are as follows:

- Reason for admission
- Planned/unplanned
- Surgical status
- Surgical site
- Infection status/presence

Acute physiological status — the worst physiologic scoring is obtained within the first hour

- GCS
- Heart rate
- Systolic BP
- Bilirubin
- Temperature
- Creatinine
- White blood cell count
- Platelets
- pH
- Ventilation support and O_2 requirements (PaO_2/FiO_2)

Sequential Organ Failure Assessment (SOFA)

Developed in 1994, this scoring system, amongst others, aimed to define the level of organ dysfunction rather than predict relative mortality. A score is applied to six systems:

- Respiratory
- Cardiovascular — score adjusted if inotropes are required

- Hepatic
- Coagulation
- Renal
- Neurological

A grade of 0–4 is applied relative to the level of failure, which is gathered within the first 24 hours of admission to the ICU. A score of 2 or more, an increase from baseline, is an indicator for organ dysfunction and possible sepsis (Table 2.1). This required review and essential monitoring.

The quick Sepsis-related Organ Failure Assessment score was introduced in 2016 as a tool to rapidly identify potentially at-risk septic patients outside the ICU. This was in line with the revision of the sepsis definition. This tool is considered be more specific than the systemic inflammatory response syndrome to support: the identification of potential organ failure, escalating or prompting timely sepsis management interventions and the potential mobilization of patients to an appropriate setting, usually ICU, for ongoing management. However, its effectiveness as tool alongside other risk tracking methods has yet to be validated. The model gathers physiological data on the following system as a possible indicator of infection:

- Systolic BP ≤ 100 mmHg
- Increased respiratory rate ≥ 22 bpm
- Altered mental status − GCS <15

Derangements in these recordings of ≥ 2 prompted the need for senior review and initiation of relevant treatment once formally assessed. This may require the movement of patients/clients to an appropriate area for closer monitoring. The benefits of this tool boast its swift simplicity and repetitive use. Patients who are assessed and suspected or identified as infected should promptly receive the appropriate sepsis management bundles.

Trauma Revised Injury Severity Score (TRISS)

The Trauma Revised Injury Severity Score methodology uses a combination of:

- Anatomical scores outlined in the Injury Severity Score (ISS),
- Physiological measurements presented in the Triage Revised Trauma Score (T-RTS)
- Trauma type
- The patient's age

The ISS introduced in 1987 uses these indices as a monitor of care, predictor of trauma injury survival and how future trauma care can be improved. The limitations of the ISS, due to its recording of only one trauma injury, led to its revision and introduction of the New Injury Severity Score (NISS) in 1997 to provide a more accurate measurement of mortality probability.

TABLE 2.1 Sequential organ failure assessment.

Score	0	1	2	3	4
Respiratory P/F ratio (mmHg)	400	400	300	200[a]	100[a]
Cardiovascular MAP (mmHg)	No hypotension	MAP 0.70	Dopamine 0.5 mcg/kg/min or dobutamine (any dose)	Dopamine 0.5 mcg/kg/min or noradrenaline (norepinephrine), 0.1 mcg/kg/min	Dopamine 0.15 mcg/kg/min or noradrenaline (norepinephrine) 0.1 mcg/kg/min
Neurological GCS	15	13–14	10–12	6–9	6
Renal creatinine (mg/dL) or urine output (mL/d)	1.2	1.2–1.9	2.0–3.4	3.5–4.9 or 500	5.0 or 200
Hepatic bilirubin (mg/dL)	1.2	1.2–1.9	2.0–5.9	6.0–11.9	12.0
Haematological platelet count (×10³/mm³)	0.150	150	100	50	20

GCS, Glasgow Coma Scale; MAP, mean arterial pressure.
[a]with ventilatory support.

NISS, includes the Abbreviated Injury Scale (AIS15), to score the three most severe anatomical injuries. The AIS score incorporates an excess of 200 anatomical injuries and is classified according to the severity of the injury on a 6-point scale (1 = minor and 6 = severe). A score >15 indicates the severity of the patient's condition as major, a score of 9–14 classified as moderate and ≤8 will fall in the minor trauma category. The NISS score is based on the level of severity and calculated as the sum of the squares in each of the highest three AIS categories:

- Head or neck
- Face
- Chest and thoracic spine
- Bony pelvis and limbs/extremities
- Abdomen, lumbar spine or pelvic contents
- Body surface
- T-RTS used for trauma triage uses the following physiological categories and scored accordingly (Table 2.2):
  - GCS
  - Systolic BP
  - Respiratory rate

The parameters are coded to a value between 0 and 4. The respective values are then multiplied by a weighted coefficient/measurement before they are added together to provide the total T-RTS. The score obtained will be between 0 and 7.84 (Tito et al., 2018).

Patient's age and the trauma mechanism, whether blunt or penetrating injury, are also weighted and contribute to the score. Overall, the TRISS score is generated using the American-based Major Trauma Outcome Study-derived coefficient.

However, whilst this scoring system amongst others have been validated internationally and proven useful in managing and prognosticating the demographic outcome of the trauma patient, additional factors are significant. This includes preventative measures, access and timeliness to acute specialized services, rehabilitation and outcomes in combination with the collation of mortality and morbidity statistics to inform future practices (Lecky et al., 2014).

It is essential that these scoring tools are periodically revised to reflect the evolving demographics, therapeutic interventions, evidence-based practice and prognostics techniques.

The Intensive Care National Audit and Research Centre (ICNARC)

Intensive Care National Audit and Research Centre was developed specifically by researchers in the United Kingdom as a tool, which would score patients

TABLE 2.2 Revised trauma score (RTS).

	Measure	Coded value	Score weighting
GCS	13–15	4	X 0.9368
	9–12	3	
	6–8	2	
	4–5	1	
	3	0	
SBP	>89	4	X 0.7326
	76–89	3	
	50–75	2	
	1–49	1	
	0	0	
RR	10–29	4	X 0.2908
	>29	3	
	6–9	2	
	1–5	1	
	0	0	
		Total combined RTS	

GCS, Glasgow Coma Scale; *SBP*, systolic blood pressure: *RR*, respiratory rate.

who were specially admitted to the ICUs within the United Kingdom (except for Scotland). An outcome prediction scoring system is applied and calibrated using components from the APACHE, SAPS and Mortality Probability Model systems. It has been validated and proven to be an effective in predicting outcomes for the UK population and provides a database to critically explore standards of care and patient outcome (Harrison et al., 2014).

Therapeutic Intervention Scoring System (TISS)

Rather than predicting mortality outcome, this scoring system focuses primarily on indirectly categorizing the severity of illness in relation to the therapeutic intervention and relative nursing workload within the critical care setting (Kiekkas et al., 2008). Developed in 1974, it has undergone several revisions resulting in a simplified and current Therapeutic Intervention Scoring System (TISS)-28. Now used universally, TISS generates a score obtained through 28 weighted items, which are divided into seven clusters. These include basics activities, and support for, ventilatory, cardiovascular, renal, neurological and metabolic support, and specific nursing interventions. The score awarded will range from 1 to 78 points. Correlated to nursing time allocated for each TISS, this equates to 10.6 minutes.

TISS scoring can be useful for:

- Index of workload activity and resourcing of nursing staff.
- Research – as a tool to evaluate its efficacy in determining workload, mortality, quality of care and comparing its use with other ICUs.
- Estimate of nursing intervention for discharge planning to stepdown units of postcritical care.
- it is important to note that TISS does not reflect accurately nursing workload, such as infection control and prevention, the weight of the patient and tasks and duties essential to nursing care (Giuliani, 2018). Therefore, it should be used cautiously as an indicator for this.

2.2 ASSESSMENT

Nutritional Assessment

Critically ill patients are at risk of hypercatabolism due to the high-energy expenditure that is synonymous with the acutely unwell. The stress and inflammatory response, altered protein and energy metabolism and the difficulty to ensure optimal nutritional intake are some of the factors. Therefore, if the nutritional status of these patients is not addressed, the risk of malnutrition may be further compounded. This is associated with prolonged length of stay and an increased risk of infection and death (Cartwright, 2004).

It is important to ensure that critical care patients continue to receive essential macronutrients whether it be orally, enterally or parentally. Food contains the nutrients essential for cell metabolism. These are subsequently digested by enzymes, which are regulated and controlled by hormones. The six principle classes of nutrients include:

- Minerals
- Vitamins
- Carbohydrates
- Fats
- Proteins
- Water

The essential function of minerals and vitamins is their regulation of physiological processes in the appropriate combination to meet the energy requirement especially in the acutely unwell. The energy-yielding nutrients are carbohydrates, fats and proteins. These nutrients provide primary and alternative sources of energy. Water is the overall vital nutrient sustaining all life processes. Nutrients collectively produce and maintain the human body's status quo by building and rebuilding tissue, providing energy and regulating metabolic processes.

Guidance on the adequacy of nutrition is required, and standards have been devised against which measured intakes can be compared. These standards are known as recommended daily amounts (RDA). However, calculating the nutritional requirements to the acutely unwell patient can be challenging. It is estimated that 250 g of lean body mass is metabolized daily in the acutely unwell patient who is unfed. Therefore, the assessment and nutrition initiation for this group of patients are essential to reduce the deleterious effects of malnutrition.

The assessment of a patient's nutritional status is essential but may often not be given priority when assessing the acutely unwell. However, whilst most critical care nurses are familiar with the use of nutrition assessment tools and protocols, the exact calorific requirements may not be so clear. Commencing nutrition administration within 24–48 hours of a patient's admission to the critical care will mitigate against protein-energy deficit and the implications this will generate. The decision of enteral or parental feeding should be considered and should take a holistic multidisciplinary approach.

Nutrition assessment can vary from basic to complex. Information collated to assist with the overall nutrition assessment should be comprehensive and include:

- Patient history
- Psychological and social status
- Physical examination
- Diet history
- Current dietary intake
- Anthropometric measurements
- Biochemical and laboratory data

The above factors will all play an important role in assessing the patient's level of nutrition and hydration.

The Patient's History, Psychological and Social Status

A concise history provides the first clues about existing or potential malnutrition. It is important, if able, to ascertain:

- If the patient has been ill at home or on the ward for a long period of time prior to admission to critical care
- Recent weight loss, intentional or unintentional
  - The age of the patient <18 or >65 years
  - Their income support
  - The accommodation they reside in
  - Social status – such as living alone or social support

- Existing medications or polypharmacy
- Their current diet (i.e. vegan, vegetarian, coeliac, allergies, how food is obtained and prepared)
- Existing diseases, which may affect their nutritional status

Observation of the Patient

- Do they look thin?
- Asses the appearance of their skin in terms of colour, condition, accumulation of fluid
- Are their clothes loose?
- Are their eyes sunken?
- Check their tongue for hydration, colour and condition
- Do their dentures fit properly?

Although not conclusive, these observations will send warning signals to the trained eye that a problem with nutrition may exist. It may also give information about any recent weight loss (Reid and Allard-Gould, 2004).

Physical Examination

A physical examination should include the following assessment:

- The oral cavity − is there a sore mouth?
- The presence of dysphagia (difficulty in swallowing) or any physical difficulties with feeding
- Any nausea, vomiting, diarrhoea − result in reduced absorption and appetite
- Any constipation will affect nutritional intake and can lead to a feeling of fullness, discomfort, depression and confusion, thereby reducing food intake
- Simple respiratory function tests can be recorded, such as vital capacity, maximum inspiration and maximum expiration, to determine respiratory muscle strength.
- Evidence of diminished functional status by measuring the strength of their hand grip

Diet History

A diet history should consist of questions about:

- Likes and dislikes
- Changes in weight
- Type, quantity and texture of food eaten since the onset of illness, as disease often alters appetite
- Has there been any changes in taste and the ability to obtain and prepare food

These factors should be noted and recorded in the patient's assessment and nursing care plan.

Anthropometric Measurements

These include noninvasive measurements of height and weight by which the body mass index (BMI) can be generated. Whilst height and weight may be distorted and difficult to accurately obtain in the critical care unit. It is sometimes easier to ask the patient how tall they are — most people have a good idea, and this is better than nothing, it is crucial in determining nutritional status. Changes in body weight do give an indication of the severity of malnutrition. The critically ill who are malnourished and have a lower BMI have an increased risk of mortality. A loss >10% is indicative of malnutrition and a loss of 6%–10% is potentially significant (BAPEN, 2018). It is important to note:

- Certain disease processes, such as cancer cachexia and oedema, may affect an individual's weight, which minimizes its usefulness as a measure of nutritional status.
- Ideal weight charts must be used with caution, as they do not consider the effects of dehydration and fluid retention on weight.
- Nutrition screening tools or charts may be limited when assessing the older patient and take no account of variations in weight due to illness or age.

Height can also be used to determine malnutrition, but it is not always possible to measure height in hospitalized patients, and it may not be an adequate guide in elderly patients. It is sometimes easier to ask the patient how tall they are — most people have a good idea, and this is better than nothing. Height and weight measurements can be used to determine BMI and together they are the most important measurement when determining nutritional status.

The use of the BMI tables to help confirm if an individual is of a healthy body weight or underweight is useful. BMI is calculated by:

$$\frac{\text{weight (kg)}}{\text{height (m}^2)}$$

The normal range is 19–25. A BMI of $<19 \text{ kg/m}^2$ could be a serious risk to health.

More complicated anthropometric measurements can be used in critical care to gain more accurate information and can be useful in oedematous or dehydrated patients where body weight figures are meaningless. Body fat content is quickly and easily estimated from skinfold thickness measurements. Most commonly used is triceps skinfold thickness. This can be obtained from different sites such as the suprailiac, subscapular, biceps and triceps. Ideally, the mean result out of three measurements should be used. This in combination with mid-upper arm circumference (MUAC) can be used in the following equation to calculate mid-arm muscle circumference (MAMC) as an absolute index of muscle mass:

$$MAMC(cm) = MUAC(cm) - 3.14 \times TSF(cm)$$

A MUAC >23.5 kg/m^2 places the patient within the healthy BMI range and therefore at a reduced risk of malnutrition. However, patients whose MUCA measurement is <20 kg/m^2 increases their predisposition to malnutrition.

These measurements can be compared with standards and, if performed serially, will reflect a change in body tissue. It is often noted that these measurements are only reliable if undertaken by a trained operator and are not always accurate or a true prediction of changes in body mass in overweight or elderly patients (BAPEN, 2018).

Table 2.2 outlines the BMI classification.

Biochemical Measurements

Biochemical measurements can be used to provide an insight to the nutritional status but should not be used in isolation in the critically ill patient as they can be of limited value (Higgins, 2013; Ojo, 2017; Weijs et al., 2014). The most common in use are as follows:

Serum Albumin

The normal range is 35−50 g/d, therefore, a level <35 g/L being indicative of protein-energy malnutrition. Low levels reflect liver and renal dysfunction and synonymous with increased mortality in the acutely unwell. It is likely to be inaccurate as conditions such as stress, nephrosis and burns, which also exhibit hypoalbuminaemia in the acute phase. This makes the measurement often misleading and not altogether reflective of nutritional deficiency in the short term. However, in the chronic situation, serum albumin remains a simple and reliable indicator of malnutrition.

Serum Transferrin

Levels could be considered a better marker of acute nutritional depletion. Interpretation of serum levels is complicated by factors such as iron deficiency, which directly affects transferrin production, and so may not be wholly appropriate as a predictor of malnutrition.

Serum Haemoglobin

Measurements will highlight the presence of anaemia, which has been correlated with pressure sore development. Anaemia can occur for a variety of reasons but may be directly related to dietary inadequacy, and questioning of dietary intake should always follow this up (BAPEN, 2018; Harrington, 2004; Rodriguez, 2004).

Identifying the high-risk patients' results in an optimization of their nutritional status and may help to ensure an uneventful recovery. The patient in critical care not only has an increased demand for energy but also, due to periods of reduction or cessation of nutritional intake, has a reduced supply of energy-containing nutrients. As a result, undernutrition or, in severe cases, malnutrition may occur.

Malnutrition

The maintenance of health depends upon the consumption and absorption of appropriate amounts of energy and all the necessary macro- and micro-nutrients. Inequity in any of these will lead to malnutrition and will have deleterious effects on the body thereby increasing the risk of mortality.

Malnutrition is defined as a state that occurs when there is an imbalance between nutritional intake and nutritional requirement. This can occur in the undernourished as well as patients classified as obese (BAPEN, 2018). Malnutrition can also be acute or chronic. Critical ill patients are at an increased risk of malnutrition by their increased metabolic demands alone due to the catabolic consumption of their protein reserves. This may be further compounded by their illness prior to admission (Griffiths and Bongers, 2005; Singer and Cohen, 2016). This places them at an increased risk of malnutrition-related disease (see below). Therefore, the use of nutrition risk assessment tools such as the Malnutrition Universal Assessment Tool (BAPEN, 2016) is amongst others, which can be used to readily identify patients who may be vulnerable to malnutrition-related complication.

Adopting an interdisciplinary approach, the appropriate intervention should follow based on the nutrition requirements of the patient (Reid and Allard-Gould, 2004).

Physiological Effects of Malnutrition

Carbohydrates are the first source of energy utilized by the body and are needed to maintain a normal blood glucose level. During starvation, carbohydrates are not available directly from the gut, but the body uses carbohydrates stored as glycogen in the liver and skeletal muscles as a source of energy.

- The body initially has a protective mechanism during a period of starvation when low glucose levels stimulate glucagon secretion by the pancreas. As a result, glycogen is converted to glucose and released from the liver. This restores blood glucose levels to normal.
- These mechanisms supply blood glucose but cannot be sustained and will soon be exhausted. In the critically ill patient, the stress response to hypovolaemia, hypertension, hypoxia and acidosis is the catalysis for catabolism when malnutrition is likely to swiftly set in.

- Fat stores are subsequently used for energy − lipolysis. This method requires a major body adjustment, as all other body tissues must reduce their oxidation of glucose and switch over to fat as their energy source.
- As the liver metabolizes fat, ketone bodies are produced in large quantities. These are oxidized by the body into carbon dioxide (CO_2), water and adenosine triphosphate (ATP).
- If fasting continues, having become deprived of glycogen stores, the brain has to gradually adapt to the use of ketone bodies as its major source of energy. When this occurs, depression of the central nervous system may ensue, leading to coma.

Always check urine for the presence of ketones.

Since other body cells are also limited in the amount of ketone bodies they can metabolize, excess ketone bodies appear in the blood, resulting in ketosis, which, if not reversed by taking food, can lead to a metabolic acidosis.

The hypermetabolic state of the patient renders lipolysis to be an insufficient source of glucose; therefore, the body will now break down large quantities of muscle protein as a source of energy to maintain cellular function. Amino acids are released and converted to glucose in the liver by gluconeogenesis, or the amino acids may be oxidized directly.

Within the dietetic arena, promising results have been shown when a detailed nutritional assessment has taken place to ensure early commencement of preoperative feeding regimens. This method of early assessment results in an optimization of the patient's nutritional status and can be seen as promoting a speedy and uneventful postoperative recovery. Therefore, the same strategies must be implemented within the critical care setting. It is important to note that malnutrition reduces the body's ability to:

- Heal wounds, which increases the risk of pressure sore development
- Manufacture haemoglobin, which reduces the O_2-carrying capacity of the blood
- Produce white blood cells, causing suppression of the immune response and reducing the patient's defence mechanisms
- Maintain adequate respiratory drive due to the reduction in pulmonary diaphragmatic muscle mass and strength, predisposing the patient to respiratory failure
- Develop muscle functioning
- Adequately contribute to the development of organs, tissues and bone

- Produce hormone, nutrients, enzymes, vitamins production and drug metabolism
- Maintain oncotic pressure − colloid osmotic pressure (OP) through the production and presence of albumin

Consequences of Malnutrition in the Critical Care Patient

- Inflammation and immunosuppression
- Opportunistic infections localized or systemically − a higher incidence of pneumonia due to an impairment in respiratory function resulting in ventilator dependency
- Catabolism, muscle wasting and weight loss are accelerated resulting in muscle atrophy, reduced muscle function and mobility
- Respiratory depression due to the reduction in diaphragmatic muscle mass and strength and cardiac failure
- Impaired gut integrity, and therefore, the patient's immune response deteriorates
- Delayed wound healing, and the prevalence of skin pressure damage
- May reduce the metabolism of drugs
- An increased risk for morbidity and mortality
- The relative costs in caring for the malnourished patient

Assessing the nutrition status of the critically ill patient and meeting their demands can be challenging. The assessment should be based on nurses' systematic observation of the patient and the collation of essential core data using relevant assessment tools and local guidelines. This will aid the appropriate initiation of a plan to meet the patients' nutrition needs to mitigate against existing or to treat malnutrition with the relevant macronutrients to promote recovery (Rodriguez, 2004).

Pressure Area Risk Assessment

Pressure sores are potentially an avoidable complication of bed rest and decreased mobility. Patients who are at more risk of developing pressure sores include:

- Those who are in a poor state of health and have numerous medical and surgical problems
- The malnourished
- The older patient
- The critically ill
- Those with neurological impairment
- Those with impaired mobility or reduced sensation
- Those with physical deformities and limited mobility or poor posture
- Those who have a pressure ulcer or a previous history
- Skin moisture

The pathogenesis of pressure sores is complex because it is affected by so many predisposing factors. However, there are three major factors identified as significant:

1. Pressure >25 mmHg will occlude capillaries. The tissues are thus deprived of their blood supply, and if the pressure is maintained for a sufficient length of time, the ischaemic tissues die. It is difficult for the acutely unwell patient to respond to the damaging pressure due to factors associated with being cared for in the ICU such as the acuity and instability of their condition, sedation, analgesia and paralysing agents.
2. Shearing or friction caused by dragging patients up the bed, which seriously damages the microcirculation.
3. Pressure and strain to structures so great that they tear the muscle, and skin fibres from their bony attachments cause shearing forces.

A patient suffering from a combination of predisposing factors is more susceptible to developing pressure sores. There is a correlation with an increased risk of infection, length of stay, mortality and morbidity, reduced quality of life, increase nursing workload and the potential need for more staffing (Sving et al., 2014). Predisposing factors can be subdivided into two main groups:

1. Intrinsic factors — aspects of the patient's condition, mental, physical, and medical states, for example, malnutrition, age, altered consciousness, immobility, adequate tissue perfusion and the age of the patient.
2. Extrinsic factors — decreased tissue perfusion secondary to external pressure to the skin, external effects of drugs, treatment regimens, patient-handling techniques, personal hygiene, weight distribution.

Pressure ulcer occurrence is a quality indicator. Therefore, patients at greatest risk from developing pressure sores may be identified using a Pressure Sore Prediction Scale. These may include the following validated risk assessment tools: the Waterlow, Braden and Norton risk-assessment scales.

- The Waterlow scale is the most widely used pressure sore risk assessment calculator in the United Kingdom.
- The Braden scale — developed in the United States — is often preferred because it has been tested and tried and found to be reliable and valid, as the Waterlow scale tends to overpredict risk.
- The Norton risk-assessment scale — although the oldest of the three tools in predicting pressure damage, it has been found not to be as reliable when compared to the Braden and Waterlow scale. Its limitation of use relates to overprediction of risk and therefore inappropriate interventions (O'Tuathail and Taqi, 2011).

Using these screening tool strategies, it is important to note that both scales are overcautious and potentially overpredict pressure sore risk. Yet, it is better to overpredict than underpredict risk, as the cost of treating pressure sores is high, while the cost of preventing them is considerably less.

All patients admitted to critical care should be assessed for risk of pressure sore development within 2 hours of arrival. It is important to realize that a risk assessment score is not a definitive answer to the question of whether an individual will develop a pressure sore. The calculator is an aid to professional and clinical judgement in determining what resources are needed. If used effectively, the calculator can be used to justify a request for resources, for example, specialized beds and/or efficient moving and handling equipment.

Specialized kinetic beds can be used to facilitate the turning process, relieve pressure and prevent pressure sore formation. These beds are very expensive and are not used routinely or to replace essential quality nursing care.

However, preventative strategies are essential in conjunction with these pressure-relieving resources. Therefore, the use of and compliance with care bundles have proven to be beneficial in the management and prevention of pressure damage in the care of acute (and nonacute) patients. This includes the combined care of:

- Risk assessment
- Skin inspection
- Pressure-relieving surfaces
- Regular position changing − at least four hourly
- Adequate nutrition and hydration
- Skin care − ensuring reinspection of the skin with each repositioning and ensuring it is kept clean and dry of moisture, faecal and urine matter. The use of barrier creams may also contribute to the prevention of skin break down.

The occurrences of pressure ulcers are usually located over the bony prominences such as the occiput, ears sacrum, ischial tuberosities, hips, heels and ankles. Pressure damage is classified into Stages I through to IV − with each stage clearly defining the severity of the damaged tissue. See table below:

Wound Assessment

The prevalence of wounds and their management are on the increase. Care may be further compounded by the aging population with existing comorbidities and those who are critically ill. Wound assessment is a complex task that requires concise information before deciding on a strategy for treatment. However, the critically ill patient should be assessed holistically. Using a measurement tool to assess wounds encourages consistent intervention irrespective of who assesses the wound at any time (Logan, 2015). A good wound assessment should include the following:

1. A body diagram to record the patient's wound sites, and in the case of multiple wounds, these should be numbered individually.

2. A separate assessment sheet should determine the site of each wound and/ or the number identified from the initial body diagram.
3. Consider the major areas in relation to the condition of any wound (Box 2.1).
4. The maximum dimensions should be an accurate record giving the length, width and depth of the wound in centimetres in order to have a standard method of measurement (Wounds, 2017).

Charting wound healing requires accurate recording of observations and wound treatment. The wound assessment tool used will be a locally practiced preference. It is important the user is aware of the tool's limitations. It is essential the patient's wound(s) are assessed as soon as possible after admission, and that the risk is reassessed whenever there is a significant change in

BOX 2.1 Major areas that should be included in a wound assessment	

Record of wound site	Body diagram from different angles:
	• Back
	• Front
	• Legs
	  • Front
	  • Back
	  • Medial
	  • Lateral

Condition of wound	• Wound dimensions • Nature of wound bed • Exudate • Odour • Pain (site, frequency, severity) • Wound margin • Erythema of surrounding skin • Condition of surrounding skin infection
Dimensions/drawing	• Length • Width • Depth • Outside tracking • Healthy granulating tissue • Sloughy areas
Documentation	All these points need to be taken into consideration when documenting nursing observations and wound treatments in relation to wound care

the patient's condition. Accurate and on-going wound assessment is a prerequisite to planning appropriate care and evaluating its effectiveness (Cook, 2014). Ensuring evidence-based interventions and treatments will contribute to the healing process.

The process of wound assessment identifies the expanding nature of nursing practice in nurse prescribing of wound-care dressings. In addition, a thorough holistic and focal assessment will highlight key points and may inevitably require a multidisciplinary approach to ensure effective treatment (Wounds, 2017).

Neurological Assessment

Neurological assessment is an essential nursing skill when caring for the critically ill adult. The detection of abnormalities will prompt timely and appropriate clinical intervention. Neurological disease may produce systemic signs, and systemic disease may affect the nervous system. However, the neurological deficits in the ICU can be multifaceted, which may influence the central or peripheral nervous system. A neurological medical health history obtained from the patient, relatives or clinical notes may provide some insight if available. In addition to this information, a complete neurologically focussed assessment should follow, but a full assessment will not be possible in the sedated or paralysed patient. The use of the relevant neurological assessment tool should be used such as:

- Alert, (new) confusion, voice, pain, unresponsive
- The GCS
- Confusion assessment method − intensive care unit
- Face, arm, speech, time
- Richmond Agitation-Sedation Scale (RAAS)

Ascertaining the level of consciousness is essential. Impairment of this may represent brain dysfunction due to direct injury or systemic problems such as trauma, neurological, infection, toxins, ischaemia, biochemical or metabolic disorders. The nurse should be mindful of the neurological abnormalities presented and those which may be reflected in the patient's overall vital signs. These provide salient information to the patient's change in clinical condition and should be dealt with promptly.

Neurological assessment includes:

- Conscious level and higher centre functions (this will include a combination of the following):
  - Attention and orientation (orientation: to time place and person; attention: complexity of repetition)
  - Mentation − memory
  - Calculation

- Abstract thought
- Spatial awareness
- Visual perception

Full assessment of the higher centre function requires the patient to communicate and will not be possible in the critically ill patient (Maher, 2016; Yogarajah, 2015). The use of the relevant tools will provide objective data.

- Cranial nerves 1−12 assessment of the cranial nerves may not always feature in the intensive care nurse's assessment, but an understanding of the relative motor and sensory impulses will contribute to the assessment process.

  Motor-sensory response - this full assessment is valid if the patient is awake and able to comply with instruction. However, assessment of the upper and lower limbs be inspected with the formal examination to establish:
  - Tone
  - Power
  - Reflexes
  - Coordination and gait
  - Sensation
- Levels of coma (Table 2.3)

  A coma relates to the impairment of the patients' arousal and conscious state and subsequent sensory and motor responses. Varying stages or states of coma have been used, and these may vary from or used interchangeably with the following states:
  - Nonconvulsive status epilepticus
  - Akinetic mutism
  - Locked in syndrome
  - Persistent vegetative state
  - Stupor minimally conscious state
  - Catatonia

  Specialist input may be required for test and investigations before a formal diagnosis. However, the use of an appropriate neurological assessment tool should be used to aid assessment (Yogarajah, 2015; Baird, 2016).

Neurological Assessment Tools
The Glasgow Coma Scale (GCS)

The tool available to assess the autonomic nervous system (ANS) is the GCS. The GCS assesses two aspects of consciousness: arousal and cognition.

1. Arousal: involves being aware of the environment.
2. Cognition: demonstrates an understanding of what the observer has said through an ability to perform tasks.

TABLE 2.3 Levels of coma.

Level	Presentation
Nonconvulsive status epilepticus	A state is only diagnosed through an EEG, which will reveal seizures but no reflected motor responses. The patient may demonstrate signs of delirium – history may reveal a recent infection, disorganized thought processes or hallucinations removal of the affecting source in addition to treatment is essential.
Akinetic mutism	Eye movement and tracking is evident. There is also a level of awareness and some communication. However, they are unable to initiate movement but will obey commands.
Locked-in syndrome	The patient will have level of cognition and therefore aware of self and environment. However, there is limited communication verbally and through body movements
Stupor/minimally conscious state	Condition of deep sleep or unresponsiveness May be aroused or caused to make a motor or verbal response but only by vigorous and repeated stimulation Response is often withdrawal or grabbing at stimulus Minimal conscious state –patients may display inconsistency in their behavioural response which may be synonymous with some awareness of the environment
Persistent vegetative state (PVS)	A chronic condition that can follow a comatosed period. Higher brain function no longer exits, and only a state of wakefulness can be observed. Patients have no awareness of environment and lack cognition. PSV is termed if this state persists for weeks or months.
Catatonia	A syndrome that may sit within the mental head field. When diagnosed and if in its extreme state, the patient may present with motor inactivity and an absence or alteration of conscious levels. Although treatable, it can be life threating.

The GCS was designed to:

- Record conscious level and the activity of the ANS or mental state
- Assess consciousness with ease and standardize clinical observations of patients with impaired consciousness

- Monitor the progress of head-injured patients and patients undergoing intracranial surgery
- Monitor neurological disorders (cerebral vascular accident, encephalitis, meningitis)
- Minimize variation and subjectivity in the clinical assessment of these patients; this estimates a patient's prognosis.
- Provide a neurological assessment that might indicate the level of patient dependency and subsequent need for nursing monitoring and interventions
- Promotes communication between healthcare professionals

It focuses on the evaluation of consciousness using three parameters: eye opening, motor response and verbal response (Table 2.4). These include:

1. The rating for eye opening based on a 4-point scale (1—4)
2. Best verbal response on a 5-point scale (1—5)
3. Best motor response on a 6-point scale (1—6)

The patient's best achievement is recorded for each parameter from a predetermined choice of options. The scores are then added together to give an overall assessment of the patient's neurological status. A score of 15 represents the most responsive, while a score of 3 is the least responsive (Baird, 2016; McLernon, 2014). However, a score of ≤8 should give rise for concern, as the patient may not be able to maintain their own airway, and an anaesthetist should be summoned if the patient is not already intubated. Ensuring the patient is stabilized, and appropriate investigations should follow to treat the underlying cause (Woodrow, 2015). Whilst the sum of the individual scores provides an overall level of consciousness, reporting the score of the individual categories would provide clarity of the neurological assessment. The GCS can also be used as part of mortality and morbidity clinical outcomes.

It is crucial not to focus on one-off readings rather a series of scores over time.

Painful Stimulus If the patient will not open their eyes or obey commands, the nurse must inflict a painful stimulus and view the response. A painful stimulus generally falls into one of two categories — central and peripheral. The brain responds to central stimulation; the spine responds to peripheral stimulation.

Central Painful Stimulation
- The trapezium squeeze and supraorbital pressure are the preferred methods when assessing motor response. The supraorbital assessment should be avoided when assessing patients with facial/periorbital fractures, whilst the sternal rub is discouraged due to the risk of bruising.

TABLE 2.4 The GCS parameters.

Parameter	Physiology	Response	Discrepancies/considerations
Eye-opening response – eye opening is closely linked to being awake and alert.	When the set of neurons are impaired, it will require a greater sensory input to produce the same response of eye opening. A best eye-opening response will show that arousal mechanisms located in the brain stem are functioning.	Spontaneous eye opening is when the eyes are opened without any stimulation from the nurse. If patients have their eyes closed, their state of arousal can be assessed by the degree of stimulation that is required to get them to open their eyes, e.g. painful stimuli – finger-tip pressure	The patient may not be physically able to open their eye: ptosis or swelling. This should be documented that it is not testable.
Best verbal response – if patients are unable to open their eyes spontaneously, then eye opening is assessed to speech.	The best verbal response assesses two aspects of cerebral function: • Comprehension or understanding of what has been said – reception of speech • Ability to express thoughts into words – expression of speech.	Speak to the patient in a normal voice and ask simple questions. Never ask yes or no questions. A person who is orientated knows who he/she is (name) where he/she is and what time it is (month, the year, date and day of the week are not required).	Discrepancies may occur between confused conversation and inappropriate words (e.g. swearing). The patient can be scored as confused if the question is misinterpreted or not understood: • Foreign language • Hearing deficit • Damage to the speech centres in the brain • The patient may be awake but cannot talk – aphasic: Scores 1 on GCS Other factors such as dysphasia, presence of an endotracheal or tracheotomy tube, fractured mandible or maxilla should be considered at the time of assessment; otherwise, the patient will seem worse than they are. Document that this area is not testable

Best motor response – the ability to obey simple commands such as 'put out your tongue'.	To indicate how the brain is functioning as a whole, the best motor response is used. The addition of motor power or strength of the limbs provides information on motor movement, which is assessed through the patient's ability to overcome resistance.	The request to 'squeeze my fingers' should be avoided; if used, the patient must also be asked to release their grip. It is much safer to ask him/her to 'hold up two fingers', 'hold up your right hand' or 'touch your right ear'. Painful stimuli can be used to assess motor response in the unresponsive patient using the trapezius pinch or pressing on the supraorbital notch – be mindful if patient has facial fractures- this assessment should not be used.	Area for consideration when assessing best motor response is the presence of a drift in the patient's upper limbs. Another area for consideration is posturing, previously known as decorticate and decerebrate movements, now known as abnormal flexion and extension. If patients require paralysing agents – this area is unable to be tested and should be clearly documented.

GCS, Glasgow Coma Scale.

- For best results, the stimulus should last between 10 and 15 seconds with increasing pressure to elicit a response.

Peripheral Painful Stimulation
- Used to assess eye opening, as central painful stimuli may cause eye closure by inducing a grimacing effect.
- Using a pen or pencil pain applied directly to the tip of the nail bed or to the lateral outer aspect of the nail bed of a finger to avoid causing no damage to the structures under the nail bed.
- It will initiate a spinal and cranial nerve reflex, and the patient will pull the stimulated part away.

Be aware of the degree of painful stimulus as this may amount to battery.

Inflicting a painful stimulus may not always be needed, as the patient may find objects such as nasogastric tubes (NGTs) and O_2 masks irritating and may localize spontaneously to such sources. A grimace might be useful as a means of indicating that the patient is receptive and responsive to pain. It is important to remember that the nurse's goal is to assess the brain's best response to stimulation in order to catch early deterioration, not to 'cause pain' for no reason.

Pupil Size and Reaction to Light Assessment of pupil size and reaction to light is done by shining a torch into the patient's eye. It is important to note whether the patient has any pre-existing irregularities with their pupils which are normal for them, for example, previous eye injury, cataracts, blindness in one eye, unequal pupils. Any abnormalities should be escalated. It is important to note:

- The pupil size — average pupil size is 2—5 mm
- The pupil reaction to light — is the constriction: brisk, sluggish or fixed
- The shape of the pupil — should be round
- If both pupils react equally to light and are equal in size

Special Care Considerations When undertaking the pupillary response, the following should be observed:

1. The light should not be shone directly into the patient's eyes; rather, a torch should be shone from the outer aspect over the pupil and beyond it. Otherwise, by the time the observer assesses the pupil, it would have already responded.

2. It is best to carry this out in dim lighting, as one then sees the eyes constrict better when light is shone on them or it should be agreed among staff to eliminate any inconsistencies in the patient's score (discrepancies of not dimming the light could occur during the night).
3. Progressive dilatation and loss of pupil reaction on one side occur as a result of pressure on the third cranial nerve, on the same side, indicating an enlarged intracranial mass (haematoma).
4. Progressive cerebral oedema eventually leads to compression of the third cranial nerve on the other side, so neither pupil then reacts to light (severe brain injury).
5. Some drugs, for example, atropine, dilate the pupil; opiates, for example, morphine, constrict the pupil.

Observation of Vital Signs The last section of the GCS is the observation of vital signs, which are not strictly part of the GCS but are important and can provide essential additional information as changes in a patient's neurological condition can result in alterations in vital signs:

1. A high temperature can be due to damage to the hypothalamus, which increases cerebral metabolic O_2 requirement. This is an unwanted complication when oxygenation of the brain may already be depleted; the patient may also show signs of desaturation.
2. Control centres for BP, heart rate and respiration are all located within the brain stem. Damage to this area of the brain can affect their control, and can lead to:
   - Changes in rate, depth and pattern of breathing due to increases in CO_2. Other changes in breathing due to hypoxia, deterioration of brain stem function (Cheyne–Stokes respirations and/or central neurogenic hyperventilation).
   - A decrease in heart rate due to deterioration of the brain stem (bradycardia).
   - An increase in BP, occurring when there is an increase in intracranial pressure (ICP). Cerebral resistance occurs and, to maintain cerebral perfusion, BP is raised.
3. Neurological observations should be recorded at frequent intervals, 1 hour being the maximum time allowed, but the recordings should be determined by practitioners' professional judgement.
4. Cushing's triad − this is linked to cerebral oedema, and its presence in the vital signs includes:
   - Hypertension (raised systolic with a wide pulse pressure)
   - Bradycardia
   - Hyperventilation/irregular respiration

The GCS provides a quick guide for the evaluation of the acutely ill patient. The primary purpose of the GCS is to alert medical and nursing staff to deterioration in a patient's neurological status. Signs of deterioration in a neurological patient are:

- Increased drowsiness, restlessness, confusion
- Fits
- Changes in speech ability
- Fixation in one or both pupils
- Increase in pupil size
- Deterioration in motor power
- Change in respiratory rate
- Increase in BP, decrease in heart rate
- Cardiac dysrhythmias
- Increase in ICP
- Nausea and vomiting
- Changes in body temperature

A general examination of the patient should accompany the GCS (Box 2.2), and other signs and symptoms should be taken into consideration (Table 2.5).

Anxiety

A person's response to anxiety is due to activation of the sympathetic nervous system, potentiated by adrenaline and noradrenaline from the adrenal medulla

---

BOX 2.2 The interrelationship between H^+, CO_2 and HCO_3^- in acid–base balance

$$CO_2 + H_2O H_2CO_3 H^+ + HCO_3^-$$

CO_2, carbon dioxide, HCO_3^-, bicarbonate, H_2CO_3, carbonic acid, H^+, hydrogen ions, H_2O, water.

The CO_2/HCO_3^- buffer system is important in acid–base balance, but the H^+ concentration of body fluids is influenced by both PCO_2 and HCO_3^- concentration. The equation demonstrates that the lungs and the kidneys largely determine acid–base balance. The lungs maintain acid–base balance through control of PCO_2 and the kidneys through the excretion or re-absorption of HCO_3^-. It should also be noted that this equation is completely reversible. Therefore, increases in CO_2 can be converted into H^+, and H^+ can be converted to CO_2 for excretion – depending upon the presence of the enzyme carbonic anhydrase.

Modified from Marieb, E., 2017. Human Anatomy and Physiology. Benjamin/Cumming, San Francisco CA.

TABLE 2.5 Signs and symptoms of neurological conditions.

Sign or symptom	Considerations
Headache	Onset (gradual, sudden), frequency, duration, severity character (aching, throbbing) Associated features (vomiting, visual disturbances) Site (area affected − right/left) Relieving factors (analgesia) Precipitating factors (stooping, coughing) Timing (when it occurs, night/day, any time)
Visual disorder	Onset, frequency, duration Impairment (one/both eyes, total/partial) Diplopia (double vision): this will be reported by the patient and could be secondary to a corneal problem such as cataracts. However, additional information needs to be elicited. Hallucinations (formed images, unformed shapes) Precipitating factors
Loss of consciousness	Onset, frequency, duration Tongue biting, incontinence, limb twitching (epilepsy) Alcohol/drug abuse Head injury Cardiovascular or respiratory symptoms (chest pain, thumping in chest, breathlessness) Precipitating factors (stress, headache)
Speech disorder	Onset, frequency, duration Difficulty in forming words, expression or understanding
Motor disorder	Onset, frequency, duration Lack of co-ordination − balance (cerebellum, inner ear) Involuntary movement Weakness (progression, clumsiness, difficulty in walking and leg stiffness) Relieving factors (rest) Precipitating factors (walking)
Sensory disorder	Onset, frequency, duration Pain (lack of sensation, different types, severity) Numbness/tingling Site Relieving factors (rest) Precipitating factors (walking, neck movement)
Sphincter disorder	Onset, frequency, duration Difficult in control (incontinence, retention) Anal Bladder

Continued

TABLE 2.5 Signs and symptoms of neurological conditions.—cont'd

Sign or symptom	Considerations
Lower cranial nerve disorder (IX, X, XI, XII)	Onset, frequency, duration Balance/staggering Swallowing difficulties testing the gag response Voice change/quality Tongue movement (XII) responsible for speech, swallowing and food manipulation Precipitating factors (neck movement, head positioning) Vertigo (rotation of surroundings)
Mental disorder	Onset, frequency, duration Memory/intelligence deterioration Personality/behaviour change

(Frazier et al., 2012; Pritchard, 2010). There are many factors in everyday life that provoke anxiety, and hospitalization can be counted as one of them. Anxiety is difficult to define mainly because it is often explained as a vague, uneasy feeling, the source of which is often nonspecific or unknown to the individual.

Anxiety may be both positive and negative:

1. Positive in relation to learning ability, as a high anxiety level may have a motivating function.
2. Negative in relation to particular experiences, for example, hospitalization.

Coping with the anxiety of hospitalization can sometimes lead to aggressive behaviour because of anger and frustration. Alternatively, coping strategies may take the form of escape from the anxiety-provoking situation, resulting in withdrawal due to the person's feelings of helplessness and inability to gain control over events.

Anxiety is present in at least some hospitalized patients. This may be more prevalent in the critical care patient. The physiological effects of anxiety are linked to an increased mortality and morbidity. Therefore, it is important that the critical care nurse recognizes how anxiety may be displayed and have an impact physiologically, psychologically and behaviourally when assessing their patients (Frazier et al., 2012; Pritchard, 2010). Failure to do this and to respond appropriately can have deleterious effects on the patients clinical or postintensive care stay outcome. Equally important are the strategies taken to alleviate or mitigates against these factors. The assessment of anxiety may rely on listening and talking to patients, questioning, and discussions with family/friends and through observation.

The use of tools such as those outlined below may assist in the assessment process:

- Linear analogue scale
- Visual analogue scale
- Graphic anxiety scale
- Hospital anxiety and depression scale
- General anxiety disorder assessment

Stress

Stress is seen in terms of an individual's interactions with events. The concept of 'stress' is seen as an interaction process between the individual and his or her environment, rather than a single event or set of responses. Stressors make physical and psychological demands, which require individuals to assess and understand the situation and then respond to it.

In situations when a person can understand and react to the circumstances in a satisfactory manner (e.g. studying for exams), it is unlikely to be perceived as stressful by that individual. However, if the stressors demand new responses or ones which are undeveloped (e.g. illness), then it is likely that the experience will lead to stress.

Hence 'stress' is taken to be an absence of, or a deficiency in, the individual's ability to cope with current environmental demands. The resulting illness caused by stress is linked to increased sympathetic nervous system arousal. The body's response to a stressor is reflected by a reaction, which involves the whole body and generally consists of three distinct response phases:

1. The alarm reaction — widespread physiological response, which includes a large outflow into the bloodstream of adrenal hormones in an attempt to defend the body from the stressor.
2. The stage of resistance or adaptation — where an attempt is made by the body to reestablish equilibrium and to regain control to maintain homeostasis. If the body is unable to reestablish homeostasis because of persistent exposure to the stressor, then the third phase will result.
3. Exhaustion — ending in death.

The acutely ill individual in hospital is exposed to many stressors simultaneously. These act synergistically rather than cumulatively.

There are a number of events that make significant emotional demands upon the person while in hospital, for example:

- Hearing the initial diagnosis may be a difficult and stressful process; the fear and anxiety generated by the news may be disruptive and debilitating to its recipient, making it more difficult to absorb further information or to make informed choices.

- Perception of the situation itself is an intricate concept, which may in turn be affected by past experiences, genetic predisposition, values and beliefs, self-concept and the level of anxiety at the time the stressor is perceived.
- Some treatments use powerful drugs, accompanied by side effects, which may include nausea and vomiting.
- Continued exposure to stressors can result in the development of stress ulcers, reduced wound healing, reduced cardiac function and a reduced immune response to infection, among other physiological and psychological sequelae.
- Coping with specific life events such as marriage, divorce, bereavement, redundancy, accidental injury or long-term illness.

Therefore, the implications of stress for the nurse in caring for a patient in hospital is that they understand the relationship between the individual and his or her environment, life-events and acute illness and as such take the following into consideration:

- Assessment of recent and current major life events and/or crises, as these may have accumulated to predispose to the acute illness.
- Assessment of the individual's normal coping mechanisms and support networks, so that these can be enhanced, reinforced and/or improved.
- Recognition that the present acute illness may cause stress in itself, particularly with regard to potential impact on employment, dependent family members and financial insecurity, thus making the patient more vulnerable to infection, depression and slower recovery.
- The need to assist the patient's family members with positive coping mechanisms in a situation that may be perceived as stressful for them.

The ANS controls many other body functions, and the physiological responses to stress can influence the measurements frequently undertaken by the nurse during his or her daily work. The physiological responses to stress involve neuroendocrine activation and increased sympathetic activity, which stimulates:

1. The cardiovascular system
2. A highly complex series of events that leads to stimulation of the peripheral sympathetic system
3. The adrenal medulla, resulting in the release of numerous substances into the circulation (Table 2.6):
   - Catecholamines
   - Glucocorticoids
   - Mineralocorticoids
   - Antidiuretic hormone (ADH)

The secretion of these stress hormones prepares the body for fight or flight from the insult and can influence measurements such as the temperature,

TABLE 2.6 Substances released during stress.

Substance	Action
Catecholamines	Adrenaline – increases heart rate, cardiac output, metabolic rate and blood glucose levels, causes dilatation of bronchioles. Noradrenaline – peripheral vasoconstriction, increases blood pressure.
Glucocorticoids	Cortisol from the adrenal cortex leads to gluconeogenesis, glycogenolysis, proteolysis and lipolysis, enhances adrenaline's vasoconstrictive effects.
Mineralocorticoids	Aldosterone – increases sodium reabsorption in the renal tubules, resulting in a reduction in urine output and increase in intravascular volume, providing compensation for stress and fluid/blood loss.
Antidiuretic hormone	Targets kidney tubules and inhibits or prevents urine formation; as a result, less urine is produced, blood volume increases and the thirst response will be aroused.

pulses, electrocardiogram (ECG), BP, central venous pressure, respiration, UO, blood analysis, O_2 saturation and pain. The nurse needs to be aware that ultimate control lies with the brain, and, as such, a reduced level of consciousness or an increased level of anxiety and/or stress can lead to inaccurate measurements. The effects of these stressors may follow the patient and family once discharged from the ICU and their ongoing recovery in the short- and long-term. Therefore, the need for a period of ongoing structured support is essential in the recovery process and as they readjust to normality (Elliot et al., 2016).

Ensure that you implement stress-relieving strategies in patients and their families.

Pain Assessment

Pain is one of the main symptoms that cause people to seek medical advice. The presence of pain can interfere with obtaining accurate and reliable measurements; therefore, pain should be treated at an early stage.

A regular assessment of pain contributes to the quality of relationship between critical care nurses and patients and is beneficial in the treatment and monitoring of pain levels. Effective treatment of pain is essential in the critical care setting and is undoubtedly compounded by the fact that often patients are unconscious. Additional barriers to effective pain assessment and management in this setting may be secondary to difficulties in communication because of endotracheal tube (ETT) or tracheostomy tube, medications or the patients' clinical condition that may affect cognition. Therefore, it is often difficult to adapt an applicable and working pain assessment tool for the critical care setting because often patient participation is either absent or limited.

Steps to Pain Assessment

Obtaining the Pain Story

- Assessment of the physical component of the pain:
  - Initial assessment − pain assessment tools
  - Ongoing assessment
  - Response to treatment
- Assessment of the nonphysical aspects of pain:
  - Anxiety − about treatment and meaning of pain
  - Helplessness and depression
  - Social worries

It is important that the nurse assesses the location, type and intensity of patient's pain in order to select the appropriate treatment. There are many simple pain assessment tools:

1. The visual analogue scale − a straight line, usually 10 cm in length, with one extreme marked 'no pain at all' and the other end marked 'worst possible pain'; descriptive words may be added.
2. Numerical rating scales are marked between 0 and 10, with 0 signifying 'no pain' and 10 meaning 'unbearable pain'.
3. Verbal rating scales or verbal descriptors use four or five preset categories and consist of a list of adjectives that describe levels of pain intensity by extremes ('no pain', 'mild pain', 'discomfort', 'severe/distressing pain', 'excruciating/very severe pain').
4. The Bourbonnais pain assessment tool − two pain assessment tools designed to complement each other. The tool, a 'pain ruler', consists of two parts: a scale ranging from 0 (reflecting no pain) to 10 (reflecting excruciating pain), and a list of adjectives, which describe different perceptions of pain. The person experiencing pain is then asked to match the word or words that describe his or her pain to the number which corresponds to the intensity of the pain.
5. The London Pain Chart − the chart includes a body chart to record the site(s) of pain, a verbal descriptor scale for intensity, and measures to relieve pain.
6. The Abbey pain scale is used for the measurement of pain in individuals with dementia who cannot verbalize and gives a score using six questions

on vocalization, facial expression, change in body language, behavioural change, physiological change or physical changes.

7. The pain and function assessment tool combines the verbal descriptor scale using a scale of 1–10, 1 being no pain and 10 worst possible pain, with the Wong-Baker facial grimace scale

Once assessed, it is imperative that the pain is treated; a failure to relieve pain is morally and ethically unacceptable (see Section 5 for pain relief). Pain can have a detrimental effect on a patient's condition and can significantly slow recovery. The undertreatment of pain can lead to:

- Decreased tidal volumes and alveolar ventilation, leading to decreased O_2 delivery to organs
- Preventing the patient from coughing, resulting in an increase in the collection of secretions contributing to atelectasis and chest infections
- Avoidance of movement, leading to an increase in risk of deep vein thrombosis (DVT) and pulmonary embolism (PE)
- Increased stress response and sympathetic stimulation, resulting in vaso-constriction and tachycardia, raising BP, increasing the workload of the heart
- Stress – interferes with intestinal smooth muscle and causes an increase in metabolic rate, leading to difficulties in meeting nutritional needs and may lead to loss of weight

It is important that the same pain assessment tool is used throughout and that the tool used is the most appropriate for the patient's needs at that particular time. Also, when assessing patient's pain, it is vital to listen to what the patient is saying about their pain. Interestingly, nurses generally rate patient's pain lower than it actually is.

The use of pain assessment tools in the unconscious patient can prove to be ineffective and inapplicable, as patient co-operation is required to evaluate their degree and level of pain. The critical care nurse may also encounter challenges to effectively assess pain when caring for the following patients: the older patient, those with intellectual disabilities, the patient with delirium, pregnancy, burns, chronic pain and those with dementia. It is therefore paramount that the critical care nurse takes pain assessment to the next level of specialized care. Within a critical care setting, the bedside nurse must be adequately equipped to take into account and interpret the patient's physiological parameters as an early indicator of pain – for example, elevated BP, tachycardia and sweating are all recognized signs of pain as well as working closely with the wider multidisciplinary team for appropriate and effective management.

Pain is a complex and controversial issue; it involves many body structures and is much talked about in relation to its origin and theory. There is no doubt that pain management in critical care is the role of the nurse. Pain can be avoided, leading to better patient satisfaction and quality of life. Critical care nurses must move towards effective care in this important area of clinical practice.

Posttraumatic stress symptoms are prevalent in the post-ICU patient.

Respiratory Assessment

Respiration is an essential body function necessary for the diffusion of gases between the alveoli and blood as well as the maintenance of blood pH. Ventilation is the mechanical movement of gas or air in and out of the lungs. The respiratory rate is the ventilatory rate and is recorded in breaths per minute. Effective respiration is dependent on many factors, both nervous and chemical in nature — including the chemoreceptors and lung receptors, which control depth, quality and pattern of breathing.

Rate

The normal rate at rest is approximately 12–20 breaths per minute in adults and is faster in infants and children. Changes in the rate of breathing are defined as tachypnoea (an increase in respiratory rate >20 breaths per minute) or bradypnoea (a decreased respiratory rate <12 breaths per minute).

Depth

This is the volume of air moving in and out with each respiration, normally measured as the tidal volume of about 500 mL, which is constant with each breath. Normal relaxed breathing is effortless, automatic, regular and almost silent. Dyspnoea is breathlessness and an awareness of discomfort with breathing.

Pattern

The pattern of breathing changes in disorders of the respiratory control centre. The respiratory pattern is normally regular and consists of inspiration, pause, longer expiration and another pause. In certain diseases, the pattern changes.

- Hyperventilation — an increase in both the rate and depth of respiration to about 20–30 breaths per minute.
- Apneustic — a pattern of prolonged, gasping inspiration, followed by extremely short, inefficient expiration.
- Cheyne–Stokes — periodic breathing characterized by a gradual increase in rate and depth of respiration followed by a decrease, resulting in apnoea.

Ensure that you know your patient's normal breathing pattern.

Undertaking a Respiratory Assessment

Sight, hearing and touch all play an important part in undertaking a respiratory assessment. In order to carry out an efficient assessment of the respiratory system, a systematic approach should be adopted. This should include:

1. Read and familiarize yourself with the patient's past medical history and critical care admission notes. This will give you useful information and underpin your respiratory assessment strategy.
2. Observe the patient:
   - If they are breathing spontaneously, note their respiratory rate, rhythm, depth and equality of movement from both sides of the chest.
   - Note whether the patient appears comfortable or not.
   - Are they able to speak coherently?
   - What is their central and peripheral colour?
   - If the patient is mechanically ventilated, note whether the ventilator settings correspond to the recorded settings.
   - Check and record the length of the tracheal tube at the lips.
   - Check $SpaO_2$ recordings and interpret arterial blood gases (ABGs).
   - Listen to (auscultate) the lung fields using a stethoscope.
   - Check for equal air entry sounds and note if they are absent.

In addition, observations should include:

- Cyanosis − lips, toes, fingers − lack of O_2 or due to peripheral shut down ($\downarrow$ tissue perfusion)
- Inability to talk − due to shortness of breath
- Use of accessory muscles − pectoral or sternocleidomastoids; these are used to increase thoracic size in an attempt to improve ventilation.
- Cough − effectiveness, sputum production, colour, consistency
- Chest movement:
  - Is it bilateral?
  - Can sputum rattle be felt?
  - Is the patient confused?
  - Are there signs of wheezing?
    - Pursed lips
    - Nasal flaring
    - Mouth breathing

The respiratory rate is a good indicator of respiratory function, for example, if a respiratory rate is >30 or <12 breaths per minute; this is likely to be indicative of a respiratory problem. In the spontaneously breathing patient, those who are experiencing a tachypnoea >30 bpm or bradypnoea <12 bpm need to be reviewed by medical staff because nontreatment may result in the form of respiratory failure. In ventilated patients who are breathing in a spontaneous mode and have an increased respiratory rate, this may indicate that they are distressed and struggling to oxygenate effectively.

Apart from rate, the rhythm and depth are also informative indicators of how a patient is breathing. Irregular breathing or the appearance of excessive respiratory muscle effort can both be considered as indicators that the patient is not oxygenating effectively.

It is important to note that these indicators alone are not conclusive; without change in O_2 saturation and deterioration in ABGs, they cannot alone be guaranteed indicators of potential respiratory failure. Symmetry in the patient's chest movement is paramount in the effectiveness of oxygenation, as an asymmetrical movement may indicate an underlying problem with ventilation — for example, tension pneumothorax, pleural effusion or the endotracheal tube (ETT) has slipped into the right main bronchus.

Interpreting Auscultation of the Chest

Auscultation is the skill of listening to a patient's breath and heart sounds through a stethoscope. When undertaking auscultation, you should ensure that you can hear air entry to both sides of the chest.

In a normal chest, you are likely to hear three types of air entry sounds as you move around the chest. These are as follows:

- *Bronchial* — These sounds are loud and high pitched and sound like air being blown through a hollow pipe. The expiratory phase is longer and louder than the inspiratory. Normally, they are heard only over the upper part of the sternum. They are only heard elsewhere in the lungs when there are respiratory problems.
- *Bronchovesicular* — These sounds are a combination of vesicular and bronchial and are heard mainly in the first and second intercostal spaces near the sternum. The inspiratory and expiratory phases are about equal and — such as bronchial sounds — they are not normally heard elsewhere unless there are respiratory problems.
- *Vesicular* — These sounds are normally described as relatively soft and low pitched, with sighing or gentle rustling sounds heard over the peripheral parts of the lung. Another characteristic is that the inspiratory phase is longer than the expiratory phase, and there is no pause between each of these phases.

A high percentage of critical care patients present with an abnormal chest X-ray, and this will make auscultation of the chest important in aiding chest diagnosis. Chest sounds can be divided into two main groups, and these are as follows:

- *Adventitious sounds* – These are crackles, wheezes and pleural rubs.
- *Abnormally transmitted sounds* – These include bronchial breathing and diminished breath sounds.

Bronchial breathing is caused by the transmission of bronchial sounds through consolidated lung tissue to a part of the lung where they are not normally heard. It is commonly associated with *atelectasis* or *acute respiratory distress syndrome* (ARDS).

Crackles are short, explosive and nonmusical and can be either coarse or fine. They can vary in quantity from scanty to profuse, can occur during either inspiration or expiration, and can be heard early or late in the respiratory cycle. Crackles are caused by sputum in the bronchi and trachea or by the uneven opening of the alveoli during inspiration. Coarse crackles are often found in critical care patients with bronchiectasis, while fine crackles are often associated with pulmonary fibrosis.

Early inspiratory crackles are often scanty and can be heard at the lung bases. They tend to be indicative of severe airway obstruction, for example, chronic bronchitis, asthma and emphysema. Furthermore, coughing and postural changes do not affect them. On the other hand, late inspiratory crackles are usually present in restrictive diseases, for example, pneumonia, right-sided heart failure, and are more numerous than early inspiratory crackles. The late inspiratory crackles do vary with patient position.

Wheezes are associated with musical noises. They can consist of monophonic (single), multiple short or long 'notes' (polyphonic) of a high or low pitch and can occur during inspiration or expiration. Monophonic wheezes are not consistent or regular and often present in critical care patients with asthma symptoms or pulmonary obstructions, for example, bronchial tumours, whereas polyphonic wheezes consist of different notes starting and finishing at the same time and are often associated with acute and chronic obstructive airways disease.

Stridor is a particular type of wheeze, which originates from a laryngeal or tracheal obstruction. It is distinctive and can be heard without the aid of a stethoscope, from a distance. In the ICU setting, it is most commonly heard in patients postextubation who have developed laryngeal oedema, but it can also be heard in patients with a partial upper respiratory obstruction.

Pleural rubs are present in patients whose normally smooth and well-lubricated pleural membranes have become inflamed or thickened and can no longer pass easily and silently over one another. The sound is often longer and lower pitched in comparison to a crackle. Pleural rub sounds vary depending on whether a large section of the chest wall is involved, and they have the ability to reverse their sounds between inspiration and expiration.

Ensure that you are familiar with respiratory sounds as they play an important role in nursing assessment.

Assessment of the Skin

Loss of homeostasis in body cells and organs reveals itself on the skin. The skin is an organ from which a great deal of information can be obtained:

- Nutritional status
- Fluid balance
- Circulation
- Emotional state and age

The skin can provide clues leading to the diagnosis of a patient's health problems and to an evaluation of the effectiveness of the patient's care, both nursing and medical. Assessment of the skin involves consideration of:

- Age — skin tends to become drier or more wrinkled with age.
- The general state of grooming gives a clue to the patient's physical or mental state.
- Toenails may be neglected because of arthritis, which makes it difficult for the patient to reach them.

Observation of the Skin

- Indication as to the patient's physical condition.
- It may indicate signs of shock, anaemia, high temperatures, reduced O_2, or a particular disease or condition.

Skin Colour

This is of great importance in assessment of the critically ill patient:

- Pallor
  - Skin is dependent on blood flow through the surface vessels; when blood flow is reduced, pallor will occur due to the vasoconstriction in response to stimulus.
  - Occurs in other conditions such as myocardial infarction (MI) and exposure to a cold environment.
  - During stress, adrenaline causes selective vasoconstriction, and noradrenaline causes the blood vessels of the systemic circulation to vasoconstrict.
  - Anxiety and pain may also lead to the appearance of pallor.

- Anaemia
  - Surface vessel blood flow is adequate, but the haemoglobin concentration of the blood is low.
  - O_2 saturation monitor is not a good estimate — all haemoglobin present in the blood will be fully saturated, giving a normal reading.
  - Look at the mucous membranes, for example, inside the lips or lower eyelid — blood vessels lie nearer the surface; therefore, colour can be observed.
- Flushing
  - An increased blood flow of normal haemoglobin content to the surface of the skin — a red appearance of the skin.
  - In hot weather, cutaneous vessels will dilate to facilitate heat loss from the skin surface.
  - In inflammation, vasodilatation occurs over the affected area, and redness is a characteristic feature.
- Cyanosis
  - Occurs when there is more than 5 g/dL (0.74 mmol/L) of deoxygenated Hb.
  - Manifests as a bluish discoloration, especially of the skin and mucous membranes.
  - Occurs relatively frequently in patients with polycythaemia but is rarely seen in those who are anaemic.
  - Is difficult to assess in black patients whose skin pigments may obscure the condition. The inside of the lips, palms of the hands and soles of the feet may give some indication of the problem.
  - Occurs in individuals suffering from diseases, which result in a reduced amount of O_2 being carried by the blood (hypoxaemia), which may be:
    - Central and occur over the face or lips.
    - Peripheral, where the extremities are affected — usually indicates inadequate or sluggish blood flow in the peripheral tissues.
- Jaundice
  - An abnormal yellow skin tone — this reflects the accumulation of bilirubin in the blood this may be due to a haemolytic condition, liver disease or cholestasis.
  - Bilirubin is the waste product of red blood cell (RBC) breakdown by the spleen — 99% is excreted as bilirubin in bile; the other 1% is excreted in the urine as urobilinogen.
  - If bilirubin cannot be excreted in bile due to an obstruction, any excess is excreted in the urine or deposited in body tissues.
  - The earliest sign of jaundice can be detected in the urine.
  - A yellow discoloration is most easily recognized in the conjunctiva before leading to changes in skin colour.
  - Becomes evident when plasma bilirubin levels rise above 34 μmol/L (normal, 21 μmol/L).

- A slightly yellow appearance may be apparent in the skin in the later stages of malignant disease when cachexia exists.

Scars

- The presence of scars, striae and bruising on the skin can be significant.
- Injection marks may give a clue to drug abuse or to conditions requiring prophylactic medication by injection, such as diabetes or haemophilia.
- Small bruises or rashes such as dark purple purpura, which are evident in septicaemia, should be considered in relation to the patient's condition.

Palpation of the Skin

- The feel of the skin can give information about the patient's fluid balance, state of nutrition and health.
- Moderate and severe dehydration assessed by gently but firmly pinching up a fold of skin on the back of the hand or on the inner forearm.
- In a well-hydrated person, it will immediately return to its normal position.
- In the patient who is in an advanced state of dehydration, the fold of skin may stay pinched for up to 30 seconds.

Oedema

- Oedema is an abnormal collection of fluid in the tissues — the causes are varied.
- Oedema is a problem of fluid distribution and does not necessarily indicate fluid excess.
- It is usually associated with:
  - Weight gain
  - Swelling and puffiness
  - Tight-fitting clothes and shoes
  - Limited movement of an affected area
  - Symptoms associated with an underlying pathological condition
- Oedema is recognized by pressing firmly over a bony prominence such as the medial malleolus of the ankle for about 5 seconds — waterlogged tissue retains the imprint of the finger (pitting oedema).

Obesity

- Skinfold callipers are used to assess superfluous subcutaneous fat.
- Obese skin feels flabby and may wobble when pushed.
- An obese patient who has experienced rapid weight loss may have folds of skin on the abdomen and buttocks.

Temperature

- A relative temperature can be obtained by feeling the skin.
- Will feel warm over an inflamed area or over an area of increased blood flow.
- DVT will cause inflammation, which will increase blood to the area causing swelling and pain to the calf of the leg.
- Will feel cool or cold over an area of skin that has been shut down due to reduced blood flow.
- It is usual to employ the back of the hand for testing skin temperature – this area has a more constant blood flow.

The skin can be a powerful observation tool when assessing the critically ill patient. It requires no invasive technology – just the experience and knowledge of the nurse undertaking it. The powerful knowledge about a patient's condition that a simple skin assessment can provide requires no further discussion.

Sedation Scoring

Sedation and analgesia are administered to patients in critical care and are an essential part of modern treatment. This is because many interventions are uncomfortable, distressing and frequently painful and require patients to lie in a fixed position for prolonged periods of time, and this may exacerbate or lead to backache and discomfort. Using sedation and various analgesic preparations can lead to sleep deprivation, and efforts should be made to promote natural sleep. It is important therefore when using sedation to concentrate on the adequacy of sedation and analgesia and also to ensure the patient is getting sufficient Rapid Eye Movement sleep.

Sedation of patients' needs to be adequately assessed at regular intervals. To undertake this, the RASS has been devised (Table 2.7). The procedure for RASS assessment can be viewed in Table 2.8.

The higher the score, the more agitated or restless the patient is and is in need of intervention. Positive scores require an increase in sedation, and a negative score requires a reduction in sedation. Ideally, the patient should score 0 with the aid of nursing and possibly pharmacological intervention.

It is important to note that frequent objective sedation assessments are vital within the critical care setting, using a valid and reliable sedation assessment tool. This is vital in ensuring that the critical care nurse correctly assesses the patient's sedation depth and titrates the sedation infusion dose to avoid severe cardiorespiratory depression.

TABLE 2.7 The Richmond agitation sedation scale.

Score	Term	Description	Stimulation
+4	Combative	Overtly combative, violent, immediate danger to staff	
+3	Very agitated	Pulls or removes tube(s) or catheter(s); aggressive	
+2	Agitated	Frequent nonpurposeful movements, fights ventilator	
+1	Restless	Anxious but movements not aggressive or vigorous	
0	Alert and calm		
−1	Drowsy	Not fully alert, but has sustained awakening (eye opening/contact) to voice (0.10 seconds)	Verbal stimulation
−2	Light sedation	Briefly awakens with eye contact to voice (10 seconds)	Verbal stimulation
−3	Moderate sedation	Movement or eye opening to voice (but no eye contact)	Verbal stimulation
−4	Deep sedation	No response to voice, but movement or eye opening to physical stimuli	Physical stimulation
−5	Unrousable	No response to voice or physical stimuli	Physical stimulation

2.3 HAEMODYNAMIC MONITORING

Noninvasive Cardiovascular Haemodynamic Monitoring

Temperature

Nursing and medical interventions are commonly based on temperature recordings which, if erroneously made, can lead in extreme instances to an elevated temperature being unrecognized (Richards and Edwards, 2018). A sound understanding of temperature measurement and influencing factors is essential for nurses who care for patients in critical care.

When taking the temperature, it is the temperature set by the hypothalamus, which is attempted to be determined. The pulmonary artery temperature measurement is suggested to be the most accurate way of measuring hypothalamic set point temperature. This form of temperature measurement is available in critical care settings, and if inserted, this temperature is generally

TABLE 2.8 Procedure for RASS scoring.

	State of patient	Score
Observe the patient	Patient is alert, restless or agitated	Score 0 to +4
If not alert, state patient's name and say to open eyes and look at speaker	Patient awakens with sustained eye opening and eye contact	Score −1
	Patient awakens with eye opening and eye contact, but not sustained	Score −2
	Patient has any movement in response to voice but no eye contact	Score −3
When no response to verbal stimulation, physically stimulate patient by shaking shoulder	Patient has any movement to physical stimulation	Score −4
	Patient has no response to any stimulation	Score −5

RASS, Richmond Agitation Sedation Scale.

recorded. However, approach to temperature recording is invasive and more likely to be used the very unstable patient who may require additional monitoring of their cardiovascular status.

Other temperature sites, such as the axilla, oral, or tympanic membranes, may also indirectly reflect the brain's thermal environment. However, the rectal, bladder and oesophageal temperatures are considered to be the most accurate core measurement of hypothalamic temperature secondary to the pulmonary artery probes, when caring for the critically ill patient. However, when monitoring the acutely unwell patient, there are potential limitations of using these invasive routes.

The axilla temperature is more convenient but is generally not commonly used. This is because the axilla temperature is considered to be a skin temperature and not adequate as an indicator of core temperature. However, peripheral skin temperatures are used for determining vasoconstriction or vasodilatation to help assess the adult patient's circulation status.

The sublingual route is rarely used as patients are intubated orally or nasally and as such are unable to comply with this type of measurement. In addition, single-use chemical thermometers are also available, which work by using a chemical that changes colour with increasing temperature.

The tympanic membrane closest to the brain is the ear, a temperature site that is popular in critical care unit. It uses tympanic membrane thermometry and is known as the infrared light reflectance thermometer. It detects the temperature within the eardrum. This site of measurement has clear advantages: the close proximity of the measurement site to the hypothalamus, convenience, comfort, rapidity and acceptance by the patient. It registers in a matter of seconds with little inconvenience and no discomfort to the patient. Inaccurate readings usually occur due to inconsistent measurement techniques by clinicians. A temperature is recorded to determine if it is normal, high or low. It is often assumed that, when it is high, the person has an infection, but this is not always the case (Uleberg et al., 2015; Schell-Chaple et al., 2018).

With the popularity of electronic thermometer and the obsolesced mercury-filled device, nursing staff should be aware of the limitations of the different types of thermometers in use.

With the advancement of technology, the introduction of less invasive but equally accurate devices will contribute to effective monitoring and detection of changes in the acutely unwell.

Many standard thermometers do not record temperatures below 35°C, so for an accurate measurement of hypothermia a low-reading thermometer is necessary.

Skin/toe Temperature

When patient's circulation is impaired, there are changes to the peripheral circulation to the body's extremities (Edwards, 2003a). This will be reflected in the peripheral skin temperature, as it gives a good indication of the presence and severity of a circulatory defect. The toe temperature gradient provides a valuable, inexpensive and noninvasive monitor of tissue perfusion.

Skin temperature can be used to determine the severity of shock:

- During hypovolaemia circulation to the major organs and central temperature needs to be maintained.
- Under ANS control improves the circulation through:
  - Baroreceptor activity − vasoconstriction and
  - Noradrenaline − receptors cause further vasoconstriction.

The end result is:

- Heat conservation
- Cool extremities that feel cool to touch
- An increase in BP
- Improved circulation to the body's major organs

Pulse

The rhythmic contraction of the left ventricle of the heart results in a transmission of a pressure impulse through the arteries. This pulse is customarily palpated at the radial artery in the wrist. The important factors to consider in relation to the radial pulse are:

- Rate
- Rhythm
- Pressure (volume)
- Deficits with apex rate

The pulse rate is an important component of cardiac output (CO). Fluctuations of pulse rate in the well individual normally occur together with fluctuations in stroke volume (SV) to maintain optimum CO for the activity being performed, for example, rest or exercise. In the resting adult, the pulse rate would normally be about 70 bpm. A rate >100 bpm is termed a tachycardia, and a rate <60 bpm is termed a bradycardia.

If an altered pulse does not produce signs of haemodynamic changes, it is not necessary to treat it, but if the patient does show such signs, for example, volume depletion, immediate treatment is indicated. This may include drug or intravenous (IV) infusion therapy or nonpharmacological measures can be used, such as the Valsalva manoeuvre or the physician may perform carotid sinus massage.

The rhythm of the pulse may vary normally with respiration, especially in young adults, so that the pulse is irregular, speeding up at the peak of inspiration and slowing down with expiration; this is termed sinus arrhythmia. An irregular pulse is commonly categorized into the following rhythms:

- Regularly irregular
- Irregularly irregular

A regularly irregular pulse is most likely to be caused by ectopic beats (a beat originating from a site other than the sinoatrial node), which occur prematurely. If they persist in an acutely ill person, the medical staff will require notification, as they can be indicative of increased cardiac irritability. This may be due to ischaemia or drugs (such as digoxin), increased sympathetic activity as a result of stress (for example hypoxia), or they may be related to potassium imbalance, all of which require further investigation. An irregularly irregular pulse usually indicates atrial fibrillation where atrial behaviour is chaotic and disorganized, and the transmission of impulses to the ventricles is irregular.

The importance of using the pulse as an early reliable indicator of physiological change is often overlooked and a greater significance put on the BP. Yet, assessing the pulse rate through palpation is less invasive, less time-consuming and can be measured more accurately.

Pulse Pressure

This is a wave of pressure caused by a sequence of distension and elastic recoil in the wall of the aorta, which forces blood rapidly down the systemic arterial system. It determines the strength of force of the pulse, and it can be defined as the difference between the systolic and diastolic BPs. The normal values are <40 mmHg.

When the pulse pressure is low, the strength of the pulse may be feeble and thread, for example, in hypovolaemia. When the pulse pressure is high, the pulse strength may be bounding, and the person experiencing this may feel palpitations or a pounding heart (Al-khalisy et al., 2015):

- increased by increased SV during exertion
- increased by arteriosclerosis (loss of elasticity)

The pulse deficit is the difference between the heart rate counted at the apex of the heart using a stethoscope, and the pulse rate counted simultaneously at the wrist. For the majority of patients, the heart rate and pulse rate will be the same, but a deficit will occur in:

- Atrial fibrillation
- Multiple ectopic beats.

Peripheral Pulses

There are many pulses in the body where an artery surfaces over a bony protrusion. The main pulses are apical, radial, carotid, femoral, brachial, aortic, popliteal and dorsalis pedis. The femoral and carotid pulses are important when establishing the adequacy of CO, for example, in someone who has suddenly lost consciousness due to possible cardiac arrest. The brachial pulse is used to measure BP; and the pulses of the lower limbs, the popliteal pulse located behind the knee and the dorsalis pedis and posterior tibial pulses in the feet are important in determining adequacy of perfusion to the lower limbs.

By feeling these pulses, a critical care nurse can determine if a pulse is present, absent, strong and equal, faint and equal, any weakness or a bounding feeling as if there is a great pressure within the artery, whether it is fast or slow or irregular. These will all give the nurse indications as to whether perfusion is inadequate or oversupplied, each giving the nurse clues to the overall circulation of each individual area of the body.

Use a Doppler if difficult to palpate a limb pulse.

Blood Pressure

By definition, BP is the force exerted by the blood on the walls of the vessels in which it is contained (Richards and Edwards, 2014). It varies with age, gender, weight, stress level, mood, posture, physical activity. BP also varies through the heart and vascular system. It is the highest and most variable in the aorta and other elastic arteries, decreasing through arterioles and capillaries. A number of factors, most significantly CO, peripheral resistance, elasticity of vessels and hormonal and chemical control mechanisms determine it. Maintenance of an adequate BP is essential to permit perfusion of the brain and the coronary arteries and the production of urine by the kidneys. A MAP of 70 mmHg is required for adequate organ perfusion.

However, in the person admitted to critical care, the homeostatic mechanisms, responsible for maintaining optimum BP (Table 2.9) may be stretched to their limit, fail to function, or be interfered with by drugs. The consequences of not being able to maintain an adequate BP may lead ultimately to cerebral hypoxia, cardiac failure, acute kidney injury and multisystem failure. These states occur as a result of prolonged hypotension (a low BP) or hypertension (a high BP).

Hypotension will only occur when all the homeostatic mechanisms are exhausted. It may occur in hypovolaemia where there is a diminished circulatory fluid volume. Hypovolaemic shock is the state that results from hypovolaemia and is a further decrease in the circulating fluid volume so large that the body's metabolic needs cannot be met.

Hypertension is a consistent elevation of systemic arterial BP. This can be equally harmful to the patient in the acute setting, especially if it results in the breakdown of a recent surgical anastomosis or increases the work of a

TABLE 2.9 Summary of homeostatic mechanisms that govern BP.

Control	Action
Control of resistance via the sympathetic nervous system, maintains vasomotor tone in all vessels	Directly via baroreceptors Indirectly via chemoreceptor
Chemical control Adrenaline and noradrenaline ADH Angiotensin II Atrial natriuretic peptide Inflammatory mediators	Vasoconstriction Vasodilation Sodium regulation — removes excess Water regulation
Renal autoregulation	Renin Aldosterone ADH
Capillary dynamics	Pressures exerted within the capillaries: Filtration Absorption/osmosis/diffusion

ADH, antidiuretic hormone.

damaged myocardium. The generally agreed values for the upper limits of a normal BP is 140 systolic and 90 diastolic. Hypertension can affect the circulation by damaging the wall of the systemic blood vessels, stimulating the vessels to thicken and strengthen to withstand the stress; this gradually narrows the lumen of the blood vessels and can lead to heart and renal disease or intracerebral haemorrhage (stroke).

An increasing hypertension can also be indicative of raised ICP (when combined with a simultaneous decrease in pulse rate). The increasing BP in this instance is a protective measure to maintain cerebral perfusion if the ICP increases following head injury, anoxia or space-occupying lesions.

Monitoring BP is an important facet of the critical care nurse's role as systolic pressure reflects the adequacy of CO, and diastolic pressure reflects the peripheral resistance exerted by the arterioles, measured in millimetres of mercury. Measuring the BP remains one of the most important and widely used assessment tools in hospital, as from this one test, much information can be gleaned about the patient's state of health.

In critical care areas, the majority of patients will have an arterial pressure monitor inserted, whereby the patient has a needle inserted into an artery. The radial, brachial or femoral artery may be used which then is attached to a transducer and plugged into the monitor. This produces an arterial pressure waveform and a continuous readout of BP (see later). This line is attached to normal saline 0.9% and a pressure bag set at 300 mmHg. This will provide a continuous infusion of 3 mL/h of normal saline into the artery to maintain patency. The arterial line is also used as access for blood analysis.

Respiration

The respiratory rate in adults is normally between 12 and 20 breaths per minute. Counting should be over a minute and takes place when the patient is resting and unaware of the observation since conscious awareness of breathing can lead to alteration in rate and pattern. This is because breathing is under the control of both the involuntary and voluntary nervous system.

Control of Respiration

Neural mechanisms and generation of breathing rhythm:

- Medullary respiratory centres
  - Medulla oblongata
    - Dorsal respiratory group inspiration
    - Ventral respiratory group − inspiration and expiration
  - Pacesetting centre normal respiratory rate and rhythm of 15−20 breaths per minute − eupnoea.
- Pons respiratory centre
  - Influence and modify activity of medullary neurons

- Pneumotaxic centre
  - Inhibitory impulses to inspiratory centre of medulla
  - Fine tune breathing rhythm
- Apneustic centre
  - Inspiratory drive
  - Prolongs inspiration
  - Breath holding in inspiratory phase
  - Breathing deep and slow
  - Apneustic centre inhibited by pneumotaxic centre

Factors influencing the rate and depth of breathing:

- Changes in response to body demands.
- Inspiratory depth is determined by the respiratory centre.
- The greater the frequency, the greater the force of respiratory muscle contraction.
- The rate of respiration is determined by how long the inspiratory centre is active or how quickly it is switched off.
- Irritating reflexes
  - Vagal nerve − respiratory centres
    - Constriction of air passages.
    - Mucus, debris, cigarette smoke, noxious fumes.
    - Same irritants stimulate cough in trachea, bronchi; sneeze in nasal cavity.
- Inflation reflex
  - Hering−Breuer reflex ends inspiration, so expiration can begin
- Influence of higher brain centres
  - Hypothalamic controls
    - Emotions and pain can modify respiratory rate and depth
    - An increase in temperature and increase in respiratory rate
    - A decrease in temperature and decrease in respiratory rate
  - Cortical controls
    - Conscious control over rate and depth of breathing − medullary centres bypassed
    - This process limited − why?
  - Chemical controls
    - Central chemoreceptors in the medulla
    - Peripheral chemoreceptors in vessels in the neck − mildly sensitive
  - Chemoreceptors
    - CO_2:
      - Located primarily in the central chemoreceptors
        - Hypercapnia → hyperventilation
        - Hypocapnia → hypoventilation → apnoea
    - O_2:
      - Found in the peripheral chemoreceptors

- Arterial O_2 must reduce substantially before O_2 levels increase ventilation
  - Arterial pH
    - Effect on central chemoreceptors is insignificant compared to the effect of hydrogen ions generated by elevations in CO_2
    - Mediated through the peripheral chemoreceptors
    - Changes in CO_2 and hydrogen concentration are interrelated but distinct stimuli

Interactions of CO_2, O_2 and Arterial pH

- Every cell in the body must have O_2 to live; the body's need to rid itself of CO_2 is the most important stimulus for breathing in a healthy person.
- CO_2 does not act in isolation, and various chemical factors enforce or inhibit one another's effects:
  - Rising CO_2 levels are the most powerful respiratory stimulant; low partial pressure of CO_2 levels depress respiration.
  - Low O_2 tensions augment partial pressure of CO_2 effects; high partial pressure of O_2 levels diminishes the effectiveness of CO_2 stimulation.
  - When arterial partial pressure of O_2 falls below 8 kPa (60 mmHg), it becomes the major stimulus for respiration, and ventilation is increased via reflexes initiated by the peripheral chemoreceptors. This may increase O_2 loading into the blood, but it also causes hypocapnia and an increase in blood pH, both of which inhibit respiration.
  - Arterial pH does not influence the central chemoreceptors directly.

Urine Output

The process of passing urine or emptying the bladder is called micturition also known as voiding or urination. Occurs generally when about 200 mL of urine has collected in the bladder activating stretch receptors. The average urinary output should be between 30 and 70 mL or more per hour. This should be regularly monitored by UO, either from collecting the patient's urine in a bedpan or urinal or by a catheter inserted into the bladder and collected in a bag and charting it on a fluid chart. The minimum UO is ø30 mL/h; some practitioners prefer 50–70 mL/h. Strict documentation on a fluid balance chart will measure or take into consideration a patient's:

- Fluid intake (IV, oral, enteral feeding)
- Fluid output (urine, wound/chest drains, vomiting, diarrhoea, insensible loss)
- UO reduces during:
  - Stress to increase BP
  - Loss of circulating volume

- Renal failure, hypoxic injury to the kidney (ATN), retention of urine
- Heart failure (left ventricle function, coronary heart disease, congestive heart failure [CHF], MI)
- UO increases:
  - In diabetes insipidus
  - Diuretic phase of renal failure
  - Following the administration of diuretics
  - In hypothermia (massive diuresis, due to extreme cold)
  - In fluid intake

If there are concerns about the patient's kidney function, overall fluid and electrolyte balance, quality of urine and circulatory status, then urinary output should be measured at regular intervals and accurately recorded. If UO falls below 0.5 mL/kg/h for more than 2 hours, the medical team should be informed as fluid administration may need to be increased or diuretics prescribed. UO is measured at hourly intervals and accurately recorded. Interpretation of UO is always considered as an overall fluid balance over a 24-hour period.

Urine Testing

The kidney has a prime role in maintaining normal healthy life, and many early changes that occur in the body may be reflected in the urine well before they become clinically obvious. A critical care nurse is usually the first person to deal with a patient admitted to the unit and has the most opportunity of contact with, and a chance to observe, the patient. Thus, nurses are well placed to aid in the detection and diagnosis of disease, as they may be the first to be aware of the patient's clinical condition. Often there are some clues (Table 2.10), which can suggest a few simple preliminary tests that may easily show whether to pursue a particular line of investigation and these tests can be performed by the critical care nurse on a urine sample.

Urine examination can yield important information about the early signs of disease, as many life-threatening conditions of insidious onset such as diabetes, cancer of the bladder or renal disease may be revealed by the analysis of the constituents of the urine (Table 2.11). Taking notice of some of the areas measured in routine urine tests helps to provide valuable clues to the patient's condition or the effectiveness of treatment. It is unfortunate that urine testing is described as 'routine' and generally undervalued. Urine testing is a simple procedure, which is low in cost and can diagnose many conditions early. It is fast, easy to interpret and nonintrusive to patients (Higgins, 2013).

TABLE 2.10 Clues suggesting preliminary urine tests are required.

Symptom or sign	Possible diagnosis	Tests to consider
Weight loss	Malnutrition	Look for ketones
Weight loss, perhaps with an increase in thirst	Diabetes	Look for glucose and ketones
Frequency of micturition	Infection	Test for bacteria (i.e. nitrites) or protein and blood
	Renal disease	Test for specific gravity, protein, blood
Yellow tinge to skin	Jaundice	Test for increases in urobilinogen and urine bilirubin

Appearance of Urine and Cause

- Colour
  - Yellow-orange to brownish green — bilirubin from obstructive jaundice
  - Red to red-brown — haemoglobinuria
  - Smoky red — unhaemolysed RBCs
  - Dark wine colour — haemolytic jaundice
  - Brown-black — melanoma
  - Dark-brown — liver infection
  - Green — bacterial infection
- Odour — infection, diabetes, anorexia, diet

The significance of the urine test strip results can be found in the:

- Specific gravity 1005–1035 (state of hydration)
- pH 4.5–8 (acid–base balance)
- Blood (cancer of the bladder, stones, infection, trauma)
- Protein (renal disease, urinary tract infection [UTI], hypertension, pre-eclampsia, CHF)
- Bilirubin and urobilinogen (liver disease, haemolytic anaemia)
- Nitrates (UTI)
- Leucocytes (UTI)
- Glucose (diabetes mellitus, stress, Cushing's syndrome, acute pancreatitis)
- Ketones (fasting, uncontrolled diabetes mellitus).

Taking note of some of the constituents measured in a routine urine test may

- allow evaluation of a person's fluid balance;
- aid diagnosis;

TABLE 2.11 Urine testing: significance of results.

Measure	Interpretation	Significance in disease
Specific gravity determines hydration and the amount of waste products to be excreted in relation to water; dependent on state of hydration and the amount of waste products to be excreted. One way to determine if hydration is adequate.	SG gives a good indication of the net fluid balance and is of particular value in patients where there is an unquantifiable loss, such as in burns cases, breathing difficulties, diarrhoea or fever. In healthy adults, SG varies between 1005 and 1035 (pure water is the standard, with an SG of 1000).	Urine with a persistently low SG is suggestive of diabetes insipidus or renal damage. An increase in specific gravity will indicate dehydration, perhaps due to bleeding, vomiting, diarrhoea, reduction in fluid intake or fever.
The pH should reflect the acid–base balance of the body, as excess hydrogen or bicarbonate ions are excreted by the tubules to maintain the normal status.	Under normal circumstances, the urine has a pH of around 6, but it can range from about 5 to 8.5.	Metabolic acidosis from starvation, high protein diets or diabetic ketoacidosis will lead to an acid urine but diets including a lot of vegetable, mild or even bicarbonate-based antacids can cause an alkaline urine, when the pH will rise.
Blood A potentially serious sign and needs thorough and rapid investigation.	Positive results must be followed up to determine where the blood is coming from. False-positive results may occur, from containers contaminated with bleach, skin preparation with povidone iodine, or from the use of stale urine.	Asymptomatic haematuria is usually the earliest sign of cancer of the bladder. It can also be due to trauma, infection or stones. The blood will disappear with resolution of the infection, or stone.
Protein: In early renal disease, the glomerulus and tubules may leak small amounts of protein into the urine.	As renal disease progresses, detectable levels of protein will be found in the urine.	A number of diseases are associated with proteinuria including renal disease, urinary tract infection, hypertension, pre-eclampsia and congestive heart failure. When testing for urinary protein, a morning specimen of urine is recommended to ensure sufficient concentration.
Bilirubin and urobilinogen: In normal health, bilirubin is not found in the urine As it is excreted via the bile duct into the gut.	When the liver is diseased or there is obstruction to the flow of bile into the gut, Bilirubin or its metabolites are likely to be found in significant quantities in the urine.	Urobilinogen is normally present in urine, but elevated levels may indicate liver abnormalities or excessive Destruction of red blood cells, such as in haemolytic anaemia.

Continued

TABLE 2.11 Urine testing: significance of results.—cont'd

Measure	Interpretation	Significance in disease
Nitrites: urine normally contain nitrates from dietary metabolites, and some of the common bacteria responsible for urinary infections will convert these nitrates to nitrites.	Nitrites are not normally present in urine but are produced in increasing numbers when gram-negative bacteria such as *E. coli* convert dietary nitrates (found in the preservatives in meat products and cheese and smoked food) to nitrites. It would be appropriate to send the specimen to the laboratory for culture and sensitivity and refer the patient to the doctor for treatment.	As *E. coli* is responsible for 80% of urine infection the presence of nitrites is strongly suggestive of urinary tract infection. Visible signs may also be present – for example, is the specimen clear or cloudy? Cloudiness should be noted. If the specimen is turbid and one or more of the four tests are positive, there is a 50% chance that the urine is infected.
Glucose: not normally found in urine.	There are two categories of urine tests for glucose, the Clinitest and impregnated test strips.	The presence of glucose may be due to raised blood glucose levels (hyperglycaemia). It can be associated with many medical conditions such as diabetes mellitus, stress, Cushing's syndrome and acute pancreatitis.
Ketones: when the body metabolizes fat waste, the breakdown products are the ketones – excreted in the urine. In good health, they are not detectable in urine.	There are two tests available for ketones: Acetest, which is a tablet test, and a strip test.	Usually ketones may be found in people who are fasting but can also be present in excessive amounts in people with uncontrolled diabetes. Ketones are acidic substances and when present in excess can lead to metabolic acidosis, which, if untreated, can cause death.
Odour: A urine specimen should be noted before further testing.	Normal, freshly voided urine has very little smell but develops an ammonia smell on standing. Infected urine smells foul and may have a characteristic fishy smell on voiding and the smell worsens on standing.	Ketoacidosis in patients who have been starving or suffering from anorexia or diabetes gives urine a characteristic smell. Eating fish, curry or other strongly flavoured foodstuffs can also make the urine smell.

- assist in monitoring circulatory status and
- help to provide valuable clues to the effectiveness of treatment.

The results of a urine test should be recorded accurately in the critical care patient's records, as soon as possible after testing. A negative test result may not only point to an alternative diagnosis, but it is also a valuable baseline indicator to be referred to later in evaluating the progress of a patient during the course of his or her illness. A negative result should always be recorded even if at the time it appears unimportant, or irrelevant.

O_2 Saturation

Adequate tissue oxygenation depends on a balance between O_2 supply and delivery, and the tissue demands for O_2. When O_2 demand exceeds O_2 supply, hypoxia occurs. Hypoxia can cause vasoconstriction of blood vessels and thus redistribute the circulating volume. Most cells require O_2 to survive, function correctly, and maintain tissues.

Hypoxia can occur from:

- A blockage whereby the tissues become hypoxic due to a reduced blood flow, as in arteriosclerosis
- The loss of RBCs, which carries O_2 to the cells, often observed in haemorrhage
- The inability to get O_2 into the circulation, seen in patients with impaired respiratory function.
- Reduced circulation seen in the shocked patient

Always check the O_2 saturation site for tissue perfusion – especially after prolonged usage.

Hypoxia may be observed in several ways such as changes in behaviour and level of consciousness. This is because the brain continuously needs a steady supply of oxygenated blood flow, and this is why the brain is a sensitive indicator of a patient's perfusion status. A family member may need to be called upon for documentation of the patient's normal personality and intellectual status.

The critical care nurse is frequently the first to observe the presence of hypoxia and the one who can intervene to correct the problem with oxygenation. Very early signs of cerebral underperfusion include:

- The inability to think abstractly or perform complex mental tasks
- Restlessness
- Apprehension

- Uncooperativeness
- Irritability
- Short-term memory may also be impaired

During the hypoxic state there may be changes in BP, pulse, and colour of mucous membranes. This may lead the nurse to extend the assessment for hypoxia by obtaining an O_2 saturation measurement or obtaining arterial blood from the arterial line for blood gas for analysis (see later).

O_2 Saturation Monitoring

O_2 saturation is the measure of molecules of O_2 attached to haemoglobin and is widely used in many patient care settings. There are four molecules of O_2 attached to each haemoglobin; when this occurs, blood is fully saturated at the normal percentage of 98%. O_2 monitoring uses pulse oximetry, which is a noninvasive technique to measure the saturation of blood in the arterial capillaries. It is a spectrophotometric measurement of the proportion of oxygenated haemoglobin in the arteries. The absorption of light by desaturated, and fully saturated haemoglobin is different.

This light absorption is measured by a special light detector and appears as the percentage O_2 saturation of the haemoglobin in the arteries. The light detector of the oximeter is attached to a tissue that is reasonably transparent to these wavelengths of light. This may be the:

- Finger
- Toe
- Ear lobe

As such, it is very useful in following changes in arterial oxygenation. There must be:

- A good flow of blood to the area (it is not effective if severe vasoconstriction is present)
- No mechanical movement of the probe — this will cause interference
- No nail varnish — this will affect the normal haemoglobin saturation measured

Pulse oximetry is used:

- to estimate arterial O_2 saturation ($SpaO_2$) and
- to monitor changes in arterial O_2 saturation.

Limitations of O_2 Monitoring

It is important for practitioners to note that the O_2 saturation monitor can give misleading information regarding the true nature of the patient's O_2 status. This is due to how O_2 is loaded onto haemoglobin:

- Each haemoglobin molecule can combine with four molecules of O_2.
- After the first molecule binds the haemoglobin, molecule changes shape.

- Haemoglobin more readily takes up two more molecules − uptake of fourth is further facilitated.
- All four are bound − fully saturated.
- One, two, three − partially saturated.
- The unloading of one O_2 molecule enhances the unloading of the next and so on.
- This gives rise to the O_2 disassociation curve, which plots the relationship between the:
  - amount of O_2 bound to haemoglobin (O_2 saturation) and
  - partial pressure of O_2 (PaO_2) in the blood.
- The S-shaped curve shows the relationship between O_2 saturation %, and PaO_2 is not linear because of O_2 loading mentioned above.
- The curve highlights that at a normal PaO_2 of 13.3 kPa, O_2 saturation is 100%.
- If the drops to 8 kPa, the O_2 saturation will remain within acceptable limits − 90%.
- Thus, even if PaO_2 drops to 8 kPa, 90% of the Hb will be saturated. Hb is almost completely saturated at a PaO_2 of 9 kPa.
- At a further drop of just 1.7 kPa, the O_2 saturation will drop from 90% to 70%.
- Thus, the upper part of the curve provides an excellent safety factor in the supply of O_2 to the tissues.

Critical care nurses need to be made aware that:

- An O_2 saturation of 90% may not indicate to the nurse there is a low O_2 supply in the blood, which is determined by the partial pressure of O_2. In this way, a patient's partial pressure of O_2 can be deteriorating but not register on the O_2 saturation monitor.
- If the O_2 saturation falls below 85%, the pulse oximeter may become progressively less accurate.
- Pulse oximetry cannot be used in any form of carbon monoxide inhalation. This is because carbon monoxide has a greater affinity to haemoglobin than O_2. The O_2 saturation monitor will read the haemoglobin as fully saturated, but not with O_2, but fully saturated with carbon monoxide giving a normal reading between 98% and 100%.
- In anaemia, there is a reduction in haemoglobin; those available will be fully saturated.
- In compensated asthma with a high respiratory rate (hyperventilation) and a respiratory alkalosis, the bond between O_2 and haemoglobin is strengthened (the Bohr effect), and this will maintain O_2 saturation, but not cellular O_2 delivery.

When using pulse oximetry in practice other observations should be undertaken with it:

- Colour
- Pulse rate
- Breathing pattern and rate
- Arterial blood gases (which gives partial pressure of O_2)

An awareness of these principles will ensure that O_2 saturation monitoring is safe and minimize the potential for unrecognized hypoxaemic episodes.

Always check an abnormal reading twice; try repositioning the probe initially then reassess the patient.

End-tidal Carbon Dioxide ($P_{ET}CO_2$) Monitoring

The $P_{ET}CO_2$ monitors exhaled CO_2 on both intubated and nonintubated patients using a capnograph. The normal range for expired $P_{ET}CO_2$ is generally between 4.5 and 5.7 kPa (34–45 mmHg).

A decrease can indicate:

- PE
- Any condition that leads to a decrease in CO because of decreased alveolar blood flow

An increase can indicate:

- Respiratory conditions that lead to airway narrowing
- Lung disease that is associated with respiratory changes in the mechanical properties of the lungs

The $P_{ET}CO_2$ method of expiratory gas analysis can be undertaken through a nasal cannula, which simultaneously delivers supplemental O_2. Its use is common practice in the ventilated patient. It is positioned within the ventilator circuit providing a continuous measurement of CO_2 in a graphic wave format. In the lungs, ventilation is uniformly distributed and closely matches perfusion end-tidal CO_2 ($P_{ET}CO_2$) and thus reflects partial pressure of arterial CO_2 with a difference of up to 0.6 kPa (5 mmHg). The benefits of using a $P_{ET}CO_2$ device include the following:

- To verify correct placement of the ETT and to avoid oesophageal intubation, this will be evidenced by wave formation.
- It may be used during cardiopulmonary arrest and can reflect the effectiveness of chest compressions and spontaneous return of circulation.
- As a measure of effective ventilation

- Aid in weaning patients from ventilator support
- Evidences mechanical or physiological problems such as poor respiratory effort, poor position of ET tube
- The transportation of patients (Rowan et al., 2015)

This method of expiratory gas analysis is advocated in respiratory management of mechanically ventilated patients.

A false reading may be given if the probe is in contact with water.

Invasive Cardiovascular Haemodynamic Monitoring

Invasive cardiac monitoring gives a much clearer picture of a patient's haemodynamic state; however, it is invasive and therefore has numerous complications attached.

Arterial BP Monitoring

This involves a needle being put into a patient's artery, generally the radial or brachial. This measure of BP is determined in a different way. Arterial BP is measured using the pressure exerted on the sides of the blood vessels unlike the manual BP, which uses Korotkoff sounds. Therefore, the two measures cannot be compared. To produce an effective BP, the transducer attached to the arterial line reflects:

- Compliance (distensibility of the elastic arteries
- SV
- Rises during ventricular systole, decreases during diastole
- Systolic pressure (P_S) − pressure in arteries during ventricular systole (cardiac contraction)
- Diastolic pressure (P_D) − pressure in arteries during ventricular diastole (resting period)

Regularly recalibrate the transduced presser via the patient monitor.

Systolic and Diastolic Pressures

- Systolic pressure (P_S), 110−120 mmHg
  - Semilunar valves open and blood is ejected
  - Compliance decreases pressure needed to eject blood into arteries
  - Increased SV (amount ejected) → increased pressure

- Diastolic pressure (P_D), 70–80 mmHg
  - Semilunar valves closed and
  - Elastic recoil of arteries contributes to continued pressure → movement of blood.

Mean Arterial Pressure

- Average pressure in main arteries
- Heart spends more time in diastole
  - Therefore, MAP = diastolic pressure (P_D) + (pulse pressure [P_P] divided by 3); MAP = P_D + (P_P/3)

Capillary BP

- Pressure in capillaries
- Pressure drops from 35–40 mmHg (at arterial end) to 15–20 mmHg (at venous end)
- Lower pressure helps prevent breakage of capillary walls and decreases fluid loss to tissues

Venous BP

- Low, steady pressure of around 15 mmHg
- Venous return supported by:
  - Valves – prevent backflow: varicose veins and the failure of these valves allows blood to accumulate in veins; especially common in legs
  - Respiratory pump – changes in thoracic and abdominal pressures during breathing
  - Thoracic pressure decreases and abdominal pressure increases during inspiration
  - Muscular pump 'milking' by skeletal muscle promotes return – prolonged inactivity or prolonged contraction causes blood to pool (this may allow clots to form)

Maintaining BP

BP varies directly with:

- CO
  - Controlled by cardiac centres in the medulla oblongata
  - Sympathetic outflow
  - Parasympathetic outflow
- Blood volume (BV)
- Peripheral resistance (PR)

Based on controlling blood vessel diameter. The mechanisms include neural and chemical controls alter distribution to meet demands of various organs/tissues to maintain overall MAP through vasomotor tone (Comissio and Lucchini, 2018).

Neural Control of Resistance

- Vasomotor centre (VMC) controls vasomotor tone
  - Located in medulla oblongata (as part of cardiovascular centre)
  - Maintains vasomotor tone in all vessels
- Reflexes initiated by baroreceptors or chemoreceptors integrated into medulla oblongata (reticular formation)
- Vasomotor tone
  - Vasomotor fibres (sympathetic outflow)
    - Most fibres use noradrenaline
    - Increased sympathetic activity $\rightarrow$ vasoconstriction $\rightarrow$ increased BP
  - Fibres to vessels serving skeletal muscle use acetylcholine (Ach)
    - Increased sympathetic activity $\rightarrow$ vasodilation $\rightarrow$ increased flow to skeletal muscle

Baroreceptors

- Baroreceptors (pressoreceptors) present in carotid sinus, aortic arch, most other elastic arteries of neck and thorax
- Increased BP stimulates baroreceptors
  - Increases impulses to inhibit VMC
  - Decreased sympathetic outflow
  - Vasodilation
  - Decreased BP
- Concurrent impulses from baroreceptors (stimulated by increased BP) to the coronary intensive care cardiac centre of the brain to increase parasympathetic outflow to heart; as a consequence, there is also a decrease in sympathetic outflow.
- Prolonged hypertension causes baroreceptors to 'reset' to higher pressure.
- Decreased BP detected by baroreceptors, as sympathetic nervous system impulses decrease as a result:
  - Stimulates a sympathetic nervous system response.
  - There is a release of adrenaline and noradrenaline.
  - Increase of heart rate and contractility with bronchodilation $-$ β_1 and β_2 receptors.
  - Vasoconstriction secondary to α_1 and α_2 response.

Chemoreceptors

- The peripheral chemoreceptors are located in the aortic arch and carotid arteries.
- Connected to CAC cardiac centre of the brain and the VMC by afferent fibres.

- Respond to O_2, pH (hydrogen ion), CO_2 levels.
  - Decreased O_2 or pH, or increased CO_2 → increases impulses to CAC and VMC → increased sympathetic outflow → increased heart rate and vasoconstriction → increased BP → helps move blood through system faster → gets blood to lungs faster.

Chemical Control of Resistance Chemicals that act on vessels, heart or blood volume (BV):

- Noradrenaline (norepinephrine; from adrenal medulla) → vasoconstriction
- Adrenaline (epinephrine; from adrenal medulla):
  - Vasodilation
  - Nicotine (in tobacco) − stimulates sympathetic ganglionic neurons and adrenal medulla
- ADH (a.k.a. vasopressin; released from the neurohypophysis)
  - stimulates water reabsorption and
  - at high levels, causes vasoconstriction.
- Angiotensin II
  - Angiotensin I is produced from angiotensinogen in response to renin from kidney. This is then converted by the angiotensin-converting enzyme to produce angiotensin II.
  - causes intense vasoconstriction and
  - stimulates secretion of ADH and aldosterone (long-term control).
- Atrial natriuretic peptide (from atria of heart) − antagonizes aldosterone and causes general vasodilation, regulation of sodium and volume through the excretion of urine
- Alcohol
  - inhibits ADH secretion and
  - depresses VMC.
- Endothelium-derived factors − affect vascular smooth muscle
  - Inflammatory chemicals − vasodilation
    - Histamine, prostacyclins, kinins and others
    - Released during inflammatory response
  - Endothelin − potent vasoconstrictor, released in response to low blood flow
  - Nitric oxide−a powerful vasodilator released in response to high blood flow; causes systemic and local vasodilation

Regulation of BV

- BV important to venous pressure, venous return, end diastolic volume (EDV), stroke volume (SV), cardiac output (CO) control:
  - Direct renal control − responds to both increased and decreased BP
    - Increased BP → increased filtration → increased water loss → decreased BV
    - Decreased BP → decreased filtration → decreased water loss → increased BV

- Indirect renal control — renin-angiotensin pathway — responds to decreased BP (Fig. 2.1)
  - Decreased BP → juxtaglomerular cells of kidney tubules secrete renin → converts angiotensinogen to angiotensin I → II
  - Kidney also releases renin in response to sympathetic impulses
- Angiotensin II
  - Stimulates aldosterone secretion
  - Stimulates ADH secretion
  - Causes vasoconstriction

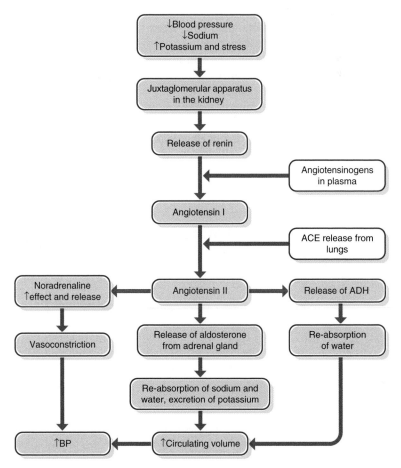

FIGURE 2.1 The renin—angiotensins—aldosterone system. *ACE*, angiotensin-converting enzyme; *ADH*, antidiuretic hormone; *BP*, blood pressure.

Capillary Dynamics

- Movement across capillary is based on gradients (Fig. 2.2)
  - Solute gradient (diffusion)
  - Water gradient (osmosis)
  - Pressure gradient (hydrostatic pressure [HP])
- Forces moving fluid out of capillary − moving fluid into the interstitial space
  - Capillary HP
    - Also called capillary BP (or blood HP)
    - 38 mmHg at arterial end of capillary (average)
    - 16 mmHg at venous end of capillary (average)
  - Interstitial fluid OP
    - Proteins in interstitial fluid (ISF) exert OP on plasma
    - Pulls fluid out of capillary into tissues
    - But normally very little protein present in ISF
    - Average value is 1 mmHg
- Forces moving fluid into capillary
  - Interstitial fluid HP − physical pressure pushing ISF into the capillary
    - Ranges from slightly negative to slightly positive
    - Generally 0 mmHg used in equations
    - Fluid removed by lymphatic system

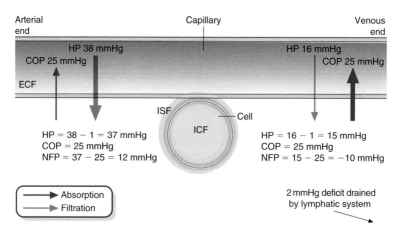

FIGURE 2.2 Normal capillary dynamics and pressures, which allow the normal movement of fluid across a semipermeable membrane (filtration) to nourish the cell; most of the fluid is absorbed (absorption) back into the circulation. The remaining excess is drained by the lymphatic system. The dynamics can be changed to demonstrate the formation of oedema (see text). *COP*, colloidal osmotic pressure; *ECF*, extracellular fluid; *HP*, hydrostatic pressure; *ICF*, intracellular fluid; *ISF*, interstitial fluid; *NFP*, net filtration pressure.

- Capillary OP — pressure due to presence of large, nondiffusible molecules (e.g. plasma protein) that draws fluid into the capillary from the ISF
  - Average value is 25 mmHg
  - Little change along capillary from arterial to venous end

For a summary of homeostatic mechanisms to control BP, see Table 2.9. Therefore, due to the many mechanisms that control BP, it is a poor indicator of shock. A falling BP is a late sign of shock. For early detection of changes:

- Tachycardia, in high temperatures and raised blood glucose level due to stress and the release of catecholamines
- Pale skin colour, cool to cold skin due to redistribution of blood
- Reduction in UO, due to selective vasoconstriction of the renal bed, actions of ADH and aldosterone
- Absent bowel sounds
- An ↑or → in BP and rate and depth of breathing
- Mental state alterations ranging from restlessness to coma
- Complaining of thirst

These are much more reliable, as the body will maintain BP at all costs.

Central Venous Pressure Monitoring

The measurement of the central venous pressure (CVP) provides important haemodynamic information to guide the therapy of patients. CVP is indicated:

- To obtain blood for laboratory estimation
- To administer parenteral nutrition
- Administration of hypertonic or irritating solutions
- Administration of vasoactive or inotropic agents and monitor effect
- As a venous access when all other routes exhausted
- Where a large fluid replacement is required — it is essential to monitor effect
- Acute circulatory failure

The CVP normally reflects the volume of blood returning to the heart, which exerts a pressure on the walls of the right atrium and measuring it can provide information about:

- The adequacy of the body's volume of blood in relation to circulatory capacity
- The effectiveness of the right side of the heart as a pump
- Vascular tone
- Pulmonary vascular resistance

Measurements on critical care are usually made using a CVP placed within the subclavian vein or internal jugular vein attached to a transducer and then plugged into a monitor. However, a CVP line can also be placed in the external jugular or femoral vein. The insertion of a CVP is a strict aseptic procedure. The patient should be in the supine position. If breathlessness occurs when lying flat, the CVP readings may need to be taken with the patient lying at a greater angle no more than 30 degrees, in which case the angle used should always be indicated alongside the recorded CVP measurement. The monitor has to be zeroed at regular intervals. The CVP is a dynamic measure and as such differs between individuals; the average is 3–10 cm H_2O when measured electronically or manually. The manual water manometers are now rarely used within the ward environments.

It is not the single CVP reading that is important but the trend demonstrated by a series of readings over time. Therefore, each time a CVP measurement is made, it is essential that it is made under identical conditions so that all possible variables (such as patient position) remain constant. Patient management should not result from the information received from CVP measurements alone. The wider clinical picture needs to be considered, for example, BP, CO, heart rate, respiratory characteristics, UO.

Complications of a CVP

- Air embolism — the lines used to measure CVP are central venous lines and thus present the inherent danger of air embolism. All IV administration equipment should, therefore, possess Luer lock connections to minimize accidental disconnection.
- Pneumothorax — damage to the apices of the lungs, leading to pneumothorax when using the subclavian route for insertion.
- Irritation of the atrial muscles of the heart causing arrhythmias.
- Risk of infection and subsequent septicaemia; maintenance of asepsis is therefore essential.

Changes in the CVP Reading

Generally, there is an overestimation of the value of the CVP reading. If a fall in CVP occurs, this is proposed to indicate a moderate fall; for example, in patients who bleed following surgery or because of extreme vasodilatation, whereby the capacity of the circulation is increased but the circulating volume remains constant, as in patients with a pyrexia or from the excessive use of vasodilator drugs (Hill, 2018).

A consequent rise in CVP is proposed to give rise to concerns about fluid overload. This can lead to circulatory collapse, whereby the left side of the heart becomes dysfunctional. The consequences will be that the heart is unable to effectively pump blood, leading to a low CO and an increase in right and left ventricular (LV) filling pressures. It is presumed, therefore, that the CVP can be used as a guide both to determine severity of fluid loss and measure when too much fluid has been administered and to ascertain cardiac instability.

This, however, is an overestimation of the value of the CVP reading, as a reduction in CVP will occur in hypovolaemia, during hypervolaemia and left-sided cardiac failure. In the instance of hypervolaemia and the CVP, it may take nearly 24 hours for events occurring in the left side of the heart to reflect through the lungs into the right ventricle, atria, and superior vena cava and be mirrored as an increased CVP reading.

A common problem caused by hypervolaemia is cardiac failure, and in this instance, the left side of the heart generally fails first. This will cause severe systolic dysfunction of the left ventricle and eventually a consequent reduction in SV. As a result, there is a decline in the amount of blood returning to the heart (venous return) and a reduction in CVP will be recorded. Other factors, which may distort and elevate CVP measurements may include the ventilated patient and a pneumothorax. This implies that CVP readings are not completely reliable in estimating circulatory function. Therefore, a more accurate measure should be used to determine the pressure in the left side of the heart (Comissio and Lucchini, 2018).

Always look at the overall trend rather than a one-off reading.

Pulmonary Artery Pressure Monitoring

In 1970, the first flow-directed catheter measuring cardiac status, function and systemic O_2 transportation was developed. The pulmonary artery pressure (PAP) catheter measures right atrial (RA) pressures, right ventricular (RV) pressures, PAPs, pulmonary artery wedge pressure (PAWP), systemic vascular resistance (SVR), CO, cardiac index (CI), core temperature and mixed venous O_2 saturation (SvO_2).

A special catheter tip (e.g. Swan Ganz or thermodilution pulmonary artery catheter) that sits at the distal port of the pulmonary artery and includes a balloon obtains these measurements. When the balloon is deflated, the pressure reflected is the PAP. The PAP indirectly measures the left ventricle's end-diastolic pressure (LVEDP) and is an invaluable assessment. The normal systolic pressure is 20−30 mmHg, and the diastolic is 8−15 mmHg.

When the balloon is inflated or 'wedged', the right pressures become blocked by the inflated balloon and the PAWP is recorded, and the tip indirectly reflects left atrial pressure, LVEDP, and LV preload. The PAWP is a much more reliable measurement than the CVP in determining cardiac function. The normal PAWP is 5−12 mmHg, but many patients may require a much higher pressure − 15−20 mmHg − to achieve optimal preload.

If the PAWP is high and CO low, this may indicate hypervolaemia, giving rise to LV insufficiency and cardiac dysfunction. If hypovolaemia is present, both PAWP and CO would be reduced. Hypervolaemia and hypovolaemia require different therapies to maintain adequate cardiac function.

The use of a PAP is a highly invasive technique with a potential risk of morbidity and mortality because it involves the threading of a catheter from a central vein through the right atrium and right ventricle and into the pulmonary artery. The critical care nurse should be aware of the potential implications and complications when patients require PAP monitoring. This is included either during insertion or use such as:

- Catheter migrating (this will be evident on the change in wave formation on the monitor)
- The risk of ischaemic should the catheter/balloon 'lodge' in the pulmonary artery
- Atrial or ventricular arrhythmias on advancement of catheter to obtain a wedge pressure
- The use of PEEP may distort readings
- The risk of infection
- Air emboli
- Bleeding
- Damage to valves
- Haemothorax
- Heart blocks
- Perforation

There is an increase in the use of other techniques that adequately and relatively less invasive in measuring cardiac function. These have become more frequently incorporated into critical care haemodynamic monitoring practice such as echocardiography using oesophageal, transthoracic, supra-sternal or transtracheal dopplers; the use of the pulse wave contours (i.e. LiDCO, Pulsion Medical System, PiCCO).

Indications for Use

- Acute cardiac failure.
- Shock.
- Diagnosis of tamponade.
- Mitral regurgitation.
- Ruptured ventricular septum.
- Management of high-risk obstetrical patients.
- Intraoperative and postoperative management of high-risk patient, such as those with:
  - Respiratory failure
  - Pulmonary hypertension
- The CVP fails to give accurate or sufficient detail regarding cardiac function.

The PAP Measure

- When the balloon is deflated, the pressure reflected is the PAP. The normal systolic pressure is 17−32, the diastolic is 7−13, and the mean is 9−19 mmHg (these measures may vary in the literature).
- The PAP catheter measures RA pressure or CVP, RV pressure (PAP), PAWP, SVR, and CO.

The PAP is Elevated in

- Pulmonary hypertension caused by tension pneumothorax, haemothorax, chronic obstructive pulmonary disease (COPD)
- Left-sided heart failure
- Mitral stenosis/insufficiency
- Fluid overload
- Tamponade
- Pulmonary emboli
- MI
- Cardiomyopathy

The PAP will be decreased in:

- beta-adrenergic stimulation and
- hypovolaemic shock.

Pulmonary Artery Wedge Pressure

When the balloon is inflated, the inflated balloon blocks the right pressures and the PAWP is recorded:

- indirectly reflecting left atrial pressure
- LVEDP
- LV preload

The PAWP is a much more reliable measure in determining the circulating volume. The normal PAWP is 5−12 mmHg, but many patients may require a much higher pressure, 15−25 mmHg (Comissio and Lucchini, 2018).

Changes in PAWP The PAWP will be Elevated in:

- Valvular-dependent cardiac dysfunction in mitral stenosis insufficiency or severe aortic stenosis
- Left-sided heart failure

- Decreased LV compliance by cardiac tamponade
- PEEP
- MI
- Vasopressors
- PE, hypoxia, ARDS
- Acute mitral valve regurgitation
- Acute cardiac tamponade
- Acute ventricular septal defect

The PAP will be decreased in:

- hypovolaemia and
- after load reduction caused by vasodilating agents.

Cardiac Output This is the amount of blood pumped by the heart per minute (L/min) and determines the function of the heart and cardiovascular system.

The CO changes according to different needs of the body; it is generally about 4–8 L/min. Two variables contribute to CO —SV and heart rate (HR) — mL/beat. The SV is the volume of blood pumped by the heart in a single systolic contraction of the LV and remains stable at 75 mL/beat. The product of the SV and the HR is equal to the CO or:

$$CO(mL/min) = SV(mL/beat) \times HR(bpm)$$

Cardiac Index

- A CO value is dependent on body size
- To account for changes in CO that occur in patients with different body size, CO is divided by body surface area (units are square metres)
- Body surface area is automatically calculated by the software from the values for height and weight of the patient or nomograms can be used
  - CI is approximately 60% of the CO
- Normal range 2.5–4.2 L/min/m^2

$$CI = CO/BSA$$

CO and PAWP

- If the PAWP is high and CO low, this may indicate hypervolaemia, giving rise to LV insufficiency and cardiac dysfunction.
- If hypovolaemia is present, both PAWP and CO would be reduced.
- Hypervolaemia and hypovolaemia require different therapies to maintain adequate cardiac functioning.

Systemic Vascular Resistance This is the average or total resistance to blood flow in the entire systemic circulation. Lower values indicate vasodilatation (sepsis), while higher values indicate vasoconstriction (stress, hypothermia, hypovolaemia). Most patients have a range of 9.6−18.8 min/L (770−1500 dyn/s/cm^{-5}).

$$SRV = (\text{Mean arterial pressure} - \text{central venous pressure})/80$$
$$\times \text{ cardiac output(L/m)}$$

Factors that decrease SVR:

- Vasodilator therapy
- Hyperdynamic septic shock
- Cirrhosis
- Aortic regurgitation
- Anaemia
- Anaphylactic and neurogenic shock

Factors that increase SVR:

- Hypovolaemia
- Hypothermia
- Cardiogenic shock
- Vasopressors such as noradrenaline, vasopressin

CO and SVR In sepsis, the CO may be normal or high due to changes in HR, despite a reduced SVR due to the severe vasodilatation from the increase in body temperature. In this instance, CO is not a good indicator of circulatory function; however, an increased CO and reduced SVR should determine treatment, for example, noradrenaline.

Mixed Venous O_2 Monitoring

The SvO_2 or the percentage of saturation of venous haemoglobin reflects the overall balance between O_2 delivery and O_2 consumption of perfused tissues (Richards and Edwards, 2018). Measurement of SvO_2 is determined by the saturation of haemoglobin in the pulmonary artery. It reflects a mixture of venous saturation from various organ systems and represents O_2 saturation of the body, rather than one organ or area. The normal value for SvO_2 is 75%, with a range of 60%−80%.

A decrease in SvO_2 is an early indication that O_2 transport and uptake may be inadequate, and interventions may be necessary. Low values (<40%) may result from increased O_2 demand or decreased O_2 delivery. This may also be evident in the anaemic patient or the catabolic patient. Abnormally high SvO_2

(>80%) levels can be caused by high FiO_2 rates or decreases in O_2 demand, such as with hypothermic patients or those who are anaesthetized.

Any changes in SvO_2 outside the normal range of 60%−80% or a trend of deviation from the baseline that is >10% should be considered for further assessment or intervention. Nevertheless, continuous SvO_2 monitoring can be used as an indicator of the adequacy of O_2 supply to the tissues and as an early warning sign of cardiopulmonary changes and pathophysiological events.

Mixed SvO_2 is used as a measure of adequacy of tissue perfusion. It varies directly with CO, haemoglobin and saturation of arterial blood, and inversely with metabolic rate. Normal is 75%. Decreases occur when O_2 delivery falls or tissue O_2 demand increases:

- All types of shock
- Pyrexia, for example, hyperpyrexia/hyperthermia
- Hypoxia
- When it drops as low as 30%, O_2 delivery is insufficient to meet tissue O_2 demand leading to anaerobic metabolism and lactic acidosis.

Increases are more difficult to interpret but are observed in conditions such as:

- Arteriovenous fistulae
- Cirrhosis
- Left to right cardiac shunts
- Cyanide poisoning
- Hypothermia
- Unintentional PA catheter wedging

Increased readings reflect a failure of cells to take up and utilize O_2. This can be measured continuously using a fibreoptic PA catheter or from inter-mittent blood sampling.

Always remember to enter the patient's weight and height details for cardiac calculations.

Transoesophageal Echocardiography

This uses an ultrasound probe attached to the end of a flexible endoscope, which is introduced into the oesophagus. It is possible to measure CO via an ultrasound probe in this way, as the oesophagus runs parallel with the descending aorta at the level of the fifth and sixth thoracic vertebra. The aorta crosses the oesophagus anteriorly at the arch, and it is because of this that the probe placed into the oesophagus requires an angled tip. The probe emits a beam of ultrasound waves of known frequency from the oesophagus across the descending aorta.

The ultrasound waves are reflected off moving objects, for example, RBCs, and back to the probe. During diastole when the blood is not moving, the reflected wave is at the same frequency as the emitted wave. During systole, the blood is moving away from the probe, and the frequency of the reflected wave is lower. The faster the blood is moving away, the greater the drop in frequency. Thus, the Doppler measures the velocity of the blood flow in the descending aorta.

The oesophageal Doppler technique has the advantage of being continuous and relatively noninvasive – it involves no skin punctures:

- The probes are simple to insert and information on cardiac function is instantly available.
- The oesophageal doppler monitor (ODM) has the ability to evaluate cardiac anatomy and performance, together with the facility to accurately estimate volume status.
- The estimation of pulmonary pressures has been shown to have a high degree of correlation with simultaneous invasive measurements.
- The shape of the waveform provides valuable information on circulating BV and heart contractility. The probe determines CO and other haemodynamic changes by assessing size, shape and changes in shape of the velocity waveforms of the descending aortic blood flow, which demonstrates increases in resistance.
- Patients with transoesophageal echocardiography (TOE) often show haemodynamic improvement after fluid loading.
- TOE gives a visual display of the heart and blood flow in the descending aorta allowing noninvasive assessment of CO and recognition of overfilling of the left ventricle. Changes in CO can be more accurately followed.

TOE is used to determine:

- Cardiogenic shock – a high diastolic pulmonary venous flow pattern into the left atrium is observed, which is reflected by elevated left atrial pressures. Cardiogenic shock is therefore recognized as a reduction in ejection fraction, and the pulmonary venous flow pattern will show predominantly low flow state as evidence of elevated LA pressure.
- Severe fluid overload – there may be evidence of RA and ventricular distension with a poorly functioning right ventricle.
- Cardiac tamponade – which is specific for the diagnosis of tamponade.
- Assessment of LV function.
- Myocardial ischaemia and infarction.
- Complications of cardiac surgery.
- Valvular heart disease.
- Aortic dissection.
- Suspected endocarditis.

- PE.
- Thoracic trauma.
- TOE can also determine:
  - RV infarction
  - RV dilatation
  - RV anterior wall hypokinesis
  - Paradoxical septal motion and small LV dimensions
  - Differential diagnosis as well as diagnosis, where the origin of cardiac dysfunction is uncertain

This technique holds some obvious advantages over pulmonary artery catheter insertion, namely:

- A reduction in the risk of complications, which have been quoted up to 7.2% for the more invasive procedure.
- Ease and minimal expertise required for insertion of the probe and acquisition of signals.
- Negligible running costs after the initial capital expenditure with the transducer reusable after sterilization in a suitable detergent.
- Prolonged usage in the same patient.
- Continuous appreciation of circulatory changes, ventricular function, and the effects of therapies by both medical and nursing staff.

However, the patient may require sedative or mild anaesthetic for this procedure. Whilst a pulmonary artery catheter or alternative cardiac function measuring devices may still be necessary for absolute measurements of CO, PAWP, SVO_2, and SVR, especially in situations such as septic shock. Therefore, to obtain clear picture of the haemodynamic status and to assist in the determination of support therapies, a measure of SVR is necessary.

To determine hypervolaemia does not necessarily require a definite measure of SVR. It could prove useful in patients who it is felt did not warrant the invasive PA technique and is an attractive proposition for critical care areas possessing neither equipment nor experience in invasive monitoring or concerned about the potential hidden risks.

Haemodynamic information only previously obtainable by pulmonary artery catheterization is now available from this relative noninvasive technique.

Gastric Intramucosal pH

The gut is sensitive to decreases in O_2 delivery. Vasoconstrictors are secreted (angiotensin II and vasopressin) causing redistribution of blood flow to the heart and brain; the gut mucosa is in danger from hypoxia. If O_2 is reduced, gut cell respiration switches to anaerobic metabolism, and lactic acid is formed − which is buffered by bicarbonate causing CO_2 and water to be released. Therefore, the CO_2 levels in the gastric mucosa determine the degree of perfusion.

Gastric tonometry determines gastric intramucosal CO_2 and is compared to arterial bicarbonate (assumed to be the same) into an equation to determine pHi. Low intramucosal pHi values are associated with worse prognosis.

ICP Monitoring

The skull and meninges contain three major components:

- Brain tissue (80%)
- Cerebral spinal fluid (CSF; 10%)
- Cerebral blood flow (CBF; 10%)

The pressure these three components exert in the rigid skull is termed the ICP. The normal range of ICP is between 0 and 15 mmHg; above 15 mmHg is determined a raised ICP. The brain maintains this normal pressure by compensation mechanisms known as autoregulation, which occurs following an insult or injury leading to increased brain, blood or CSF volume. To compensate, the following occurs:

- Displacement of CSF from the cranial subarachnoid (SA) space, spinal and lumbar space; CSF production decreases and CSF absorption increases.
- Reduction in CBF − venous blood is shunted away from the affected areas. A widespread reduction in CBF to compensate can lead to further brain insult or ischaemia due to the reduced cerebral perfusion, an increase in CO_2 and therefore acidosis.

Always remember to calibrate the machinery before taking a reading.

These compensatory mechanisms may become exhausted and an increase in ICP above 15 mmHg may occur. This may occur due to:

- Trauma
- Hydrocephalus
- Infection
- Tumours
- Metabolic disorders
- Cerebrovascular accident
- Encephalopathies

In certain injuries, monitoring techniques can be employed to measure the ICP. There are three types of ICP monitoring device – all monitor but only one can drain. These include:

1. Fluid-coupled systems with external transducers:
   - Ventriculostomy (intraventricular catheter [IVC]), able to drain excess CSF to control increased ICP
     - Placed in the lateral ventricle
     - Considered reliable and accurate in measurement
     - A high risk of infection
2. Fluid-coupled surface devices:
   - SA bolts devised because of the concern for infection with IVCs – unable to drain CSF
   - Are only a monitoring instrument
     - Easy to insert
   - Can be inaccurate and tend to underestimate the ICP due to occlusion by tissue or clot formation
     - Leakage of CSF is likely
3. Solid state systems include the fibre optic system and cable:
   - Can be combined with IVC for simultaneous ICP monitoring and CSF drainage
   - Solid-state systems are not always directly compatible with common critical care bedside monitoring – a separate system for recording and trending may be required. Can be placed in the:
     - Lateral ventricle
     - Brain parenchyma
     - Epidural space

Complications of IVC/ICP monitors are the risk of infection such as meningitis or ventriculitis, which is related to the duration of catheter insertion. SA bolt infection is rare, and generally, infections are superficial and rarely involve the brain or the meninges. Injury to the brain due to ICP monitoring includes direct brain puncture, parenchymal or subdural haemorrhage but is uncommon.

Close recording of observations is necessary, especially of MAP. This is necessary to determine adequate CBF and to calculate and record ICP and cerebral perfusion pressure (CPP). CPP is the pressure needed to perfuse the brain, and the normal range is 60–90 mmHg aiming for >70 mmHg in patients with brain pathology. It is calculated by subtracting the ICP from the MAP:

$$CCP = MAP - ICP$$

CBF is compromised if the CPP is below 60 mmHg. Reduced CPP may result in irreversible brain damage or death. It is thought that the threshold for mechanical brain injury is an ICP between 20 and 30 mmHg.

Factors that reduce the ICP:

- Position — head elevated by 30 degrees.
- Fluid restriction — slightly dehydrated state.
- Temperature control — hypothermia.
- Drugs:
  - Diuretics
  - Corticosteroids
  - Anticonvulsants
- Hyperventilation — reduced partial pressure of CO_2 will cause cerebral vasoconstriction and a reduction in ICP — hypercarbia is important to avoid in patients with increased ICP.
- A reduced level of O_2 will increase ICP and hypoxia or cerebral ischaemia should be avoided.
- Removal of the cause, for example, surgery.

2.4 DIAGNOSTIC PROCEDURES

The Electrocardiogram Rhythm Strip

The ECG is a record of the changes in electrical activity occurring within cardiac muscle. The cardiac cells involved in the contraction are specialized and are unlike any other cells in the body, as each individual cell can initiate its own electrical impulse (Richards and Edwards, 2014). Although cardiac muscle has this special property, hormones and chemical transmitters are important in producing the finer control of the heart and maintenance of homeostasis.

Bipolar and unipolar electrodes provide an ECG rhythm known as the PQRST waves, which detect the electrical charges within the cardiac cell. The ECG can provide information about the heart rate and rhythm, the effects of electrolytes or drugs on the heart and the electrical orientation of the cardiac muscle. The normal ECG trace should record between 60 and 100 complexes (PQRST) per minute (Allen et al., 2011).

What is an ECG?

The action potentials transmitted through the heart during the cardiac cycle can be recorded on the surface of the body. The recording can be obtained by electrodes on the body, connected to an ECG machine. The voltage changes are fed to the machine, amplified and displayed visually on a screen, graphically on ECG paper, or both.

Terminology

- Isoelectric line — baseline
- Positive — upward deflection

- Negative − downward deflection
- Voltage − height and depth of a wave
- Time − measured along horizontal axis; 1 second = five large squares
- Cardiac cycle − represented on ECG by P wave, QRS complex, T wave
- Bi-phasic − deflection which is both positive and negative

ECG Leads

The ECG leads provide a variety of views of the heart's electrical activity from different angles. An ECG lead consists of two surface electrodes of opposite polarity either one positive and one negative or one positive surface electrode and one reference point. A lead composed of two electrodes of opposite polarity is called a bipolar lead and constitutes the standard limb leads (I−III); these:

- Record the difference in electrical potential between the left arm, the right arm, and the left leg electrodes and
- Represent the axis of the heart.

A lead composed of a single positive electrode and a reference point is a unipolar lead which makes up the:

- Augmented limb leads (aVR, aVL and aVF) and
- Precordial leads (V1−V6).

The various leads produce different ECG tracings.

Routine monitoring of ECG is usually obtained in lead II, as it is in the direct line of positive axis.

ECG Paper

ECG paper moves at 25 mm/s and consists of small and large squares (five small squares). ECG measures time and amplitude:

- Time is measured on the horizontal plane;
- Small squares are 0.04 s in time and 1 mm in voltage and
- Large squares are 0.2 s in time and 5 mm in voltage.

Amplitude is measured on the vertical axis of the graph paper:

- Small squares equal 0.1 mV
- Large squares equal 0.5 mV

Methods of Calculating Heart Rate

- 25 mm × 60 = 1500 divided by five small squares = 300.
- Count the number of small squares between R waves, divide these into 1500, for example, 18 small squares divided into 1500 = 83 bpm.
- Count the number of large squares between the R wave and divide into 300, for example, four large squares divided into 300 = 75 bpm.

During a period of acute illness, the sequence of the ECG can be affected. The rate may increase due to heart failure, hypertension, blood loss, pain, stress or anxiety or reduce its rate due to overprescription of certain drugs (digoxin) or a lack of O_2 supply. Abnormal rhythms can occur from heart failure, coronary artery disease, MI (Edwards, 2002), and fluid overload (Edwards, 2000) and fluid and electrolyte imbalance (Edwards, 2001).

Sinus Rhythm

The P Wave

- Atrial depolarization and it is the first positive deflection seen.
- It should be no longer than 0.11 seconds, or three small squares, amplitude is normally 0.5−2.5 mm.
- It should always be followed by a QRS complex unless conduction disturbances are present.

The PR Interval

- Measured from the beginning of the P wave to the beginning of the QRS complex irrespective of whether the QRS complex begins with a Q or an R wave.
- It varies between 0.12 and 0.20 s, or three to five small squares.
- Dependent on the heart rate and conduction of atrioventricular (AV) node.
- Normal tracing indicates electrical impulse has been conducted through the correct conduction pathways.

The QRS Complex

- Usually follows the PR interval.
- Consists of three waves, Q, R and S.
- Should be narrow and sharply pointed.
- Represents ventricular contraction (depolarization), marking the beginning of ventricular systole, and can be:
  - Predominately positive (upright);
  - Predominately negative (inverted) and
  - Biphasic (partly positive, partly negative).
- Varies between 0.04 and 0.11 s, or two to three small squares; amplitude varies from <5 mm to more than 15 mm.

The ST-segment

- It is the resting period between ventricular contraction and the returning of the cardiac muscle to its resting stage.

- Early repolarization should always return to the baseline; depressed or elevated in abnormalities:
  - A depressed segment indicates ischaemia
  - An elevated segment (1 mm abase baseline) may represent injury

The T Wave

- Represents repolarization of the ventricular myocardial cells.
- Usually slightly rounded.
- Deep and symmetrical inverted T waves suggest cardiac ischaemia.
- T waves elevated more than half of the height of the QRS complex (peaked T waves) could indicate hyperkalaemia.

The QT Interval

- Is the period from the beginning of ventricular depolarization (onset of the QRS complex) until the end of ventricular repolarization or the end of T wave.
- During this period, the heart is fully refractory (the absolute refractory period).
- During the latter period of the interval (from the peak of the T wave onward), the conduction system is relatively refractory.
- Drugs may prolong the QT period.

The Diagnosis of Arrhythmias

Some of the important features that can be looked for in an ECG in its interpretation are the:

- Rate of discharge — is the rate 60 or above 100
- Rhythm or regularity of the complexes
- Duration of the PR interval
- Whether each P wave is followed by the QRS complex
- QRS complex — width, configuration, deep Q waves in leads
- T wave — are they inverted throughout, only in certain leads, or more prominent in others
- Interpretation

Normal Sinus Rhythm

- Rate: 60–100 (Fig. 2.3)
- Rhythm: regular
- Pacemaker site: SA node
- P waves: normal in shape, upright

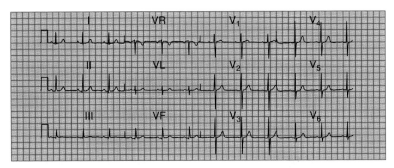

FIGURE 2.3 Normal sinus rhythm.

- PR interval: normal, 0.12—0.20 seconds
- QRS: normal, 0.14—0.12 seconds
- Clinical significance: none, normal rhythm

Sinus Bradycardia

Aetiology: vagal tone, disease, drugs, IMI (Fig. 2.4)

- Rate: <60
- Rhythm: regular
- Pacemaker site: SA node
- P waves: upright, normal in shape
- PR interval: 0.12—0.20 seconds
- QRS interval: 0.14—0.12 seconds
- Clinical significance: can result in reduced CO, hypotension
- Management: nothing if fit young person, atropine, internal pacing wires

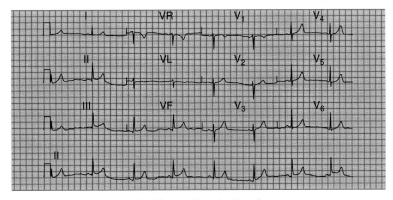

FIGURE 2.4 Sinus bradycardia.

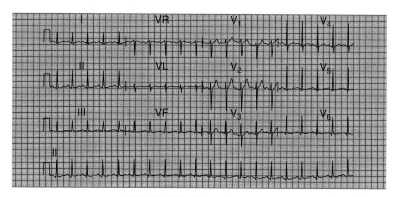

FIGURE 2.5 Sinus tachycardia.

Sinus Tachycardia

- Aetiology: exercise, anxiety, homeostatic compensation, hypovolaemia, cardiac failure (Fig. 2.5)
- Rate: >100
- Rhythm: regular
- Pacemaker site: SA node
- P waves: upright, normal in shape
- PR interval: 0.12−0.20 seconds
- QRS interval: 0.14−0.12 seconds
- Clinical significance: can result in decreased CO, increases myocardial O_2 demand
- Management: none required, normal compensatory mechanism to stress

Supraventricular Tachycardia

- Aetiology: re-entry tachycardia, circulate around AV node, occurs at any age, not fully understood, rare in patients with MI, precipitated by stress, tobacco, caffeine etc. (Fig. 2.6)
- Rate: 150−250 beats per minute
- Rhythm: usually regular
- Pacemaker site: may vary from SA node to AV node
- P waves: may be upright, normal if pacemaker at SA, inverted if near AV junction
- PR interval: usually shortened, possibly normal
- QRS interval: 0.14−0.12 seconds
- Clinical significance: can occur in healthy hearts, can be well tolerated, accompanied often by palpitations, dizziness, anxiety and nervousness. CO can be compromised. May increase myocardial ischaemia

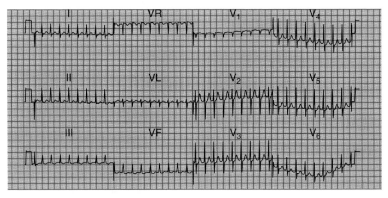

FIGURE 2.6   Supraventricular tachycardia.

- Management: vagal manoeuvres, Valsalva, adenosine, amiodarone, verapamil, cardioversion

Atrial Flutter

Aetiology: rapid re-entry focus, conduction through AV node may vary, seen in middle age to older adults, with advanced cardiovascular disease: cardiomyopathy, hypertrophy, heart failure, cardiac infections (Fig. 2.7)

- Rate: 150–300 beats per minute
- Rhythm: atrial rate regular, ventricular rate usually regular
- Pacemaker site: reentry
- P waves: 'saw-tooth' pattern unless in 2:1 block conduction when difficult to see – can appear to be sinus rhythm
- PR interval: usually constant

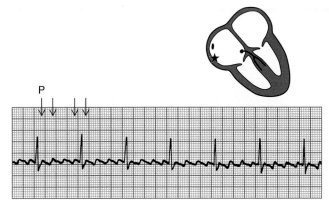

FIGURE 2.7   Atrial flutter.

- QRS: 0.04−0.12 seconds
- Clinical significance: usually well tolerated if reasonable ventricular rate, but may ultimately reduce CO, loss of atrial 'kick' occurs
- Management: as per SVT, with the addition of digoxin

Atrial Fibrillation

Aetiology: multiple areas of re-entry and/or from ectopic pacemakers in atria outside of SA node, AV conduction becomes random, more often chronic, associated with heart failure, cardiac disease, may be on digoxin, calcium channel blockers or beta blockers (Fig. 2.8).

- Rate: atrial rate cannot be counted, 350−700, ventricular rates vary according to AV node conduction
- Rhythm: irregular
- Pacemaker site: ectopic pacemakers or multiple re-entry pathways
- P waves: not visible, fibrillation waves
- PR interval: none
- QRS: 0.04−0.12 seconds as long as no ventricular conduction disturbances
- Clinical significance: atrial kick can be lost, CO reduced by up to 15%, may precipitate angina, MI, cardiac failure
- Management: may not require treatment if tolerated, if haemodynamically unstable will require cardioversion, amiodarone, beta blockers, digoxin, anticoagulants

Idioventricular Rhythms

Aetiology: dying heart/agonal impulses from higher pacemakers fail to fire or reach ventricles, and the AV nodes intrinsic rate does not meet that in the

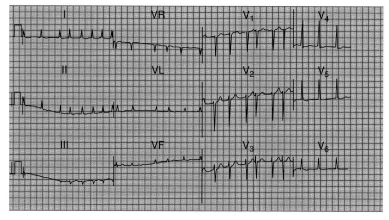

FIGURE 2.8 Atrial fibrillation.

ventricles; therefore, the ventricles become responsible for the dominant pacemaker generated by the Bundle of His and Purkinje fibres. Often seen after defibrillation or secondary to myocardial damage, failed pacemaker or drug toxicity.

- Rate: 20−40
- Rhythm: usually regular but may be irregular
- Pacemaker site: ventricular
- P waves: usually absent
- PR interval: none
- QRS: wide and bizarre, >0.12 seconds
- Clinical significance: usually very significant, hypotension, dizziness, palpitation, poor output, may present as a prearrest rhythm
- Management: O_2, pacing, atropine, if rhythm is nonperfusing treat as an emergency

Premature Ventricular Contractions

Aetiology: ectopic pacemaker site (or sites) that originates from ventricles, occurs in many underlying rhythms, alters sequences of ventricular depolarization. Often followed by a compensatory pause. Premature ventricular contraction (PVCs) may be unifocal (from one ectopic site) or multifocal (from several ectopic sites). Multifocal are more dangerous than unifocal with a risk of R on T phenomenon. PVCs may be caused by myocardial ischaemia, hypoxia, acid−base and electrolyte imbalance, heart failure, hypokalaemia, hyperkalaemia, hypomagnesemia, hypocalcemia, drug toxicity, stimulants, sympathetic drugs.

- Rate: depends on underlying rhythm and number of PVCs
- Rhythm: when a PVC present, irregular
- Pacemaker site: ectopic focus in ventricles/bundle
- P waves: present in normal beat, undetectable in PVCs
- PR interval: none in the PVC, present if interrupted by normal rhythm
- QRS: ≥0.12 seconds, wide and bizarre
- T wave after the PVC may be deflected in opposite direction due to altered depolarization sequence
- Clinical significance: usually significant if appear in runs of five or more, hypotension, poor output, may present as a prearrest rhythm
- Management: O_2, antiarrhythmics, possibly lidocaine, possibly amiodarone, check potassium levels.

Ventricular Tachycardia

Interpretation: three or more consecutive ventricular complex occurring at rate over 100, which override primary pacemaker. Usually triggered by PVC. Atria and ventricle activity asynchronous (Fig. 2.9).

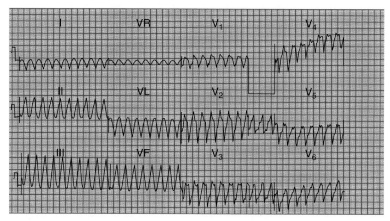

FIGURE 2.9   Ventricular tachycardia.

- Aetiology: cardiac ischaemia, hypoxia, electrolyte imbalance, heart failure, drug toxicity, sympathetic drugs, stimulants.
- PR interval: none in the PVC, present if interrupted by normal rhythm
- Rate: 100−250
- Rhythm: regular or slightly irregular
- Pacemaker site: ventricles
- P waves: not related to QRS (if seen)
- PR interval: none
- QRS complex: wide and bizarre >0.12 seconds
- Clinical significance: reduced CO, life-threatening
- Management: O_2, antiarrhythmics, possibly lidocaine, possibly amiodarone, check potassium levels, if pulseless treat as VF

Ventricular Fibrillation

Chaotic ventricular rhythm results in quivering ventricular movements and pulselessness. Does not allow sufficient mass of myocardial muscle to fully depolarize and repolarize, so organized ventricular contraction does not take place. Most common presenting rhythm in cardiac arrest (Fig. 2.10)

- Aetiology: coronary artery disease, ischaemia, hypoxia, acidosis, electrical injury, electrolyte imbalance, drugs and toxicity, MI
- Rate: not determined
- Rhythm: not determined
- Pacemaker site: numerous in ventricles
- P waves: not determined
- PR interval: not determined
- QRS complex: wide and bizarre and not determined

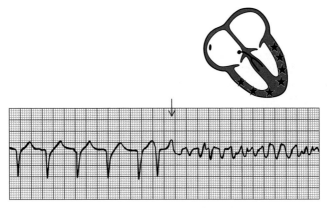

FIGURE 2.10   Ventricular fibrillation.

- Clinical significance: a lethal dysrhythmia, with lightheadedness, followed by loss of consciousness and cessation of circulation and breathing
- Management: an emergency, begin BLS, administer O_2

Asystole

Absence of all Ventricular Activity (Fig. 2.11).

- Aetiology: may be primary event in cardiac arrest or subsequent to VT, VF, asystolic, pulseless electrical activity (PEA) arrest. Associated with global myocardial ischaemia and necrosis.
- Rate: none
- Rhythm: none
- Pacemaker site: none
- P waves: none
- PR interval: none
- QRS complex: none
- Clinical significance: a lethal dysrhythmia, with a poor prognosis, should be confirmed in three leads, maximum gain check patient and connections
- Management: cardiopulmonary resuscitation (CPR) and advanced life support, administer O_2, adrenaline, possible pacing

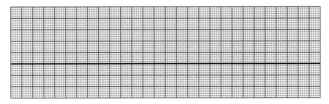

FIGURE 2.11   Asystole.

Pulseless Electrical Activity

- PEA for short
- There is electrical activity without any resulting mechanical output
- Rhythm can be any: often bradycardia or agonal
- Prognosis is poor, various causes:
  - Hypoxia
  - Hypothermia
  - Hypovolaemia
  - Hypo/hypercalcaemia
  - Tension pneumothorax
  - Tamponade
  - Toxins
  - Thromboembolic disturbances
- Management: CPR and advanced life support, adrenaline, atropine, if slow rate, treat reversible causes

Heart Blocks

First Degree AV Block

- Delay in conduction at the AV node, within an underlying rhythm (Fig. 2.12)
- Aetiology: associated with myocardial ischaemia, MI, increased vagal tone, digoxin toxicity
- Rate: generally sinus or rate of underlying rhythm
- Rhythm: regular or that of underlying rhythm
- Pacemaker: SA node
- P waves: normal
- PR interval: prolonged >0.20 seconds
- QRS: usually normal
- Clinical significance: little, rarely may progress to other AV blocks
- Management: generally none required

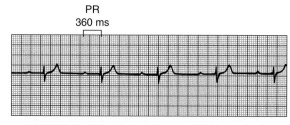

FIGURE 2.12 First-degree AV block. *AV*, atrioventricular.

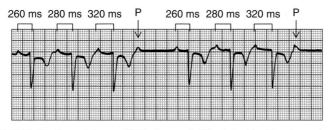

FIGURE 2.13 Second-degree AV block, type 1 (Wenckebach). *AV,* atrioventricular.

Second Degree AV Block, Type 1 (Wenckebach)

- Intermittent block, at level of AV node. Conduction delay at the PR interval progressively increases until conduction is blocked (Fig. 2.13)
- Aetiology: occurs often in MI and myocarditis, as well as increased vagal tone, ischaemia, drug toxicity, electrolyte imbalance
- Rate: atrial rate is that of underlying sinus or atrial rhythm; ventricular rate is normal or slow but slightly less than atrial rate
- Rhythm: atrial rhythm is regular; ventricular rhythm is irregular
- Pacemaker: SA node
- P waves: normal
- PR interval: progressively lengthens before nonconducted P-wave
- QRS: usually normal
- Clinical significance: usually transient and reversible, may develop into more serious block. If dropped beats are regular, patient may become haemodynamically unstable
- Management: if symptomatic atropine or pacing

Second Degree AV Block, Type 2

- Intermittent block when impulses are not conducted by AV node. Normal conduction occurs followed by a nonconducted impulse; the ratio of conducted to nonconducted is usually constant. Usually occurs below the bundle of His (Fig. 2.14)

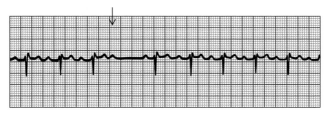

FIGURE 2.14 Second-degree AV block, type 2. *AV,* atrioventricular.

- Aetiology: usually associated with MI and septal necrosis, does not result solely from increased parasympathetic tone or drug
- Rate: atrial rate is unaffected that of underlying rhythm ventricular rate less, may be bradycardic
- Rhythm: regular or irregular, depending on whether conduction ratio is constant or variable
- P waves: upright and uniform, some P waves not followed by QRS complexes
- PR interval: usually constant for conducted beats and may be >0.20 s
- QRS: may be wider than normal due to bundle branch block
- Clinical significance: this is a serious dysrhythmia which may severely compromise the patient's haemodynamic state; there is a risk of developing third-degree heart block; therefore, intervention is required
- Management: if symptomatic atropine or pacing

Third-degree AV Block (Complete Heart Block) Complete block at AV node, SA node activates artia and ectopic pacemaker serves ventricles. Atrial and ventricular electrical activity completely unrelated (Fig. 2.15).

- Aetiology: increased septal necrosis, acute myocarditis, digoxin overdose, beta blocker or calcium channel blocker, vagal tone, electrolyte imbalance
- Rate: atrial rate of underlying atrial or sinus rhythm, ventricular rate 40−60 typically if in junction, may be lower if in ventricles
- Rhythm: atrial and ventricular rhythm regular but independent of each other
- P waves: present, unrelated to QRS complexes
- PR interval: no relationship between atrial and ventricular activity
- QRS: usually wide and bizarre especially if pacemaker site in ventricles, occasionally normal duration
- Clinical significance: severe bradycardia and cardiac compromise, may be very unstable and is potentially lethal
- Management: pacing

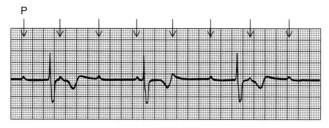

FIGURE 2.15   Third-degree AV block. *AV,* atrioventricular.

The 12-lead ECG

After only 30—60 seconds of hypoxia, changes can be observed on an ECG rhythm strip and/or a 12-lead ECG. An ECG is often the first diagnostic procedure to yield results. It is designed to record the electrical impulses produced by the heart with the use of electrodes on the skin and generates a waveform that is described as the PQRST (Fig. 2.3); the:

- P wave represents atrial activity.
- P—R interval represents the period of delay within the AV node.
- QRS complex is the wave of depolarization down the bundle of His, the left and right bundle branches and the Purkinje network.
- T wave represents ventricular repolarization.
- The flat line between the end of the T wave and the beginning of the next P wave is the resting or filling phase.

Changes to an ECG rhythm can be determined by interpreting changes that occur in time and voltage to the above waveforms (Fig. 2.3) and by using a standardized approach to the diagnosis of arrhythmias detailed previously.

However, it is a 12-lead ECG that a critical care nurse will undertake when a patient complains of chest pain. It is more useful when diagnosing an MI, despite the problems with interpretation, than the rhythm strip. It can be performed simply, quickly, and views the heart electrically in a three-dimensional manner. The limb leads are attached to the forearms and calves and allows three bipolar leads (I, II, III) and three augmented unipolar leads ([augemented vector right (AVR), augumented vector left (AVL), augumented vector foot (AVF)]) to be recorded. Chest precordial unipolar lead provide the 6 V lead positions (V_1, V_2, V_3, V_4, V_5 and V_6), and allow the heart to be viewed in the horizontal axis from the chest wall.

Thus, the 12-lead ECG produces a representation of what is happening directly underneath the electrode, whereby a nurse and/or doctor can determine whether the conduction pathway of the heart is normal or damaged. During an MI, changes on a 12-lead ECG over a period of days can be detected. These changes occur if cardiac muscle is damaged (determined in conjunction with cardiac enzymes) the electrical waves within the heart have to travel via an alternative route, and this will alter the pattern of the ECG and identify the affected area.

The Zones of Alteration

In the early stages of acute MI, there are at least three zones of tissue damage (Fig. 2.16):

1. The zone of hypoxia
2. The zone of ischaemia
3. The zone of infarction/necrosis

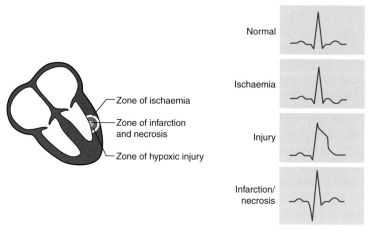

FIGURE 2.16 The zones of alteration on an ECG. *ECG*, electrocardiogram.

The first zone consists of necrotic myocardial tissue that has been irreversibly destroyed by the prolonged deprivation of O_2. It is electrically silent and does not contribute to the ECG. The second zone is hypoxic injury that surrounds the necrotic dead tissue. The myocardial cells may survive if adequate circulation to this area is revived or if not, it may progress to necrosis. The third zone is called ischaemia that is adjacent to the zone of hypoxic injury. This zone represents cells that have been deprived of some O_2 but may recover. Ischaemic and injured myocardial tissue cause ST and T wave changes on the ECG (Fig. 2.16). The ultimate size of an infarct may depend on the zones of injury.

ST Elevation

ST elevation occurs within minutes of the onset of infarction, pathological Q waves (0.40 ms in duration or 25% of the height of the ensuing R wave) may take hours or even days to develop. Elevation of the ST segments indicates the presence of ischaemic tissue, but the range and conductivity may be normal. There may be horizontal ST depression and T wave inversion lasting for 70–80 ms in V_2 through to V_4, which is also indicative of ischaemia. However, this is controversial and considered by some to be nonspecific. Richards and Edwards (2014) suggest that serial ECG changes are more helpful, as changes with time are more likely to indicate acute infarction.

The reason for ST elevation is unclear. It is proposed that it is the result of the:

- Effect of the electrical current going around the injured site to reach the uninjured muscle which alters the level of the baseline of the ECG.

- Injured cells remaining polarized, but the transmembrane potential is less than normal due to the loss of cellular potassium.
- Injured tissue conducts more rapidly than normal, and a voltage gradient develops between the normal and injured tissue; this leads to an ST elevation over the injured area.

Q Waves

An infarct is virtually certain if Q waves appear during the course of the illness. However, there has been identification of non-Q-wave infarctions. Diagnosis of non-Q-wave infarction relies on a combination of the history, increased serum cardiac enzymes and ECG changes. These patients are often considered for angioplasty, for even though associated with smaller amounts of myocardial damage, a substantial amount of heart muscle may still be at risk.

The Four Stages of an MI

To use an ECG as a diagnostic tool for an MI, a sequence of readings needs to be taken, as not every change is evident immediately. These are known as the four stages of an MI (Fig. 2.17).

Localizing an MI on a 12-lead ECG

The 12-lead ECG can localize the area of heart muscle damage, although indication of the infarction site is not uniformly accurate. An anterior MI may be identified by observing ST elevation and inverted T waves, in particular, the leads of a 12-lead ECG (AVR, V_1, V_2, V_3, V_4). An inferior MI will have ST elevation in leads II, III and AVF. When looking at a 12-lead ECG, leads II, III and AVF can show signs of an MI most clearly. Often, the infarction involves more than one discrete region of myocardium, for example, anteroseptal, inferolateral (Allen et al., 2011; Table 2.12).

Pleural Effusion

This is an excessive collection of fluid in the pleural space. The fluid may be serous fluid, blood, pus or lymph. A pleural effusion on a chest X-ray is best seen with the patient in the erect position. A computed tomography (CT) scan may help to identify underlying lung pathology and possible sites for diagnostic aspiration.

Causes:

- Heart failure
- Hypoproteinaemia
- Pneumonia
- Carcinoma of the bronchus
- Tuberculosis

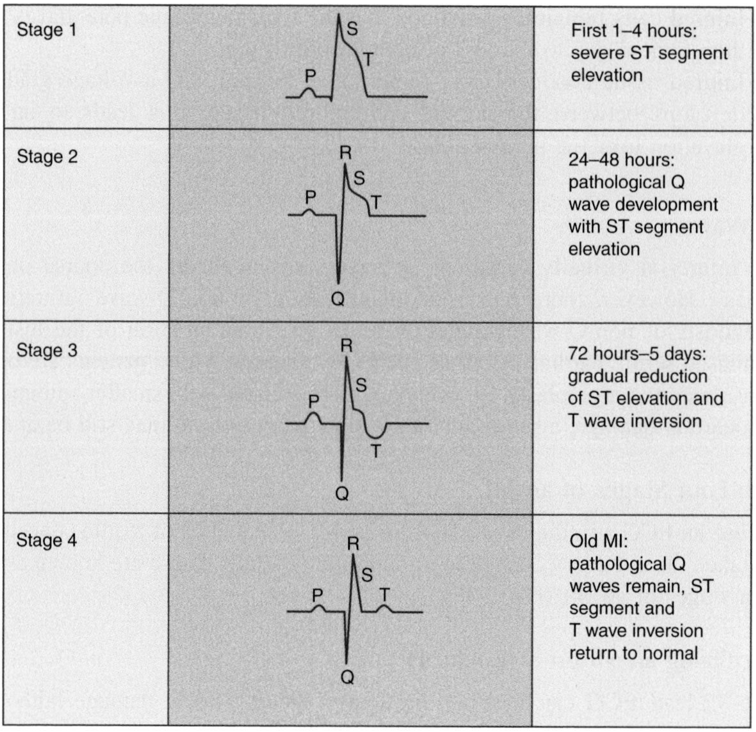
Stage 1
S
T
P
First 1–4 hours: severe ST segment elevation
Stage 2
R
S
P
T
Q
24–48 hours: pathological Q wave development with ST segment elevation
Stage 3
R
S
P
T
Q
72 hours–5 days: gradual reduction of ST elevation and T wave inversion
Stage 4
R
S
P
T
Q
Old MI: pathological Q waves remain, ST segment and T wave inversion return to normal

FIGURE 2.17 The stages of a myocardial infarction. *Adapted from Edwards (2002).*

TABLE 2.12 Locating an MI on a 12-lead ECG.

MI location	Leads with indicative changes, e.g. ST elevation
Inferior	II, III, AVF
Anterior	V_1, V_2, V_3, V_4, AVR
Lateral	I, AVL, V_5, V_6
Anterolateral	I, AVL and all chest leads
Anteroseptal	I, AVL, V_1, V_2, V_3
Inferolateral	II, III, AVF, V_5, V_6
Posterior	Tall R wave in V_1, or V_7 V_8, V_9

ECG, electrocardiography.

Clinical features:

- Dyspnoea, which is variable dependent upon the size of the effusion.
- Dull chest pain
- Symptoms due to the underlying cause, for example, carcinoma of the lung.

The effusion will be seen on a chest X-ray as a water-dense shadow with a concave-upwards upper border. If the effusion is causing dyspnoea, it should be drained. The fluid is best removed slowly, and an indwelling chest drain may be inserted.

Lumbar Puncture

In this procedure, cerebrospinal fluid (CSF) is withdrawn following the insertion of a hollow needle into the lumbar SA space. It will give information on the presence of:

- Meningeal inflammation
- Haemorrhage, infection
- Cerebrospinal fluid cytology

The needle is usually inserted between the second and third or third and fourth lumbar vertebrae (L2 and L3 or L3 and L4). This is below the level of the spinal cord, which extends to L1 or L2, and is in the region of the cauda equina. The fluid obtained is examined for diagnostic purposes and may be required:

- To record the pressure of the CSF using a manometer
- In suspected meningitis or encephalitis to look for bacteria in the CSF
- In suspected malignant tumours to look for cancer cells (cytology)
- To aid diagnosis in SA haemorrhage when there would be blood in the CSF
- To introduce intrathecal medication such as antibiotics or cytotoxic drugs
- To introduce contrast media for radiological examination

A lumbar puncture is contraindicated in the following circumstances:

- In critical care patients with papilloedema or deteriorating neurological symptoms, where raised ICP is suspected
- In the presence of infection, as this may lead to meningitis or abscess formation, for example, localized skin infection around the insertion site
- The presence of frontal sinusitis
- Middle ear discharge
- Congenital heart disease or prosthetic heart valves
- In patients who are unable to cooperate or who are too drowsy to give a history
- In patients who have severe degenerative spinal joint disease

- In those patients undergoing anticoagulant therapy or who have coagulo-pathies or thrombocytopenia

A doctor carries out the procedure using an aseptic technique. The position of the patient is vitally important, and the critical care nurse may be responsible for helping the patient to maintain this position during the procedure:

- The patient should be in the left lateral position, with maximum flexion of the spine and as near the edge of the bed as possible.
- There should be one pillow under the patient's head.
- To gain maximum stretching of the lumbar vertebrae the patient should flex the head to the chest and draw the knees to the abdomen, holding them with their hands.
- The nurse may help by supporting the patient behind the knees and neck, thus ensuring the widening of the intervertebral space.

Careful positioning is necessary so that the doctor can feel the lumbar spine more easily and so insert the needle accurately. It is imperative that the lumbar puncture is performed below the first lumbar vertebra where the cord terminates.

When the needle is in position, the stylet is removed, and a manometer is attached to record the pressure of the CSF. The normal pressure of the CSF is 60–180 mm H_2O. For laboratory analysis, approximately 5–10 mL of CSF is withdrawn. The nurse should note:

- The colour of the CSF – it should be colourless.
- The presence of blood in the CSF – the first few millilitres may be bloodstained due to trauma following insertion of the needle, but after this, the fluid should run clear.
- The consistency of the CSF – it should be like water.
- The opacity of the CSF – it should be clear; cloudy CSF is typical of bacterial meningitis.

The Queckenstedt's test is done when an obstruction to the flow of CSF in the spinal pathway is suspected. Pressure is recorded using the manometer while jugular compression is applied. Normally, the pressure of the CSF would rapidly rise when jugular compression is applied and just as rapidly released. If an obstruction such as a spinal tumour or dislocated vertebra is present, the rise and fall of pressure will occur much more slowly. Pressure is applied for a maximum of 10 seconds, and recordings taken via the manometer. Further recordings are then taken for 10 seconds when the pressure is released. When pressure recordings are complete, the specimens of CSF will be collected in culture bottles.

Following the completion of the procedure:

- The needle is withdrawn, and the wound sealed with a plastic sealant dressing.

- The patient is asked to lie down flat in bed for 6–12 hours. This should prevent the development of a headache.
- Observation for leakage from the puncture site together with neurological observations should be continued for up to 24 hours.

Patient positioning is paramount.

Radiography (X-rays)

An X-ray can give a variety of information about the lungs, heart, pleura, bones and mediastinal structures. X-rays are electromagnetic vibrations of short wavelength produced by passing a high voltage through a cathode ray tube. The beam crosses the patient and is partially absorbed in the process. Those energy waves (photons) that leave the patient are captured by an image receptor. The energies of the photons are decreased by differing amounts as they pass through different tissues in the body. The remnant radiation that leaves the patient produces the photographic image on the radiographic film.

- *Radiolucent* materials allow X-rays to pass through them easily; air is radiolucent.
- *Radiopaque* materials do not easily allow light to pass; bone is a relatively radiopaque material.
- On a plain radiograph, gas and fat absorb few X-rays and appear dark.
- Bone and other calcified regions absorb most of the X-rays and appear white.
- Some foreign bodies such as metal and some glass are radiopaque, but wood and plastic cannot be seen.

Chest X-rays

The chest X-ray is by far the commonest type of X-ray to be taken. The different types of chest X-ray are:

- Posteroanterior – standard department film, the plate is in front of the patient's chest, with the X-ray tube 6 feet behind the patient.
- Anteroposterior – usually a portable film, the plate is behind the patient's chest, and the X-ray tube is closer to the patient. The positioning of the patient is often inconsistent, and often the film will not show full inspiration.

- Lateral — departmental film, difficult to take as a portable film due to the added difficulties in positioning the patient. Helpful to show specific areas of consolidation.

Examination of a Chest X-ray The examination must be carried out in an orderly sequence, identifying normal anatomical structure and any abnormal shadows:

Normal anatomical structures:

- Labelled to identify left and right, if it is not, the aortic knuckle and the stomach air bubble appear on the patient's left.
- With the correct exposure, the vertebral bodies should be visible through the upper part of the heart shadow but not the lower. An overexposed film will appear very dark. The degree of exposure should always be taken into account when comparing successive films.
- Patient in straight position — the medial ends of each clavicle should be evenly disposed on either side of the adjacent vertebral spinous process. If the patient is rotated to the left, the medial end of the left clavicle will be further from the midline than the right.
- Depth of inspiration — determined by the position of the diaphragm and the ribs.
- Soft tissues — in women, the breast and nipple shadows should be noted, and in men, those of the pectoralis muscle. Horizontal lines caused by folds of flesh may be seen in the obese patient.
- Thoracic cage — symmetry of the skeleton should be noted, and the width of the intercostal spaces should be equal on both sides. Unilateral crowding of the ribs will be seen in kyphoscoliosis or loss of lung volume through collapse or resection of lung tissue. Rib margins should be examined for irregularities caused by trauma and fractures etc. It is important to identify the margins of the scapula.
- Diaphragm — each hemidiaphragm should be evenly curved with a clear outline. Both the costophrenic and cardiophrenic angles are clear and sharp.
  - Position — on full inspiration:
    - Right — anterior end of the sixth rib in the midclavicular line
    - Left — 1–2 cm lower than the right.
- Heart shadow — the transverse diameter of the heart should be less than half the maximum diameter of the thoracic cage. The outline should be clear.
- Trachea — this is visible as a vertical translucent band overlying the spinous processes of the upper thoracic vertebrae; should be in midline above the manubrium with the deviation of the lower one-third to the right.
- Abnormal shadows — any abnormal shadow should be analysed for its anatomical site, size and shape of its margins.

- Consolidation — is the replacement of air in the lung by tissue or fluid of greater density? Often affects part of the lobe, but if a whole lobe is consolidated, there will be no displacement of the surrounding structures. Consolidation has the following features:
  - Homogeneous shadowing, confined to segments and bounded by fissures, diaphragm, pleura and chest
  - No loss of lung volume
  - Air bronchograms
  - Relative constancy from day to day
- Collapse — this is the absorption of air with loss of lung volume. The position of the tissues is often altered with possible displacement of the heart, trachea. The mediastinal outline may be obliterated.
- Pneumothorax — air in the pleural cavity seen as an area of no lung markings, which will result in reduction of lung size. Common features are a white, visible air—lung interface, mediastinal shift to the opposite side.
- Pleural effusion — present as a uniform opacity, which extends up from the costophrenic angle. The upper margin will be concave unless air is present. If air is present in the pleural cavity, there is a horizontal fluid level with clear demarcation. In the supine position, the fluid will show as haziness over the whole lung, through which normal lung markings may still be visible. A large pleural effusion will cause mediastinal shift to the opposite side.
- Asthma — in asthma, the X-ray is often normal except during severe attacks or long-term asthma, when the following will be seen:
  - Overinflation
  - Low but curved diaphragm
  - Vessels remain normal
- Chronic bronchitis — the film may be normal even though the patient is severely disabled. Areas of infection may cause consolidation and/or collapse.
- Pulmonary oedema — may be cardiac or noncardiac in origin, may see upper lobe venous engorgement, fluffy shadows, pleural effusion may be present, cardiac enlargement may develop due to dilation of the left ventricle.
- PE — generally to exclude other pathology, patchy areas of atelectasis are often seen in submassive PE; may be confused with consolidation or collapse. May see some vascular shadowing in the affected areas; other diagnostic procedures are more reliable, for example, nuclear imaging or pulmonary angiogram.
- Positioning of invasive devices to observe the tip and position during movement or following insertion:
  - ETT
  - NGTs
  - CVP and PAP
  - Aortic balloon pumps

Portable X-rays Patients on critical care cannot often go to the radiotherapy department to have their X-rays taken and require the radiographer to come to the critical care area. In this instance, protection of the patient and staff present on the unit at the time is imperative. Exposure to radiation always involves the risk of biological changes within the body. Therefore, the patient should always be exposed to the lowest amount of radiation possible, and all individuals coming into contact with radiation should be protected.

Protection occurs by:

• minimizing the time the patient is in the path of the X-ray beam.
• maximizing the distance between the radiation source and the patient.
• shielding the reproductive organs of the patient if they are within 4–5 cm of the beam. This is extremely important in children and young adults. The shields are made of lead, which absorbs X-ray.
• improvement of X-ray machines so that there is less scatter of the radiation.

Time, distance and shielding are also used to protect staff:

• The time spent in the room where the radiation source is active should be as short as possible; the risk is only there when exposures are being made.
• Increasing the distance from the source of the beam greatly reduces the quantity of radiation that will reach the radiographer or nurse. This means that if the nurse has to hold the patient while he is X-rayed, there will be much greater exposure.
• If the critical care nurse does have to support the patient, a shield should be worn. Lead aprons or gloves are used where a fixed shield is not in place.
• Any worker regularly exposed to ionizing radiation must be monitored, usually by the use of a film badge. The film inside gets darker in response to the amount of radiation exposure, and it is analysed, usually monthly.
• Contact with X-rays should be avoided in pregnancy as exposure can lead to malformations of the foetus. There is a safe limit of 0.5 rem for a declared pregnant woman.

Angiography

• This is the opacification of the veins or arteries by the injection of appropriate contrast media.
• The femoral vessels in the groin are the favourite entry points for the catheter through which water-soluble contrast is injected; images are recorded on a video recorder.
• Obstructions due to thrombosis, atheroma or embolism can be seen.
• Clotting studies should be done first to ensure there is no bleeding tendency.

- Following cannulation, there is a risk of trauma to the vessel causing bleeding or thrombosis, and occasionally, part of the catheter has been lost into the lumen of the vessel.
- There is also a risk of allergic response to the contrast media.

Echocardiography

In recent years, a new technique has been developed where the CO and cardiac function are estimated using an ultrasound probe. It is used to examine the heart and great vessels and is invaluable in cardiac diagnosis and treatment (Table 2.13). Its advantages in critical care include its portability, ease of performance and noninvasive nature.

Types of Echocardiography

- M-mode: records a one-dimensional view of the heart; it can measure:
  - LV wall thickness
  - Cavity size
  - Valve leaflet excursion
  - Aortic root
  - Left atrial dimension
- Two-dimensional: the ultrasound beam moves continually in an arc.

Other Uses of Ultrasound

Ultrasound examination is a noninvasive form of organ imaging, with considerable appeal. High-frequency sound waves are used in diagnostic medical sonography to visualize structures in the body by recording the reflections of high-frequency pulses directed into the tissues. Ultrasound is:

- Painless and almost certainly safe
- Uses a transducer, which both emits and receives the ultrasound
- Based on the emission of sound waves and the reflections of ultrasound echoes
- The ultrasound probe containing a transducer is applied to the skin over the area of interest, and the image is displayed on a screen
- A lubricant is used to exclude air and ensure a good connection to the skin
- The probe is moved at different angles and in different directions to display any abnormalities
- 'Spot' films are also taken to record any images
- Minimal patient preparation is needed
- The bladder needs to be full of urine to examine the pelvis
- The patient should be fasted to minimize gas shadows in gall bladder studies.

TABLE 2.13 Echocardiography.

Area of importance	Role of echocardiography
Size of heart chambers	• Assesses dimensions or volume of the cavity and the thickness of the walls. • Helps identify certain types of heart disease that predominantly involve the heart muscle. • Can determine left ventricular wall thickness and stiffness with long-standing hypertension. • Serial studies can assist in gauging the response of medical treatment.
Pumping function	• Can detect the pumping power of the heart and whether it is normal or reduced to a mild or severe degree. This measurement is known as an ejection fraction (EF). • A normal EF is around 55%–65%. Figures below 45% usually represent some decrease in the pumping strength of the heart, while figures below 30%–35% are representative of an important decrease. • Can identify if the heart is pumping poorly, e.g. due to cardiomyopathy. • Can assess the pumping ability of each heart chamber, the movement of each visualized wall. The decreased movement can be graded from mild to severe. In extreme cases, an area affected by a heart attack may have no movement (akinesia), or may even bulge in the opposite direction (dyskinesia). The latter is seen with aneurysms of the left ventricle.
Valve function	• Echocardiography identifies the structure, thickness and movement of each heart valve. • Can determine if the valve is normal, scarred from an infection or rheumatic fever, thickened, calcified and torn. • Assesses the function of prosthetic or artificial heart valves. • Can diagnose mitral valve prolapse.
Volume status	• Low blood pressure, poor heart function, reduced volume of circulating blood, e.g. with diuretics. • Confusion may be caused when patients have a combination of problems. Therefore, echocardiography may help clarify the confusion.
Other uses	• Diagnosis of fluid in the pericardium. • Can determine if problem is severe/potentially life-threatening. • Other diagnoses made include congenital heart diseases, blood clots or tumours within the heart, active infection of the heart valves, abnormal pulmonary pressures.

Its advantages include minimal risk to patients, no radiation exposure and good diagnostic specificity in selected types of pathology. Ultrasound is used to examine virtually all areas of the body. It aids to:

- distinguish solid from cystic lesions;
- assess abdominal masses (difficult to see on X-ray);
- detect abnormal material in an organ, such as metastases;
- detect movement, as in the pulsation of an aneurysm;
- can measure physical dimensions, such as the diameter of the aorta;
- detect stones in the urinary bladder or the gall bladder and
- guide intervention procedures such as aspiration or biopsy.

Ultrasound may help to identify pathology in the following organs with a high degree of accuracy:

- Liver and biliary tree
- Pancreas
- Renal tract
- Pelvic structures
- Pleural, abdominal and pelvic fluid collections

Now that portable ultrasound equipment is available, these examinations may be carried out at the bedside, without the need to move the critically ill patient out of the unit.

Limiting Factors of Ultrasound

- Bone completely reflects ultrasound and obscures any tissues beyond it. This means it cannot be used to examine the brain or the spinal cord.
- Bowel gas partly reflects the ultrasound, starving the patient or using laxatives may help.
- A thick layer of fat scatters ultrasound, and so it may be better to investigate the gall bladder by other means in the very obese.

Doppler-Shift Ultrasound

This method is used to study blood flow. The beam is directed towards the artery and is reflected from the red cells. It can be used to generate an audible signal for detecting blood flow or may be processed to give information about the nature of the flow. Other uses include:

- Measuring systolic BP when low. A portable Doppler is used to detect flow beyond a sphygmomanometer cuff placed around the arm or ankle.
- Detecting the foetal heart.
- Studying flow dynamics for example in carotid artery disease.

Duration of Echocardiography

An examination in an uncomplicated case may be completed within 15–20 minutes. However, it may take up to an hour when there are multiple problems or when there are technical problems.

Transoesophageal Echo (TOE) Versus Standard Echocardiography

A standard echocardiogram is obtained by applying a transducer to the front of the chest. The ultrasound beam travels through the chest wall and lungs to reach the heart. Because it travels through the front of the chest or thorax, a standard echocardiogram is also known as a transthoracic echocardiogram.

Often, closely positioned ribs, obesity and emphysema may create technical difficulties by limiting the transmission of the ultrasound beams to and from the heart. In such cases, a TOE may be used. In such cases, the echocardiography transducer is placed down the oesophagus. Since the oesophagus sits behind the heart, the echo beam does not have to travel through the front of the chest, avoiding many of the obstacles associated with a standard echocardiography and thus offers a much clearer image of the heart.

How a TOE is Performed

The patient is made to lie on their left side. An IV sedative is given to help in relaxation, and the throat is sprayed with a local anaesthetic to numb the area. The TOE transducer is much smaller than the standard echocardiography equipment and is positioned at the end of a flexible tube. The tube transfers the images from the transducer to the echocardiography monitor for ease of visualization.

There is a risk that the patient may vomit.

On commencement of the procedure, if conscious, the patient begins to swallow the tube. The tube goes down the oesophagus. Therefore, it is important that the patient is cooperative and swallows the tube. If unconscious, the clinician advances the tube into the mouth and down the oesophagus and the procedure begins. The combined use of local anaesthesia and chosen sedative minimizes patient discomfort, and there is usually no pain experienced with this procedure.

The transducer at the end of the tube is positioned in the oesophagus, directly behind the heart. By rotating and moving the tip of the transducer, the clinician can examine the heart from several different angles. The patient's physiological signs are continuously monitored during this procedure. O_2 is given as a preventive measure and suction is used, as needed.

TOE Preparation The patient should be nil by mouth for 6 hours prior to the procedure. This will minimize any risk of vomiting and aspirating during the procedure.

Duration of TOE The actual procedure usually lasts 10−30 minutes.

Risks Associated with TOE TOE is a relatively common procedure and considered to be fairly safe. However, it does require entrance into the oesophagus and stomach. On occasion, patients may experience breathing problems; abnormal or slow heart rhythm, reaction to the sedative and minor bleeding. In extremely rare cases, TOE may cause perforation or an oesophageal tear.

Importance of TOE A TOE is an extremely useful tool in detecting blood clots, masses and tumours that are located inside the heart. It can also gauge the severity of valvular problems and infection of heart valves, some congenital heart diseases or an aortic tear. In addition, TOE is also very useful in evaluating patients who have had mini or major stokes as a result of blood clots.

Doppler Doppler helps to identify abnormal leakage across heart valves and determine their severity. Doppler is also very useful in diagnosing the presence and severity of valve stenosis or narrowing. Doppler follows the direction and velocity of blood flow rather than the movement of the valve leaflets or components. Thus, reversed blood direction is seen with leakages, while increased forward velocity of flow with a characteristic pattern is noted with valve stenosis.

Duration of Doppler Examination The additional use of Doppler may add 10−20 minutes.

Computed Tomography

CT allows the visualization of the anatomy from various sectional planes by X-raying a series of thin transverse slices of the patient's head or body that are then analysed by a computer. Very specialized equipment, which uses computerized digital imaging, as does ultrasonography and magnetic resonance imaging (MRI). A CT scan is very beneficial within critical care; however, patients need to be carefully prepared and escorted by an experienced critical care nurse.

CT scans can:

- Determine pathological anatomy, which can reveal as much as an explorative operation, especially following injury to the brain — it enables appropriate surgical intervention only when necessary.
- It is useful to explore areas of the anatomy where radiography is unsuitable:
  - The pancreas (deep inside the body)
  - The lungs and mediastinum
  - The brain and spinal cord
- It is essential in the planning of radiotherapy or chemotherapy and staging tumours.
- When planning surgery, for example, establishing the extent of invasion of oesophageal cancer.
- Assesses damage in abdominal or thoracic trauma.
- Guide needles in biopsy, drainage of fluid or aspiration.

Magnetic Resonance Imaging

Strong magnetic fields and radio waves are used along with a computer in MRI to generate sectional images of the anatomy. It is a rapidly expanding diagnostic field and involves applying a powerful magnetic field to the body, which causes all the protons of all the hydrogen nuclei to become aligned. Pulses of radio waves, which emit signals that are recorded electronically, then excite these. Images are produced using sophisticated equipment that can be viewed in any plane.

- Lipids have a high hydrogen content and so are clearly seen on MRI.
- Very useful for examining the brain and spinal cord
- Atheroma can also be demonstrated
- Can be used to investigate blood flow and cardiac function without the use of contrast media

Warn patients of noise

Endoscopy

An endoscopy is a minimally invasive diagnostic procedure, which is used to examine and evaluate internal surfaces and organs by inserting a small flexible or nonflexible tube, which not only provides an image for visual inspection and photography but also enables biopsies and retrieval of foreign objects. The endoscope has an internal camera and light, often, but not necessarily inserted through a natural body opening. Through the scope itself, lesions and other surface abnormalities or conditions can be identified.

The majority of endoscopic procedures are relatively painless and at worst associated with mild discomfort; therefore, the majority of patients receive a sedative prior to commencement of the procedure. Any method of looking into the body uses an instrument. This can either be via an orifice, such as the nose or mouth, or via an artificial opening such as an arthroscopy. Endoscopies are now illuminated by the use of fibre optics enabling accurate diagnosis to be made. There are a number of different areas that are investigated by the use of endoscopy:

- Gastroscopy, esophagogastroduodenoscopy — this enables the whole area to be viewed and peptic ulcers to be seen. The source of haemorrhage can often be identified.
- Duodenoscopy — allows the injection of contrast into the common bile duct.
- Colonoscopy — large bowel endoscopy, can be used to remove polyps and to biopsy suspicious lesions.
- Bronchoscopy — inspecting the bronchi with a narrow fibreoptic endoscope.
- Cystoscopy, cystourethroscopy — inspection of the bladder and urethra is very important in both diagnosis and treatment of diseases of the prostate, urethra and bladder.
- Ureteroscopy — can now be used to remove stones from the lower half of the ureter.
- Laparoscopy —used by gynaecologists to diagnose pelvic disorders. The abdomen is inflated with CO_2, and a scope is passed into the peritoneal cavity. Can also be used to obtain liver biopsies.
- Arthroscopy — looking at joints, range of movement.
- Thoracoscopy — organs of the chest, for example, heart.
- Hysteroscopy — used by gynaecologists to support infertility treatment and to conduct gynaecological and foetal surgery.

Endoscopic Therapy

Endoscopy can also be used for what is known as endoscopic therapy, which has resulted in a dramatic decrease in emergency surgery and reduced the mortality of ulcer bleeding. The three most popular methods are as follows:

1. Adrenaline injection: using endoscopic injection of adrenaline into and around the ulcer bleeding point.
2. Captive coagulation: this method uses direct pressure and heat energy or electrocoagulation (BiCap probe) to control ulcer bleeding.
3. Laser photocoagulation: a special laser is used for the treatment of ulcer bleeding.

Endoscope

- The endoscope consists of either a nonflexible or flexible tube containing one or more optical fibre systems and possibly a channel for mechanical devices.
- A light delivery system to illuminate the organ or object under inspection. The light source is found outside the body, and the light is typically directed via an optical fibre system.
- A lens system is also in operation whereby the image is transmitted to the operator from the endoscope.
- An additional channel is found in operative endoscopes so that the clinician can have easy access for medical instruments to biopsy the internal surface.

Risks Associated with Endoscopy

Complications associated with endoscopy are relatively rare but can include:

- Infection
- Punctured organs
- Allergic reaction to dyes used in certain endoscopic procedures
- Renal failure associated with dyes used in certain endoscopic procedures
- Respiratory depression from over usage of sedative for endoscopic procedure
- Nausea and vomiting

Fibreoptic Bronchoscopy

Indications:

- Aid difficult intubations (American Society of Anaesthesiologists III/IV)
- Clearance of secretions and direct physiotherapy
- Cleansing of bronchial areas
- Collection of microbiological and or cytological specimens
- Identify cause of bronchial/lumen obstruction
- Identify extent of inhalation injury
- Diagnose concerns with trachea and or bronchus
- Placement of catheters or balloon in pulmonary bleeding matters

Complications:

- Hypoxaemia
- Cardiovascular disturbances
- Bleeding
- Perforation

Contraindications:

- Severe hypoxaemia
- Coagulopathy

The patient may need a muscle relaxant if ventilated as they may bite on the scope.

Blood Analysis

Taking a blood sample is often the role of the doctor or phlebotomist, but the results of blood tests have a prime place in assisting the nurse to gain a full detailed assessment of his or her patient. Those that the critical care nurse may be interested in are haemoglobin, plasma osmolarity, potassium, sodium, haematocrit levels, urea and creatinine, cardiac enzymes and arterial blood gases.

False-positive results may occur from containers contaminated with bleach or from skin preparations.

Sodium

- A major cation of extracellular fluid (Edwards and Richards, 2014)
- Determines plasma osmolarity
- Major role in the movement of water and electrolytes between body fluid compartments
- Essential for:
  - Nerve impulse transmission
  - Muscle contraction
  - Movement of glucose, insulin and amino acids
- Normal — approximately between 135 and 145 mmol/L
- 2–4 g of sodium needed per day, usual intake is higher 6–10 g/d in the form of table salt

Potassium

- A major intracellular cation
- Essential for:

- Muscle contractions
- Transmission and conduction of nerve impulses
- Maintenance of normal cardiac rhythm — ECG changes if reduced or elevated
- Skeletal and smooth muscle contraction resting membrane potential
- Normal — approximately between 3.5 and 5.2 mmol/L
- ↑ will stimulate an increase excretion in urine — in renal failure K^+ increases, if not treated death will ensue
- ↓ will cause reabsorption in renal tubules to maintain homeostasis

Low- and high-potassium levels can lead to arrhythmias.

Chloride

- The main extracellular fluid anion
  - Functions in conjunction with sodium and water to maintain intracellular and extracellular balance
- Secreted by the stomach, mucosa as hydrochloric acid assisting in digestion
- Maintains acid—base balance and involved in the removal of O_2 and CO_2 from Hb in RBCs — the chloride shift
- Normal levels 95—106 mmol/L
- Balance maintained by the kidneys regulated by aldosterone and ADH

Calcium

- A necessary ion for many fundamental metabolic processes (Edwards and Richards, 2014)
- The bones contain more than 99% of the body's calcium, and the rest is in the serum and exists in two forms:
  - Ionized or free calcium (found in foods and only type that the body can use)
  - Bound to albumin — which accounts for about half of the serum calcium
- Serum levels of free calcium are 1—1.25 mmol/L, and total serum calcium including bound and free is 2.12—2.65 mmol/L
- Regulated by two hormones:
  - Parathyroid hormone (PTH)
  - Calcitonin

Phosphorus

- The primary anion in intracellular fluid
- If enough calcium is ingested, then enough phosphorus is likely, as both electrolytes are present in many of the same foods
- Normal levels 0.8−1.45 mmol/L
- Needed for:
  - Formation of stored energy in cells (ATP)
  - Assistance with the formation of bones and teeth
  - Interaction with Hb to promote O_2 release to tissues
  - White blood cell activation
  - Metabolizes fats, carbohydrates and proteins
- Contributes to:
  - The regulation of calcium
  - Muscle contraction and myocardium rhythmicity
  - Acid−base balance

Magnesium

- One of the abundant intracellular cations
- 53% in bones, and 27% in muscles
- RDA 350−420 mg/d
- Normal level 0.75−1.05 mmol/L
- Involved in:
  - Enzyme reactions resulting in ATP production
  - Right amount of excitability in nerves and muscle cells including the heart
  - Muscle and nerve function
  - Essential for the function of the sodium−potassium pump
  - Muscle relaxation by inhibiting Ach
  - Essential for the stimulation of the parathyroid hormone (PTH) secretion

Measure of Non-electrolytes

Glucose

- The final product of carbohydrate digestion and the chief source of energy in human metabolism.
- The principal sugar of the blood; insulin is required for its use.

Lipids

- Substance extracted from animal or vegetable cells
- Fatty acids, glycerides, glyceryl and phospholipids

Creatinine

- A waste product of metabolism, excreted in the urine

Urea

- The chief end product of nitrogen metabolism
- Excreted in urine

Haemoglobin Levels

The amount of RBCs in the blood. It is contained in the erythrocyte's cytoplasm and is primarily responsible for carrying O_2 and CO_2 to the body's tissues. The normal is between 11 and 18 g/100 mL of blood. A low Hb will indicate that RBCs are being lost.

Plasma Osmolality

A measure of the number of milliosmoles per litre of solution or the concentration of molecules per volume of solution, for example, the volume of water in relation to added solutes can be determined. The normal is 280–294 mOsm/L; an increased serum osmolality, >295 mOsm/L, indicates a loss of fluid and dehydration or hypovolaemia is present.

Haematocrit

The consistency of the blood, for example, thick fluids move more slowly and cause a greater resistance to flow than thin fluids, is expressed as the haematocrit, the ratio of volume of RBCs to the volume of whole blood. The haematocrit is elevated in dehydration and haemorrhage. The haematocrit is a guide for determining if whole blood or some other IV fluid should be used for volume replacement in the haemorrhagic shock patient.

Cardiac Enzymes

Cellular leak of constituents occurs when there is irreversible damage to myocardial cells. The damaged cells release a number of enzymes into the circulation known as cardiac enzymes. It could be argued that interpretation of these specialist results is the domain of the doctor. However, holistic critical care nursing care involves the identification and understanding of all aspects of illness in order to provide effective and high-quality nursing care.

The estimation of myocardial enzymes is of great diagnostic importance in an MI. The enzymes most commonly measured are aspartate aminotransferase (AST), lactate dehydrogenase (LDH), creatinine kinase (CK) and troponin T and I (Table 2.14). These enzymes are normally present in low levels in the serum of healthy people, but their rise in concentration can be used to determine the diagnosis and severity of an MI. They cannot provide

TABLE 2.14 Cardiac enzymes.

Enzyme release	Peak values	Normal values	Other situations
Creatinine kinase (CK) • released when cardiac muscle starts to die • is the first enzyme to increase after infarction	Values rise within the first 6 hours post-MI. Reach a peak between 18 and 24 hours. Values may return to normal after about 72 hours as no more cells are dying. CK levels should be measured: • at the time of patient's admission • 24 hours later • at the end of the second and third day.	Normal for men is 15–120 IU/L Women 10–80 IU/L CK values can rise 10-fold to thousands in severe cellular death.	CK is not unique to cardiac muscle. Values can rise: • during trauma • in muscle disease • in cerebrovascular damage • after muscular exercise • with intramuscular injections
CK isoforms • MB is the one related to the heart • The presence of CK-MB in the plasma indicates myocardial necrosis.	Measurement ensures levels are not confused with other muscle injury Helps to give an idea of the extent of muscle damage.	If CK-MB levels are >5% of the total CK level, the diagnosis of myocardial infarction is almost certain.	It is only found in heart muscle.
Lactate dehydrogenase (LDH)	LDH level is raised within 8–24 hours. Peaks in 3–6 days Comes back to normal in 8–14 days.	240–525 U/L	LDH release is also found in: • liver disease • renal disease • pulmonary embolism • shock • IM injection

Continued

TABLE 2.14 Cardiac enzymes.—cont'd

Enzyme release	Peak values	Normal values	Other situations
LDH isoforms: • Principally LD_1 • A rise in this isoform indicates myocardial necrosis	Has 5 isoforms Denoted as LD_1–LD_5 The pattern of LD_1 level greater than the LD_2 occurs within 12–24 hours after the attack	If there is a pattern of the LD_1 level being greater than the LD_2 level, an MI is indicated.	Released by the myocardium.
Aspartate aminotransferase (AST) • There are no cardiac specific isoforms	AST concentrations rise in 8–12 hours Approaching peak in 18–36 hours Returning to normal in 3–4 days	10–40 U/L	AST is not specific to cardiac muscle and its use in the diagnosis of MI is limited.
Troponins			

information about the location of the damage, and CK and LDH only indicate muscle tissue injury; however, a precise investigation of MI can be made by analysing the concentrations of myocardial band CK (CK-MB) and isoforms of these enzymes, for example, LD_1/LD_2 or CK-MB. In addition, also to differentiate the rise of troponin T and I from other factors and to isolate to myocardial necrosis, blood tests should be taken on admission, then 3 and 6 hours later.

Arterial Blood Gas Analysis

Blood can be taken from an artery and analysed to determine PO_2 and PCO_2 to interpret a patient's acid—base balance (Rogers and McCutcheon, 2013). Arterial blood gas analysis is part of the medical and nursing care of a patient who may have a related physiological disorder. Blood gas machines measure pH, PCO_2, PO_2, base excess (BE) and HCO_3^2 (Table 2.15). For list of chemical abbreviations related to ABG analysis, see Table 2.16. A BE is the change from normal of the concentration of bicarbonate (Richards and Edwards, 2014). With excess alkali in the blood, there is a positive BE (excess bicarbonate), whereas with excess non-respiratory acid, there is a base deficit or negative BE (reduced bicarbonate). By measuring partial pressure and these other values in arterial blood, a respiratory or metabolic acid—base disorder can be determined and whether the respiratory system or kidneys are compensating.

When attempting to analyse a person's acid—base balance, scrutinize blood values in the following order (Table 2.17). Notice that PCO_2 levels vary inversely with blood pH (PCO_2 rises as blood pH falls); HCO_3^- levels vary directly with blood pH (increased HCO_3^- results in increased pH). If any changes occur in the partial pressures of O_2 or CO_2, for example, due to respiratory disease (asthma, COPD, ARDS), metabolic disease (diabetes, renal

TABLE 2.15 The measures obtained from arterial blood gas analysis and normal values.

Measure	Normal range
pH	7.35—7.45
PCO_2	4.6—5.6 kPa (35—42 mmHg)
PO_2	12—14.6 kPa (90—110 mmHg)
HCO_3^-	22—26 mmol/L
BE (base excess)	−2 to +2
O_2 saturation	94%—98%
To convert from mmHg to kPa divide by 7.5.	

TABLE 2.16 Chemical abbreviations.

Abbreviation	Interpretation
O_2	Oxygen
CO_2	Carbon dioxide
kPa	Kilopascals
PO_2	Partial pressure of oxygen
PCO_2	Partial pressure of carbon dioxide
H^+	Hydrogen ions
HCO_3^-	Bicarbonate ions
H_2CO_3	Carbonic acid
Na^+	Sodium
K^+	Potassium
Cl^-	Chloride
NH_4^+	Ammonium

failure), or because of symptoms of disease (vomiting and diarrhoea), then the changes will be reflected in these measures.

Respiratory Disorders

- Acid–base disorders resulting from primary alterations in the PCO_2 are termed respiratory disorders.
- Any increase in concentration or retention of CO_2 (considered a volatile source of acid which evaporates rapidly in body fluids), that is, production or excretion will produce an increase in H^+ through the generation of carbonic acid (H_2CO_3; Box 2.2).
- This lowers the pH and thus promotes the development of a respiratory acidosis observed in conditions where CO_2 excretion is impaired such as COPD.
- Decreases in PCO_2 concentration, that is, if excretion is greater than production, will result in a decrease in H^1.
- The pH will rise, and a respiratory alkalosis results from a decreased concentration of free H^1.
- This is seen in conditions such as hyperventilation where CO_2 excretion is excessive.
- The lungs therefore play a major role in ensuring maintenance of H^1 ion concentration.

TABLE 2.17 Measure of arterial blood gases.

Measure	Normal limits	Interpretation
pH	7.35–7.45	This indicates whether the person is in acidosis (pH, 7.35) or alkalosis (pH. 7.45), but it does not indicate the cause.
PCO_2	4.6–5.6 kPa (35 –42 mmHg)	Check the PCO_2 to see if this is the cause of the acid –base imbalance. The respiratory system acts fast, and an excessively high or low PCO_2 may indicate either that the condition is respiratory or that the patient is compensating for a metabolic disturbance. • The PCO_2 is over 5.7 kPa (40 mmHg): The respiratory system is the cause of the problem and the condition is a respiratory acidosis. • The PCO_2 is below normal limits 5.2 kPa (35 mmHg): The respiratory system is not the cause but is compensating.
PO_2	12–14.6 kPa (90 –110 mmHg)	This does not reveal how much oxygen is in the blood but only the partial pressure exerted by dissolved O_2 molecules against the measuring electrode
HCO_3^2	22–26 mmol/L	Abnormal values of HCO_3^2 are only due to the metabolic component of an acid–base disturbance: • A raised HCO_3 concentration indicates a metabolic alkalosis (values over 26 mmol/L) • A low value indicates a metabolic acidosis (values below 22 mmol/L)
BE	−2 to +2 mmol/L	Is the amount of acid required to restore 1 L of blood to its normal pH, at a PCO_2 of 5.3 kPa (40 mmHg). The BE reflects only the metabolic component of any disturbance of acid–base balance: • If there was a metabolic acidosis then acid would have to be added to return the blood pH to normal, the BE will be positive. • If there is a metabolic acidosis, acid would need to be subtracted to return blood pH to normal, the BE is negative.

Metabolic Disorders

- Disorders of acid–base physiology of nonrespiratory origin are metabolic disorders and result from abnormal metabolism.
- Metabolic disorders may be due to excessive intake of acid or alkali or due to failure of renal function.

- If nonrespiratory acid production exceeds the excretion of acid from the body HCO_3^- decreases, and H^+ concentration increases as in a metabolic acidosis. The CO_2 yielded in a metabolic acidosis is lost via the lungs.
- This is achieved, as an increase in H^+ will reduce pH, immediately stimulating central chemoreceptors increasing rate and depth of respiration.
- This can be observed in conditions such as diabetic ketoacidosis (due to elevated H^+ production) and renal failure (due to inadequate H^+ excretion) and is referred to as 'respiratory compensation'.

If acid production is less than the excretion of acid from the body, then HCO_3^- concentration increases and H^+ concentration decreases and a metabolic alkalosis result. A decrease in H^+ will increase pH depressing central chemoreceptor response, reducing rate and depth of breathing. CO_2 is retained which generates H^+ and so reduces blood pH close to normal limits. This response is observed with severe vomiting when gastric acid loss depletes body fluid of H^+. This is another example of respiratory compensation. The rapidity of respiratory compensation is evident in these conditions, but it is also limited.

Renal Compensation

The ultimate acid–base regulatory organs are the kidneys, which act slowly to compensate for acid–base imbalance situations (Yucha, 2004). The most important renal mechanisms for regulating acid–base balance of the blood involve:

- excreting HCO_3^2 and conserving (reabsorbing) H^+ in an alkalosis
- excreting H^+ and reclaiming HCO_3^2, conserving (reabsorbing) bicarbonate ions, as in an acidosis (the dominant process in the nephrons)

This response to acid–base disturbances requires several days to be marginally effective.

Liver Function Tests

The normal level of serum bilirubin is <21 μmol/L.

- *Unconjugated bilirubin* − breakdown of RBCs in the spleen produces bilirubin; in this form, it is potentially toxic − significant in haemolytic anaemia where more is being produced or when being poorly taken up by the liver or poorly conjugated.
- *Conjugated bilirubin* − converted in the liver to a water-soluble compound, which is less toxic and excreted in bile, to the intestine. Ninety-nine percent is excreted in faeces as stercobilinogen (1% reabsorbed and excreted in the kidneys as urobilinogen) − significant when biliary vessels are obstructed in the liver, bile ducts are blocked, for example, gallstones or tumour.

A rise in both known as mixed hyperbilirubinaemia occurs in liver diseases such as hepatitis and cirrhosis as bilirubin metabolism is impaired in several ways.

Serum Enzyme Levels

During liver disease, many enzymes in high concentrations within liver cells leak across damaged cell membranes and can be detected in the blood. These levels are not measuring function but indicate damage.

Transaminases:

> Alanine aminotransferase (ALT) − is liver specific.
> AST − found also in brain, lung, pancreas, skeletal and cardiac muscle. The degree of serum elevation may range from:

- Nonalcoholic fatty liver disease <100 IU/L
  Alcoholic liver disease (100−350 IU/L)
  Acute infective hepatitis >1000 IU/L
- Paracetamol poisoning

ALT is generally greater than AST, except in alcoholic liver disease.

Alkaline phosphate (ALP) − elevated in tumours, cysts, abscesses because the locally obstructed bile canal makes more enzymes, increased in cirrhosis (2−10 times). It can arise from bone and intestinal damage. High levels generally indicate obstructive jaundice, carcinoma or tumour of the liver.

Gamma-glutamyl transpeptidase − is a microsomal enzyme, increased in hepatitis and other diseases damaging liver cells. Especially useful:

- When found together with a raised ALP suggesting liver origin.
- Follow-up marker in recovering alcoholics − increased by substances metabolized by it, for example, alcohol and phenytoin − indicates if a sober alcoholic has been drinking.

Serum Proteins

Clotting factors − factors II, VII, IX and X − these are synthesized in the liver therefore the prothrombin time (PT) will be abnormal due to the deficiency of vitamin K − the liver cannot synthesize factors. However, if is purely vitamin-K-deficient, it is likely to return to normal within 48 hours once treated. A PT more than 3 seconds longer than control (usually, 15 seconds) is lengthened in obstructive jaundice as fat-soluble vitamin K cannot be absorbed properly from the intestine in the absence of bile. A vitamin K injection in the presence of dysfunctional cells is likely to be ineffective.

Serum albumin − synthesized only by liver cells − is decreased in liver disease, during malnutrition, hypercatabolism in the acutely unwell, burns and ascites.

Serum (immuno)-globulins — reason for increase generally unknown, perhaps due to stimulation of inflammatory response or damaged liver.

- Increase in IgG — autoimmune chronic active hepatitis
- Increase in IgM — primary biliary cirrhosis
- Increase in IgA — alcoholic cirrhosis

Transport proteins — fall to low levels when liver function is impaired.

Antimitochondrial antibody (AMA) — present in critical care patients with primary biliary cirrhosis, absence excludes diagnosis.

Section 3

Critical care interventions

Section Outline

3.1 MEDIUM-TECHNOLOGY LIFE SUPPORT INTERVENTIONS

Venepuncture and Cannulation

Venepuncture

This includes a puncture into a vein for

- A blood sample for diagnostic purposes
- Monitoring levels of blood components

This is a common procedure and is more commonly performed by a phlebotomist or nurses; thus, nurses working in critical care and who are trained to undertake this procedure need to be aware of the following:

- Relevant anatomy and physiology
- Criteria for choosing a vein and the equipment to use
- Potential problems, how to prevent them and interventions
- Health and safety practices related to insertion and safe disposal of equipment
- Adherence to aseptic technique
- Comfort of the patient
- Adequate information regarding the procedure and complications

The veins used include

- Median cubital veins.
- Cephalic vein.
- Basilic vein.
- Metacarpal veins.

Choosing a vein:
Must be best for the patient. The most prominent is not always the most suitable for venepuncture; use

- Visual inspection
- Palpation

Influencing factors:

- Injury, disease or treatment may prevent the use of a limb for venepuncture
- How the patient is positioned, e.g., lying on one side
- The age and weight of the patient
- If the patient is in shock or dehydrated, poor superficial peripheral access may be present
- Medications can influence choice, e.g., anticoagulants, steroids, risk of bruising
- The temperature will influence venous dilatation, e.g., if patient is cold, no veins may be visible
- Patient anxiety about the procedure
- Venepuncture may cause a vein to collapse

Insertion:

- Choose a site for purpose, away from a joint
- Improve venous access by
  - Ensuring good lighting
  - Tourniquet needed above the venepuncture site − check local policy
  - Opening and closing the fist to force blood into the veins
  - Lowering the arm below heart level increases blood supply to the veins
  - Light tapping of the vein may be useful but can be painful and lead to haematoma
  - Immersing the arm in a bowl of warm water for 10 minutes encourages vasodilatation
  - Ointment or patches containing small amounts of glyceryl trinitrate to cause local vasodilatation to aid venepuncture
- Prevent infection from practitioner to patient, skin flora contamination of the patient:
  - Washing hands is essential
  - All wipes should be undertaken in one direction, used for at least 30 seconds, allowed to dry
- Never reinsert the device once removed as it can damage the inserted equipment
- Good fixation required; use a secure dressing, flexible, visualize the puncture site − check patency using normal saline (5 mL)

Safety of the critical care nurse during insertion:

- Adherence to universal safe technique and practice
- Gloves should be worn; however, these will not prevent a needle-stick injury and can also, due to loss of sensation caused by wearing gloves, make needle-stick injury more likely. Gloves should be worn in the following situations:
  - Inexperienced venepuncturist
  - Critical care nurse has cuts or abrasions on hands
  - When patient is restless
  - When patient is infected with HIV (human immunodeficiency virus) or hepatitis

Adopt universal precautions at all times.

Types of devices available will depend on local policy, as there are a number of new systems for collection now accessible commercially. To prevent occupational percutaneous injuries vacuum blood collection systems are commonly used.

Cannulation

A vascular device is inserted into a peripheral or central blood vessel and remains in situ to provide intravenous (IV) fluid or drug administration or continuous monitoring.

IV Cannula for Continuous Fluid and/or Drug Administration

This involves putting a devise into a patient's peripheral vein so that infusions can be given directly into the blood stream. It can be the role of a critical care nurse following appropriate training, supervision and assessment by an experienced member of staff and keeps updated. During insertion, it is importance to prevent infection; the nurse needs to pay attention to

- Preparation
- Insertion
- Aftercare

Complications

Phlebitis An acute inflammation of a vein directly linked to the presence of any vascular access device.

- Patient reports pain — the first indication of potential problems.
- If treated early enough, often the symptoms will resolve without further intervention required.
- Substances that often cause phlebitis tend to be isotonic solutions, e.g., 0.9% sodium chloride or blood products.
- Phlebitis can be further classified into mechanical, chemical and infective, depending on the cause of the problem:
  - Mechanical is predominantly due to cannula problems
  - Chemical due to the incompatibility of drugs infused
  - Infective is where infection is at the tip of the cannula (usually confirmed when blood cultures show the same microbiology as the tip which is sent for culture)
- Treatment for phlebitis is usually heat and analgesia.
- Many areas now consider it good practice to use a phlebitis scale, and this is shown in Table 3.1.

TABLE 3.1 Phlebitis scale.

IV site appears healthy	0	No signs of phlebitis — observe cannula
ONE of the following is evident: • Slight pain near IV site OR • Slight redness near IV site	1	Possibly first signs of phlebitis — observe cannula
TWO of the following are evident: • Pain at IV site • Erythema • Swelling	2	Early stage of phlebitis — resite cannula
ALL of the following signs are evident: • Pain along path of cannula • Erythema • Induration	3	Medium stage of phlebitis — resite cannula; consider treatment
ALL of the following signs are evident and extensive: • Pain along path of cannula • Erythema • Induration • Palpable venous cord	4	Advanced stage of phlebitis or the start of thrombophlebitis — resite cannula; consider treatment
ALL of the following signs are evident and extensive: • Pain along path of cannula • Erythema • Induration • Palpable venous cord • Pyrexia	5	Advanced stage thrombophlebitis — initiate treatment; resite cannula

Jackson, A. From Infection control–a battle in vein: infusion phlebitis.- Nurs Times. 1998 Jan 28-Feb 3;94(4):68, 71.

Haematoma

- This occurs when there is a sufficient leakage of blood from the vessel into the tissue surrounding the IV cannula
- This can occur on
  - Insertion when more than one wall of a blood vessel is punctured
  - Removal when not enough pressure is applied to the IV site when the cannula is removed

Infiltration/Extravasation

- This refers to the inadvertent administration of a drug into the surrounding tissues.
- Often both nursing and medical staff use the terms infiltration and extravasation to mean the same thing; classification is linked to the medication that has caused the problem.
- The clinical symptoms of infiltration are coolness, leakage at the site, swelling and tenderness.
- Local policies for treating infiltration vary, often due to the speciality, age group and medications being used.
- Often local extravasation kits may also be available to ensure quick action where necessary.
- The Intravenous Nurses Society (2016) recommends the use of the infiltration score: a score of 0 indicates no problem to a score of 4 where there is serious infiltration.

Infection Infections can cover a wide spectrum of clinical symptoms from fairly minor irritation to increased morbidity and mortality for patients. The patient may have

- A fairly minor irritation at the site (local infection)
- Bacteraemia (where bacteria are present in the blood)
- Septicaemia (systemic infection), which is more serious

Infection control should be an integral part of insertion of a cannula and all critical care nurses involved in assisting with or undertaking cannulation have a role to play in both prevention and containment of infection. Divided into two groups:

- Exogenous − where the microorganisms originate outside the patient's body (this is usually due to cross infection, e.g., hands of healthcare professionals and equipment).
- Endogenous − due to organisms already present on or in the patient's body.

Both exogenous and endogenous infection can be due to intrinsic and extrinsic contamination. Intrinsic contamination relates to infection that is present prior to use, whereas extrinsic is introduced in use. There may be increased costs of treating the infection, which then may lengthen the patient's stay in critical care and may increase the necessity for costly antibiotic therapy:

- Consider whether cannula is actually necessary. This is because some cannulae can be inserted 'routinely' and thus should be challenged.
- Ensure appropriate cleaning products are used on the skin prior to insertion of the cannula.
- Cover the cannula with a dressing, which is transparent and semi-permeable; this allows the site to be viewed easily.
- Change the cannula site every 48–72 hours – this has been shown to reduce infection rates at the cannula site.
- Use an aseptic technique and manipulations of the IV system to reduce infection.
- Site cannula avoiding lower extremities and avoid joints, nerves. Lower extremities are more difficult to view and joints/nerves will be uncomfortable and may cause patient pain and later harm.
- Try and reduce the number of attempts to cannulate as increased number of puncture sites equates to increased entry sites for infection.
- Identify 'at risk' patients and take additional precautions. At risk patients include
  - Patients who are older/younger
  - Infection already present
  - Immunosuppressed
  - Poor nutrition
  - Loss of skin integrity
  - On antibiotic therapy
  - Patients having multiple invasive procedures
- Educate staff in the portals for entry for infection so steps can be taken to directly reduce the risk.
- When using infusion equipment clean both before and after use. Check equipment to see if it is for single use only. Infection can be present on drip stands and infusion equipment.
- Good hand washing and precautions to protect self should always be employed. Infection due to health workers' hands is a major source of infection. Glove, apron and, if necessary, masks and goggles should be worn.

Flushing of Cannula

- Flushing guidance is often overlooked and is an essential component of good care.

- RCN (2016) note the flush volume should be equal to at least twice the volume of the catheter, usually 5—10 mL of 0.9% sodium chloride.
- An associated hazard is speed shock as a systemic reaction that occurs when a substance foreign to the body is rapidly introduced — occurs most commonly with rapid bolus injection.

For the gathering of data, e.g., invasive pressure monitoring. This involves the doctor inserting a special catheter for

- Central venous pressure monitoring — for the therapeutic administration of medicines and/or fluids.
- Pulmonary artery pressure monitoring — for more detailed cardiac studies.
- Arterial pressure monitoring — for access to arterial blood for arterial blood gas (ABG) monitoring.
- Intracranial pressure monitoring — for continuous measure following severe brain injury.
- These invasive pressure monitoring cannula can be attached to a transducer, which converts the pressure to a continued numerical view and waveform display. These specialist cannulae are the responsibility of the critical care nurse and are discussed in more detail elsewhere in the book.

Always be alert to the fact that when administering IV drugs to the patient they can have an anaphylactic reaction.

Blood Transfusion

The human cardiovascular system is designed to minimize the effects of blood loss:

- Average man — 5—6 L
- Average women — 4—5 L
- Forms 7%—9% of body weight
- Thicker, denser and more adhesive than water
- Flows 4—5 times slower than water
- pH — 7.35—7.45
- Temperature — 35.5—37.5°C

Blood contains many important components:

- Erythrocytes (red blood cells (RBCs))
- White blood cells (WBCs)

- Plasma, which contains:
  - Plasma proteins (albumin)
  - Electrolytes – sodium, potassium, calcium, chloride
  - Waste products – urea, creatinine
  - Vitamins and minerals
  - Glucose
  - Oxygen and carbon dioxide
  - Fats
  - Hormones
  - Clotting factors

Functions of Blood

- Distribution – it is the major transport tissue and carries everything (oxygen, carbon dioxide, hormones, nutrients) from one place to another in the body.
- Regulation – it plays a major role in maintaining homeostasis (acid-base balance and blood pH, temperature, body fluids).
- Protection – blood loss by initiating clot formation, infection via antibodies and WBCs.

There are Four Major Blood Groups

- A – contains anti-B, 42% of UK blood group
- B – contains anti-A, 9% of UK blood group
- AB – contains neither anti-A or B, the universal recipient, 3% of UK blood group
- O – contains anti-A and B, the universal donor, 46% of UK blood groups

The Rhesus factor is an antigen on RBCs divided into

- Rh+ – the individual has agglutinogen D, is dominant in Western Europe 83%.
- Rh– – has no D, 17% of Western Europe.
- Anti-D is produced if Rh+ blood is given to a Rh– individual or if Rh+ foetus is being carried by a Rh– mother) dangerous for second and consequent foetus).
- Anti-D injections are given preventing the development of Anti-D in Rh– women.

The body can compensate for only so much blood loss. Losses of 15%–30% cause pallor and weakness; a loss of more than 30% of blood volume results in severe shock and can be fatal. To treat haemorrhage whole blood should be used as routine, especially when blood loss is substantial. A blood transfusion of whole blood is required:

- To replace blood lost during an operation or after an accident
- Used to treat anaemia – iron, vitamin B_{12} or folate

- Other medical conditions:
  - Haemophilia — affects the bloods ability to clot
  - Sickle cell anaemia, thalassaemia — disruption of the normal production of RBCs
  - Leukaemia — RBCs are produced at a reduced rate
  - Malaria — RBCs are destroyed
  - Renal failure — reduction in the production of erythropoietin, which plays a key role in the production of RBCs
- Blood transfusions can cause serious reactions some of which arise from the changes that occur in stored blood

The Changes that Occur in Stored Blood are as follows

- At present blood is collected, under strict aseptic technique in a plastic vacuum container, from a donor and then mixed with an appropriate anticoagulant solution, such as citrate-phosphate-dextrose (CPD) or oxalate salts, which prevent clotting by binding with calcium ions. The blood can then be stored under refrigeration for several weeks at a temperature of 1−6°C until it is needed for transfusion.
- Various changes occur in blood as a result of its removal from the body. These changes begin within 24 hours of storage and continue throughout the entire 21 days, after which blood is considered outdated (Richards and Edwards, 2014). These changes are many and varied and have implications for nursing practice. For the specific changes that can occur in stored blood see Box 3.1.

Blood Transfusion Reactions

- When mismatched blood is infused, a transfusion reaction occurs, and the donor and recipient's RBCs are attacked by the recipient's immune system.
- A transfusion reaction can occur with the infusion of as little as 10−15 mL of incompatible blood.
- The agglutination of the foreign RBCs blocks small blood vessels throughout the body, which are destroyed. This causes a reduction in the capacity of RBCs to carry oxygen and obstruction to blood flow causing organ damage — both, which are lethal.
- Transfusion reactions can also cause fever, chills, nausea, vomiting and general lethargy, but are rarely lethal. As is commonly known, reactions do not occur immediately against the foreign antibody, but on the second occasion a transfusion is given.
- Despite blood transfusions being valuable, they are at times scarce, expensive or frustratingly slow to appear in times of crisis. Yet, there are many complications associated with blood transfusion (SHOT report: www.shotuk.org):

BOX 3.1 Changes that occur in stored blood

Acid-base changes
Because blood is stored in an air-free container, aerobic metabolism cannot take place, but anaerobic metabolism does occur, yet, the end product is lactic and pyruvic acids. Therefore, the longer a unit of blood is stored, the greater will be the amount of acid end products that it contains. The CPD solution used as an anticoagulant adds another acid component to banked blood and reduces the pH of the blood from a normal body pH of 7.4 to about 7.0.

Alterations in electrolyte concentration
When blood is stored, the sodium and potassium concentration undergoes alteration. It can be expected that a unit of stored blood will contain approximately 75–80 mEq of sodium and 5 to 7 mEq of potassium. There is also a progressive loss of red cell viability, and the red blood cells tend to take up water, causing a leftward shift in the oxy-haemoglobin dissociation curve and transfused blood cells to be less capable of releasing oxygen to the tissues than normal red blood cells.

The microaggregate load in stored blood
An increased aggregation of platelets and leukocytes occurs in stored blood, and blood has been filtered through 170 μm filters to remedy it. However, the formation of microemboli are considered smaller than 170 μm, have been identified and microfilters with pore sizes ranging from 20 to 90 μm are required. However, because those conditions that require massive blood transfusions are generally an emergency, it is extremely difficult, if not impossible, to prove that the use of microfilters during massive blood transfusions decreases the development of ARDS.

Depletion of clotting factors
Stored blood is deficient in most of the factors necessary for normal coagulation; it is specifically deficient in factors V, VIII and IX and platelets. However, the depletion of platelets and clotting factors varies from patient to patient, and it is recommended that the patient's clotting screen and bleeding status be closely monitored during transfusion.

The temperature of stored blood
Blood is stored at a temperature between 1 and 6°C which is considerably colder than human blood. The normal temperature is generally approximately 37°C. The infusion of large quantities of cold blood can cause patients to become hypothermic. This compromises the patient's heart rate, BP, cardiac output and coronary blood flow. This consequent hypothermia impairs the metabolism of citrate and lactate and increases the patient's risk of a metabolic acidosis; it increases the affinity of haemoglobin for oxygen, may impair clotting, and impairs the possibility of detecting a major transfusion reaction.

- Pulmonary damage
- Metabolic acidosis, hyperkalaemia, hypothermia
- Incorrect blood components transfused:
  - Wrong blood, patient identification errors, labelling errors, prescription errors
  - Inappropriate, unnecessary transfusion, delayed, under transfusion
  - Handling and storage errors
  - Laboratory errors
- Transfusion reactions, haemolytic transfusion reactions
- Because the administration of blood and blood products is an area of nursing practice, the nurse has to be vigilant, both in checking the correct blood group and Rh D antigen factor and in observing for any signs of transfusion reactions. Frequent observations will enable the nurse to detect any reaction at an early stage; these include discomfort, flushing, rash or pain.

Blood Products

- These are any therapeutic substances prepared from human blood. Packed red cells (whole blood from which most of the plasma has been removed) are generally only used to treat anaemia.
- Fresh frozen plasma (FFP) should never be used as a volume expander in this situation. It is better to use FFP for patients with bleeding disorders, where there is a deficiency in platelets or clotting factors, e.g., in disseminated intravascular coagulation (DIC), warfarin overdose, trauma or thrombotic thrombocytopenia.
- Preparations from human plasma:
  - Cryoprecipitate
  - Coagulation factors
  - Immunoglobulin
  - Albumin, e.g., human albumin solution (HAS)

For a more detailed account of blood products see Table 3.2.

However, there are more recent problems with blood transfusions: contracting viral infections such as hepatitis B and HIV/AIDS. Therefore, in an attempt to reduce blood transfusion reactions and the spread of viral infections, other methods of transfusion such as autotransfusion and synthetic blood products have been introduced.

Autotransfusion

To minimize the need for blood transfusion by blood donor, during surgical procedures blood can be salvaged through an autotransfusion device. This blood can either be reinfused back into the patient during surgery if blood loss is great or saved for transfusion at a later date.

TABLE 3.2 Current blood products.

Blood product	Constituents	Uses
Whole blood (510 ± 45 mL)	Use is restricted to circumstances where red blood cells as well as plasma proteins are needed, i.e., where large amounts of blood are lost.	Ideal in hypovolaemic shock, since it both increases oxygen carrying capacity and expands circulating volume.
Packed cells (280 ± 60 mL)	This is whole blood, but the majority of the plasma has been removed. It contains half the volume of whole blood, less sodium, potassium, albumin and citrate. Does contain some white blood cells and platelets.	Ideal in chronic anaemia, sickle cell disease, thalassaemia and renal disease. It is not recommended in iron deficiency and vitamin B_{12} or folate deficiency as these should be treated with the appropriate vitamin, e.g., iron tablets.
Washed packed cells	These are packed cells with all the white blood cells, platelets and plasma removed.	Indicated for patients who have a long history of transfusion reactions.
Fresh frozen plasma (FFP) (200–300 mL)	This is blood product, which is nearly always frozen and contains all the coagulation factors.	Used for the treatment of coagulation deficits. It is not recommended as a volume expander, except in certain neonatal conditions.
Cryoprecipitate (20 ± 5 mL)	Prepared from FFP and contains mainly clotting factors (factor VIII and fibrinogen).	Used to treat haemophilia or AIDS (acquired immunodeficiency syndrome) patients.
Platelets (50 ± 10 mL)	Produced from the residue left over from the production of plasma and leukocyte-depleted red blood cell concentrates.	Indications for use are thrombocytopenia, when platelet content of blood is reduced due to bleeding or diluted following massive transfusion, in acute leukaemia, aplastic anaemia, disseminated intravascular coagulation (DIC) or sepsis.

Synthetic Blood Products

Recently artificial blood substitutes, or perfluorochemicals, have become available for clinical use, often used in cases of severe anaemia when transfusion of blood products is not an option. However, the use of these products to treat blood loss is still under investigation. They work similarly to how oxygen is carried in plasma, and while only 3% of the total oxygen supply is dissolved in this way the oxygen is used. When perfluorochemical microdroplets (in which oxygen is highly soluble) are infused intravenously, oxygen is dissolved in the microdroplets and transported to capillaries for diffusion across capillary walls (Richards and Edwards, 2018).

However, synthetic blood products do have side effects, which include

- Pulmonary oedema
- Arrhythmias
- Chest pain
- Respiratory distress

In addition, it is unfortunate that the positive effects of perfluorochemicals do not endure beyond 24 hours after infusion due to their short half-life. Nevertheless, following further research these synthetic blood products may in the future:

- Reduce blood recipient adverse reactions from donor blood
- Minimize the use of and improve the cost-effectiveness of blood transfusions
- Reduce the risk of spread of infections such as HIV/AIDS and hepatitis B

Colloid and Crystalloid Therapy

The use of colloid and crystalloid therapy in emergency states is life-saving and an essential part of on going critical care nursing.

Colloids

The consideration for the use of colloids in emergency states such as trauma, shock, burns is to achieve the overall primary goal of restoring plasma volume and therefore improving or maintaining oxygen transport. According to this principle, haemodynamic stability is achieved by increasing the blood volume, which is needed for the maintenance and restoration of cellular function. This is proposed to be imperative, as inadequate circulatory blood volume causes pooling of blood in the microcirculation, the major effect being a marked decrease in venous return and a diminished cardiac output. Therefore, by administering plasma expanders there is an improvement in oxygen availability, oxygen consumption, circulating volume, haemodynamic status and tissue perfusion.

Colloids work as they contain various amounts of albumin, which gives blood its colloidal oncotic pressure (COP). This determinant pressure in capillaries holds fluid into the circulation (see Fig. 2.2). Increasing the COP in the blood will draw fluid into the circulation from the intracellular spaces, increasing circulating volume. The problems with giving too much colloid is protein/albumin is not excreted in the renal tubules so the effect of colloids can go on longer than the depletion of circulation, giving rise to fluid overload.

Despite the use of diuretics in this situation albumin is still not excreted in the renal tubules leading to continued fluid overload episodes. Table 3.3 includes a list of all colloid fluids. Therefore, there is an argument for the use of crystalloids.

TABLE 3.3 Colloid infusions available.

Colloid	Constituents	Uses
Human albumin solution (HAS) – manufactured from human blood plasma.	20% solution 50 and 100 mL bottles osmotic pressure of 100–200 mmHg; 4.5% solution 50 mL, 100 mL, 250 mL and 500 mL bottles osmotic pressure of 26 –30 mmHg.	Used in cases of hypoalbuminaemia due to renal disease, liver disease, acute pancreatitis and sepsis. Used as a plasma expander.
Haemaccel	3.5% solution of gelatine, more stable and has a longer shelf life than HAS. Generally no adverse reactions or adverse effect on coagulation.	Contains calcium and should not be given in the same line as blood as it will cause coagulation in the line. Plasma expander.
Gelofusine	Similar to Haemaccel.	Does not contain calcium and can be run through the same line as blood. Plasma expander.
Isoplex 4% solution	Similar to Gelofusine.	Contains gelatine 20 g in 500 mL of water, contains sodium, potassium and chloride. Plasma expander.
Dextran	2 solutions of 40 and 70. A polysaccharide, stable, a non-toxic and non-pyrogenic artificial colloid.	Uses are limited as it has several problems: interferes with haemostasis by reducing platelet adhesiveness, can cause disseminated intra-vascular coagulation (DIC), anaphylactic reactions, blockage of the renal tubules leading to acute renal failure.
Hespan	6% hydroxyethyl starch in 0.6% sodium chloride solution produced from corn hydrolysis, similar to Dextran 70.	A synthetic colloid, with similar uses and problems to Dextran.
Voluven	Is starch in sodium chloride.	A plasma volume substitute used to restore blood volume

TABLE 3.3 Colloid infusions available.—cont'd

Colloid	Constituents	Uses
Volulyte	Is starch in sodium chloride, sodium acetate trihydrate; potassium chloride; magnesium chloride hexahydrate.	Same use a voluven.
Perfluorocarbons (synthetic blood derivatives)	Unrelated to blood but are able to transport oxygen in solution.	Used as an oxygen-carrying substitute. Valuable in patients who refuse human blood transfusion, carbon monoxide poisoning and sickle cell crisis.

Crystalloids

Any solution that contains electrolytes will influence fluid movement; the most powerful is sodium. 0.9% normal saline is added to the extracellular fluid (ECF) compartment as in IV infusion. 0.9% normal saline is an isotonic solution, will keep sodium at a normal level, and has no effect on fluid movement. An infused solution of 0.9% normal saline will stay in the circulation and increase/maintain circulating volume and thus blood pressure (BP). 5% dextrose is not a true crystalloid, as it contains no electrolytes just glucose in water. When administered intravenously it dilutes ECF compartment sodium, intracellular fluid sodium becomes greater and fluid moves into the cells. It is good for rehydration but not for low circulating volume states. Table 3.4 includes a detailed list of crystalloid solutions.

The Colloid/Crystalloid Debate

The debate can arise whether the use of colloid solutions or crystalloid solutions should be administered.

If crystalloids are used as the primary resuscitative agents in low circulating states, the volumes required to achieve normal haemodynamic values are from two to four times those required with colloids. It is suggested that massive crystalloid fluid resuscitation predisposes the patient to adult respiratory distress syndrome (ARDS) or pulmonary oedema, which is alleged to be negligible with colloid therapy. Resuscitation with crystalloid solution alone dilutes the plasma proteins, thereby reducing osmotic pressure, encouraging fluid to shift from the extracellular to the interstitial fluid compartment, thereby predisposing to the development of pulmonary oedema and haemodilution. However, there is evidence emerging that indicates the use of albumin also puts the patient at risk of developing pulmonary insufficiency and ARDS.

TABLE 3.4 Crystalloid infusions.

Crystalloid	Constituents	Uses
0.9% normal saline	Contains sodium and chloride, no calories, has approximately the same osmolality as both intracellular and extracellular fluid.	Increases mainly extracellular volume with no significant increase in intracellular volume.
5% dextrose (not a true crystalloid as it contains no electrolytes)	Contains only 200 calories per litre, adds water to the extracellular compartment and reduces osmolality of extracellular fluid.	The water will pass into the intracellular fluid to reach equilibrium, does not stay in the circulation, good for dehydration.
4% dextrose 0.18% normal saline	Contains a combination of both of the above.	
Hartmann's solution (compound sodium lactate IV infusion or Ringer's solution)	Mixture of sodium chloride; sodium lactate; potassium chloride and calcium chloride in water.	Used to replace fluids and electrolytes due to low circulating volume or blood pressure
Plasmalyte	Is similar to Hartmann's, contains sodium, potassium, magnesium, chloride, acetate and gluconate.	A crystalloid solution used as a source of water and electrolytes

The main argument against using crystalloids to avoid blood transfusions is that it can lead to dilutional hyponatraemia or haemodilution. The blood becomes so dilute that the measured blood haematocrit becomes reduced to 17%−21% (normal range 38%−46%). Haemodilution reduces

- Colloid osmotic pressure − formation of oedema
- Haemoglobin (Hb) content − reduced oxygen carrying capacity of blood
- Coagulation factors − risk of bleeding
- Blood electrolytes − effects of low sodium, potassium, chloride etc.
- Blood glucose, other nutrients, vitamins and mineral − hypoglycaemia, and reduction in sources of energy for all body processes
- Circulating WBCs − reduced ability of the body to fight infection

In haemodilution, there is less of these elements in relation to fluid contained within blood, which can lead to serious effects on all body systems and processes, and death.

A more positive result can be obtained from using colloid supplements, as the colloid osmotic pressure is maintained and fluid shift into the interstitial fluid space is less. It is difficult to determine if the addition of colloids will in effect maintain colloid osmotic pressure and prevent fluid shift into the interstitial space. It is generally agreed that colloid supplementation, in the presence of normal kidney function, may aid in the patient's diuresis, aiding the excretion of excess interstitial fluid. If the application of haemodilution is decided and transfusion is to be avoided, the addition of colloids may allow it to be done safely. Whether this will limit the effects of haemodilution or improve patient's recovery requires further study.

Considerable controversy continues to surround the choice of colloids or crystalloid for resuscitation during low circulating volume states. Each of the fluids identified for use has physiological advantages and disadvantages. However, to make sense of this complex set of arguments and counter arguments, it is necessary to undertake an overview of the sequence of hypovolaemia.

It appears that in low circulating volume states there is

- An overall reduction in ECF volume which can be due to
  - Loss of salt and/or water − dehydration
  - Whole blood − trauma
  - Plasma − burns
  - Third space fluid shift − simulation of the inflammatory immune response

Combinations of two or three are common occurrence in any insult or injury to the body. Therefore, in low circulating volume states, it seems necessary to administer a combination of fluid replacement types, e.g., crystalloid and colloid in varying amounts depending on the patient's condition and determined by rigorous critical care monitoring:

- Blood to maintain clotting factors and Hb levels and to prevent haemodilution
- Colloids to maintain the overall circulating volume
- Crystalloids to maintain fluid and electrolyte balance, prevent the movement of water and sodium and replace fluid lost through third space fluid shift
- 5% dextrose solution to replace loss of intracellular fluid drawn into the ECF space due to the administration of colloids and/or changes in capillary dynamics

In addition, it should not be forgotten that it is also imperative that the patient's cardiopulmonary dynamics be monitored in a way that is reliable to determine physiological trends and responses to whichever therapy is finally chosen.

Rewarming Procedures

As core temperature drops below 35°C treatment becomes imperative; rewarming of the hypothermic patient is only one aspect to be considered in the care (Richards and Edwards, 2018). The nurse has a broader role in managing and caring for these patients. This should include vigilance during fluid administration; the review of blood results and an electrocardiogram (ECG); recording of urine output; and ensuring that any drugs administered during rewarming are not toxic.

Giving consideration to the patient's core temperature and the duration of their hypothermia, rewarming should be started. Rewarming methods are divided into three.

Passive External Rewarming

Once the patient's core temperature is known to be less than 35°C, steps should be taken to prevent them losing further heat to the environment. Remove all wet clothing, gently dry the patient if needed, and keep them well-insulated using blankets. The patient may then be allowed to rewarm using just normal metabolic heat production.

The patient may be covered with polythene sheeting and placed in a warm room. Space blankets prevent radiant heat loss but not that lost by conduction or convection. As these may cause sparks, they also present a hazard when oxygen is used, so are best avoided. Remember that heat is lost from the head and the back, so these should be insulated also.

This method is recommended for both mild (32.2–35°C) and moderate (28–32°C) hypothermia that have an onset of less than 12 hours. Passive rewarming treatment will not rewarm an arrested hypothermic patient and may have limited value for those who are severely hypothermic, e.g., a temperature of less than 28°C.

Close observation, cautious use of fluids and avoidance of vigorous movement to prevent cardiac arrest are essential. Movement contributes to heat loss through convection and may reduce temperature further if not closely monitored. If the patient's temperature fails to rise or they become persistently hypotensive, active external rewarming should be commenced.

Active External Rewarming

In active rewarming, the patient's skin is warmed using hot baths, hot air blowers or radiant heat. This method can also be used as an adjunct to internal active rewarming. One of the most effective methods of external active rewarming is convective warming therapy. This method uses the principles of convection, forcing heated air directly on to the patient's skin through a disposable blanket.

Active rewarming may be used when hypothermia has occurred slowly, e.g., over a 12-hour period, and is mild or moderate in nature. This method is not recommended for use alone in the treatment of patients with severe hypothermia. The patient's vital signs and peripheral temperature must be closely monitored, as rewarming shock may occur in the severely hypothermic patient, as a consequence of rewarming the peripheries before the core. Peripheral rewarming promotes vasodilatation, returning cold, acidotic blood to the heart that has significant effects on myocardial depression. To minimize this effect it is recommended that only the trunk of the body be rewarmed. If the patient is persistently hypotensive, or their core temperature continues to fall, active internal rewarming should be started.

Active Internal Rewarming

These are generally invasive procedures, whereby the deep tissues of the body are warmed. It allows the lungs and heart to be rewarmed first. Methods include using

- Warm fluid for gastric and peritoneal lavage
- Mediastinal and pleural irrigation
- Continuous arteriovenous or venovenous rewarming
- Extracorporeal rewarming
- Cardiopulmonary bypass

However, the use of warmed gases to the respiratory tract and warmed IV fluids are the easiest methods. When warming IV fluids, reference to the critical care patient's central venous pressure and urine output is necessary. If warmed oxygen is used, it should be humidified as well as warmed. The fastest method of rewarming is by cardiopulmonary bypass. However, this is not readily available in all hospitals, requires critical care input, and is thus not a method of choice for use on general wards.

The advantage of active core rewarming is that it avoids the peripheral vasodilatation associated with surface rewarming and allows correction of any fluid deficits. A disadvantage is that after-drop may be observed in patients after internal active rewarming is discontinued. A decrease in temperature of as much as 2°C may occur as blood circulates to the peripheries, re-cools, and returns to the core. Thus, when more invasive active internal rewarming methods are discontinued, attention is directed to the need for passive and active external rewarming to prevent after-drop in temperature.

Active internal rewarming is best incorporated when the hypothermia has occurred very quickly, e.g., in less than 12 hours, and is moderate or severe in nature. The treatment is to reduce the risk of cardiac arrest, by reducing the time the patient's core temperature is below 32.2°C.

Carefully monitored, non-arrested patients may be successfully rewarmed by passive or active external application of heat provided they simultaneously receive appropriate fluids to restore depleted intravascular volume. Active internal rewarming may be used as an adjunct to active external rewarming in cases of moderate or severe hypothermia, the easiest methods being warmed IV fluid and respiratory gases; the use of other methods depend on availability of facilities and/or resources. It is unfortunate there has not yet been adequately constructed research that permits the assessment of the advantages of one rewarming procedure over another. The only general agreement evident is that the patients should be rewarmed.

The process of rewarming should proceed no faster than a few degrees per hour (Richards and Edwards, 2018). If a patient is rapidly rewarmed oxygen consumption, myocardial demand and vasodilatation increase faster than the heart's ability to compensate and death can occur.

Fluid Management During Rewarming

During hypothermia, to protect the body's major organs and prevent excess heat loss from skin surfaces, the peripheral vasculature vasoconstricts. The circulating volume in the body does not change, but the changes in the peripheral vasculature cause a decrease in oxygen consumption and heart rate and an increase in BP.

When the patient is warming up consideration needs to be given to support the circulation, as blood vessels will start to vasodilate. Thus, there needs to be effective clinical management of fluid replacement therapy in response to the increasing temperature and the corresponding vasodilatation. This will ensure the maintenance of fluid volume, control circulating volume, reduce haemo-concentration and maintain arterial BP, central venous pressure and urine output. This is maintained through administering IV fluids, which are warmed before infusion and include a balanced salt solution and/or colloid solution or both.

During fluid administration to hypothermic patients, dextrose 5% and 0.9% normal saline are generally the fluids most commonly infused, but plasma and blood may also be necessary. Potassium needs to be added or contained within the bag as indicated by sequential biochemical analysis. These are needed to minimize, prevent or reverse the hypovolaemic states that may occur during rewarming. Care needs to be taken with rapid volume resuscitation, and when efforts have been made to warm fluids, this can reduce core temperature (after-drop) and cause myocardial infarction.

Enteral Feeding

Enteral feeding (EF) includes any method of delivering nutrients for gastrointestinal tract (GIT) absorption (Richards and Edwards, 2014). This generally includes feeding via the nasogastric, gastrostomy or jejunal route. There is clear evidence that long periods of time without nutrition can produce detrimental gastrointestinal responses and serious complications. It is advocated that early EF be initiated at the earliest possible point.

Advantages of early enteral feeding:

- Maintains gut integrity
- Reduces risk of bacterial translocation
- Suppresses the inflammatory immune response
- Reduces complications from sepsis
- More cost-effective in comparison to parenteral nutrition

Long periods of time without any nutrition can produce detrimental GIT responses and serious complications:

- Stress ulcers
- Production of lactic acid, as the GIT is shut down during stress and blood supply reduced leading to anaerobic metabolism of cells
- Translocation of bacteria/sepsis

It is advocated that the use of EF be early, when oral diet cannot be tolerated or is insufficient. Early EF immediately following any type of surgery is possible (i.e., within 2−6 hours of insult). Only contraindicated in complete gut failure, which is very rare. EF includes any method of delivering nutrients for absorption by the GIT, includes feeding via

- The nasogastric route
- Nasoenteric route (i.e., placed in the duodenum or jejunum)

Types of Tube

1. Nasogastric/nasoduodenal − these are the most commonly used and are suitable for short-term use such as post-operatively or during a period of critical care ventilation.
   a. The *wide-bore tube* is used initially to allow aspiration in patients with bowel obstruction or pancreatitis to easily assess gastric contents, measure and document loss and evaluate pH.
   b. The *narrow-bore* tube should replace the wide-bore tube to facilitate long-term feeding. In addition, the narrow-bore tube is more comfortable for the patient and less likely to cause oesophageal irritation or interfere with swallowing. Narrow-bore tubes are now designed to allow small amounts of aspiration for evaluation pH, which can determine if the placement of the tube is in the stomach.
2. Gastrostomy − is often used when long-term feeding is anticipated, it avoids delays in feeding, reduces discomfort, and cosmetically acceptable, when there is upper gastrointestinal obstruction.
   a. Percutaneous endoscopic gastrostomy (PEG) − the feeding tube is inserted into the stomach or intestine and sits on the surface of the skin. Made from polyurethane or silicone and held in place by an inflatable

balloon. A disadvantage of this method is that it requires local anaesthetic, sedation and radiological support to ensure tube is positioned correctly.

b. Jejunostomy tube — This is placed into the jejunum and is the preferable method if the patient has undergone upper gastrointestinal surgery or has severe delayed gastric emptying.

The Methods of Administration

- Bolus feeding — patient is restless, confused as the patient may dislodge the tube.
- Intermittent continuous feeding — feeding needs to be interrupted or discontinued to allow gastric emptying to occur, e.g., physiotherapy.
- Gravity drip — whereby it is allowed to flow through over a period of time, rarely used in critical care settings.
- Pump-assisted feeding — connected to a pump for the majority of the day and typically rested overnight. Most commonly used in the critical care setting, various flow rates per hour from 1 to 300 mL.

The Complications of Enteral Feeding

These complications can be prevented within the critical care setting. It is essential that the critical care nurse both understands and anticipates the potential problems associated with EF:

- Altered gut motility, i.e., absent bowel sounds can lead to gastric and colonic stasis
- Effects of sedation and analgesia can lead to ileus/pseudo-obstruction and distension
- Pulmonary aspiration
- Nausea and vomiting
- Diarrhoea, constipation, large aspirates
- Blockage of tube
- Trauma to the nose
- Incomplete calorific delivery due to the above
- Overfeeding

Always check the nasal area for ulceration.

Strategies to challenge complications associated with EF:

- Large aspirates — Give prokinetic agents
- Early commencement of EF — Day 1 of critical care admission, monitor feeding regimen, avoid stopping and starting feed, follow feeding regimen
- Rigorous nursing care of nasogastric tube to prevent blockages
- Bowel sounds are not required for EF to commence
- Treat diarrhoea, constipation and vomiting to aid EF

Overfeeding

The energy requirements of disease have often been overestimated to account for

- High temperature
- Increase cost of breathing

This is inappropriate as critical care patient's resting energy expenditure may represent only 20%–30%, rather than 50%, as it is offset by the decrease in physical activity. The energy requirements of patients who are unwell are usually similar to or less than those of healthy subjects. Excess carbohydrate and lipid intake can cause

- Hepatic steatosis
- Abnormal liver function
- Excess carbon dioxide production, which can precipitate respiratory failure
- Excess lipids may be deposited in the lung and impair diffusion of gases and produce infusion hyperlipidaemia

It is recommended that hypocaloric feeding be the current practice in hospital feeding regimens, especially in the early stages of injury (e.g., 1500 kcal/d for up to a week). This would reduce the risk of liver and lung complications and metabolic instability and their consequences. An increase in calorie intake would take place in the recovery phase, when nutrition level is normal and the patient is no longer at risk.

EF is the preferred route in terms of cost and the prevention of mechanical, septic and metabolic complications.

Parenteral Nutrition

Parenteral nutrition (PN) is the provision of all nutritional requirements intravenously or centrally. Therefore, instead of food being fed into and absorbed by the GIT, nutrients are infused directly into the venous circulation, thus bypassing the gut. PN contains essential nutrients in quantities to meet the requirements of the individual patient. It is administered and connected to the patient using an aseptic technique into a central venous access. PN is indicated in patients with

- Prolonged ileus
- Uncontrolled vomiting
- Chronic diarrhoea or malabsorptive states
- Severe radiation enteritis
- Short bowel syndrome
- Gastrointestinal obstruction
- Severe pancreatitis with fistula, critically ill
- Hypercatabolic states
- Patients in ITU suffering multiple trauma or burns
- Hepatic or renal failure
- Inflammatory bowel disease

Patients for Parenteral Nutrition

- Patients who are unable to eat or absorb orally for a period of 5 days (considered too long by many)
- Patients who are malnourished and unable to eat or absorb food
- Unconscious patients who may aspirate if fed orally
- To support patients who are hypercatabolic or have multi-system failure and are unable to maintain adequate nutritional intake
- Bowel rest for patients with fistulae, pancreatitis or inflammatory bowel disease

Routes of Administration

Two routes of administration:

- CVP usually subclavian vein
  - Problems with infection
  - All the complications of a CVP line
  - Limits mobility
- Skin tunnelled catheter for long-term nutrition
  - A peripherally inserted central catheter (PICC) and
  - Gets blocked very easily.

Parenteral Nutrition Solution

PN solution contains the following:

- Amino acids — both essential and non-essential 1–2 g/kg/d
- Glucose — carbohydrate energy source it provides 3.75 kcal/g — 25%–50% glucose in insulin, fatty liver

- Fat emulsion − fat energy source generates 9 kcal/g − 10 or 20% solutions ↓ insulin and in ketones
- If an insufficient energy supply from carbohydrates/fats − encourages the use of protein for energy
- Electrolytes, e.g., sodium, potassium, magnesium, calcium and phosphorus
- Vitamins, minerals and trace elements are required

The Nurse's Role

The nurse's role in delivery of PN in critical care:

- Administration sets need to be changed every 24 hours
- Feeding line should never be used for the administration of additional medicines − PN is incompatible with numerous other medicines
- Separate lumen should be used for other medicines, blood products or CVP readings
- Volumetric infusion pumps should be used
- Never attempt to catch up if the infusion is running slowly
- Incomplete bags should be discarded

The nurse's role in management:

- Aseptic conditions
- Tubing − cover these from light as many vitamins and minerals are destroyed by natural and fluorescent lighting
- Dressings to the CVP line needs to be changed regularly
- Connections of feeding solution
- Site of the subclavian catheter observed for inflammation/infection
- No blood products should be infused through the line

Aseptic conditions must be adopted when dealing with patient access and changing of PN bags.

Monitoring of Parenteral Nutrition

- TPR and BP undertaken at regular intervals to ensure complications are recognised early
- Body weight − check daily weight to monitor increases or decreases
- Fluid balance − ensure a balance is maintained; observe for positive balance as this could indicate fluid overload
- Urine testing − test for glucose and ketones
- Blood testing − creatinine, urea, glucose, sodium, potassium
- Mouth care due to limited oral intake

Complications of Parenteral Nutrition

Central line Complications

- Pneumothorax
- Arterial puncture
- Air embolism
- Sepsis
- Vein thrombosis
- Catheter blockage and accidental removal

Metabolic Complications

- Fluid overload as PN is as hypertonic fluid solution
- Hyperglycaemia due to high glucose level of PN
- Hypoglycaemia addition of insulin leads the patient with PN to hypoglycaemia
- Translocation of bacteria/sepsis if patient is NBM, gut integrity is diminished and gut flora is allowed to cross in the bloodstream
- A reduction in trace elements and vitamins destroyed in natural and artificial light and absorbed into the plastic tubing
- Metabolic acidosis − chloride/CO_2
- Refeeding syndrome − occurs during the reintroduction of food following malnutrition or starvation; there are sudden shifts in electrolytes that help the body to metabolise food
- Electrolyte disturbances
  - Hyperammonaemia
  - Hyponatraemia
  - Hypernatraemia
  - Hypokalaemia
  - Hypocalcaemia
  - Hypophosphataemia
  - Hypomagnesaemia

Required Nutritional Intake

It is important to note that overfeeding can enhance the inflammatory response and compromise respiratory function within the critically ill patients. Excessive carbohydrate and lipid intake can cause hepatic steatosis and abnormal liver function. Lipids may also be deposited in the lung, impair diffusion of gases and produce infusional hyperlipidaemia.

Overfeeding with excess carbohydrate can lead to excess carbon dioxide production, which can precipitate respiratory failure.

The energy requirement of diseases has often been overestimated. The recommendation that more energy should be produced to counteract the effects of an increased temperature is both misleading and incorrect.

A patient's energy requirements are dependent on

- Age
- Sex
- Weight
- Stress activity

Generally, 25−32 kcal/kg/d is required to maintain an adequate nutritional intake. Nitrogen intake, 0.17−0.3 g N/kg/d (maximum nitrogen intake is 18 g/d). If too much nitrogen is taken (0.0.3 g/kg/d), then this may cause a negative effect on weaning and have an effect on renal biochemistry.

The recommended protein intake is 1−1.9 g/kg/d - although consumption of this increases in the acutely unwell patient.

Carbohydrates should not exceed glucose oxidation rate of 3−5 g/kg/d. Carbohydrate overload can cause hyperglycaemia, hypercapnia, possible fatty liver and elevated triglycerides. Fibre diet is beneficial.

Pacing Techniques

A pacemaker is a small electrical device that is fitted with wires into the heart to treat some abnormal heart rhythms. Pacemakers are used for

- Complete or intermittent heart block
- Irregular heart rates or rhythm (tachycardia or bradycardia syndrome) or irregularity
- Slow natural pacemaker (sinus node disease)
- Heart failure

A pacemaker can be fitted temporarily or permanently. They are necessary when the patient's own cardiac conduction system is blocked. Pacemakers can be set to operate at a fixed rate or to operate on demand.

1. A temporary pacemaker is generally introduced by the external transvenous endocardial route. The pacing lead is passed via a vein to the endocardial surface of the right ventricle. The pacing leads are attached to a pacing box, via a small junction connection. Complications include
   a. Those associated with CVP insertion
   b. Under-sensing
   c. Over-sensing − loss of pacing stimuli
   d. Failure to capture/pace due to device defects
   e. Unstable lead positions
   f. Increased pacing threshold
   g. Right ventricular perforation
2. Transcutaneous cardiac pacing is also referred to as external transthoracic cardiac pacing, which is noninvasive. This is only a temporary measure of pacing a patient's heart during a medical emergency. Newer defibrillators can do transcutaneous pacing using pads and an electrical stimulus to

deliver pulses of electric current through the patient's chest, which stimulates the heart to contract.

3. The permanent pacemaker is a small complete electronic unit (4.5 cm × 5.5 cm × 1.25 cm), which is inserted under the skin — usually in the left mammary area, although other sites are possible. The electrodes are attached directly to the epicardial surface of the atrium and/or ventricle. The unit has a limited life and will require replacement in time, but the pacing catheter to which it is attached is usually left undisturbed. These can either be

   a. Single-chamber pacemakers and only have one lead
   b. Dual-chamber pacemakers and have two leads
   c. Biventricular and have three leads

Implantable Cardioverter Cefibrillators

Implantable cardioverter defibrillators (ICDs) are similar to pacemakers but send a larger electrical shock to the heart when the heart stops to get it pumping again. These devises can be both a pacemaker and an ICD. ICDs are used when patients are deemed at risk of cardiac arrest. A life-threatening rhythm is sensed by the ICD and delivers an electrical shock to the heart and helps restore the heart to a normal rhythm. The ICD can be implanted either

- Transvenously along a vein or
- Subcutaneously under the skin

Synchronized Cardioversion

Elective cardioversion is a timed shock, which is delivered at a certain time during the cardiac cycle. It is used to treat atrial flutter, atrial fibrillation (AF), supraventricular tachycardia (SVT) and non-pulseless VT.

- Patient should be fasted for 4–6 hours
- Cardioversion has a thromboembolic risk of 3%–7% — anticoagulation should be administered
- Serum electrolyte measurements must be checked
- Digoxin toxicity must be excluded

The procedure should be performed with

- Adequate monitoring
- Resuscitation facilities including suction
- Oxygen
- Emergency pacing
- ECG monitoring
- Noninvasive BP monitoring
- Pulse oximetry

The procedure:

- A large IV cannula is inserted
- Patient is pre-oxygenated
- Anaesthesia is administered
- Synchronization is checked before charging and discharging the defibrillator
- The amount of joules selected is dependent on the arrhythmia
- The shock is discharged; the patient goes into asystole and within 5—10 seconds sinus rhythm is restored

Ensure that you are familiar with your defibrillator before use.

Cardioversion restores sinus rhythm in a high proportion of patients.

Sengstaken-Blakemore Tube

Sengstaken-Blakemore tubes (SBTs) are inserted through the nose or mouth and used in the management of continuous upper oesophageal or gastrointestinal bleed due to oesophageal or gastric varices. The oesophageal or gastric veins swell due to portal hypertension or vascular congestion, which as pressure increases the veins are more likely to rupture, causing excessive bleeding. Therefore before deciding to insert an SBT tube, check if pharmacological and endoscopic treatments have failed to stop bleeding. The tube itself comprises of

- A large-bore rubber tube and contains two balloons, oesophageal and gastric:
  - Oesophageal balloon port, which inflates a small balloon in the oesophagus, which may not be required
  - Gastric balloon port, which inflates a balloon in the stomach, which compresses the varices
- A gastric aspiration port, which allows the removal of fluid and air out of the stomach

Sengstaken-Blakemore Tube Insertion

- Patients are often sedated or ventilated.
- Balloons are checked for patency, and the insertion end is lubricated.
- SBT is inserted orally to 55—60 cm and the gastric balloon is inflated with water once in the stomach.

- Once inflated the gastric balloon clamp must be applied.
- Tube is pulled back until resistance is felt.
- Secure SBT around mouth using counter-traction.
- X-ray SBT position.
- If bleeding persists, consider inflating the oesophageal balloon.

Sengstaken-Blakemore Tube Management

- Gastric balloon normally inflated for 12–24 hours at a time.
- Gastric balloon is deflated prior to endoscopy or sclerotherapy.
- Traction should be tested hourly.
- Oesophageal balloon should be deflated for periods of 5–10 minutes every 1–2 hours to minimize oesophageal necrosis.

Sengstaken-Blakemore Tube Complications

- Aspiration
- Perforation
- Ulceration
- Oesophageal necrosis

Keep the Sengstaken tubes refrigerated as this assists with ease of insertion.

Peritoneal Dialysis

Peritoneal dialysis (PD) is a slow form of dialysis when the kidneys to not function adequately utilizing the patient's peritoneum as the dialysis membrane. Typically, a much slower correction of fluid and electrolyte imbalance, which can be instigated in the critically ill and the need for complex equipment, is avoided, making this a possible option. However, the procedure is labour-intensive and does predispose the critically ill patient to peritoneal infection. These risk factors make PD unattractive within the critical care setting. Furthermore, with the advent of haemofiltration PD has become largely displaced within the critical care arena.

Peritoneal Dialysis Access

A trochar and cannula are inserted through a small, superficial, mid-line incision under local anaesthetic. However, a lateral approach can also be used. Once inserted, the trocar is withdrawn slightly and the cannula advanced to the pouch of Douglas. Its position may be tested by infusing fluid into the peritoneum before the final advancement of the trocar and cannula.

Peritoneal Dialysis Technique

Warmed peritoneal dialysate is infused into the peritoneum in volumes of 1−2 L at a time. The fluid is left for periods of 4−6 hours in the peritoneal cavity before draining. 500 iu heparin may be added to the initial PD cycles but is only required thereafter if the drainage fluid is cloudy or bloody.

Peritoneal Dialysate

The dialysate is a sterile balanced electrolyte solution with glucose at 75 mmol/L for standard preparation fluid or 311 mmol/L for hypertonic preparation. The preparation is dependent on whether a greater fluid removal is required. Potassium is only added if necessary as the addition of potassium within the peritoneal dialysate can cause problems as it is exchanged slowly in PD.

Peritoneal Dialysis Complications

- Fluid leak around the PD catheter
- Catheter blockage
- Infection
- Hyperglycaemia
- Diaphragmatic splinting

Most patients who start with PD will eventually observe deterioration in their general condition and need haemodialysis.

3.2 HIGH-TECHNOLOGY LIFE SUPPORT INTERVENTIONS

Haemofiltration/Haemodiafiltration

History

Haemodialysis was first used in 1960. This method was inefficient for critically ill patients due to

- The sudden changes in
  - Intravascular pressure/volumes
  - Arterial oxygen tension
  - pH and BP
- Ischaemic insult during reduced BP reduced recovery from ATN

For these reasons PD was suggested to be better, but it was not indicated where rapid correction of volume was required or metabolic abnormalities required correcting, e.g., potassium and acidosis.

Haemofiltration is whereby a simple filter was used continuously to mimic the kidney and filter the blood, a technique first used in 1977. The development of this process was fairly new, but advancements have moved on significantly.

Haemofiltration

Continuous renal replacement therapy (CRRT), which is a simple technique applying convection processes whereby there is a mass movement of plasma water and solutes across a highly permeable membrane.

Methods of Therapy:

- Slow continuous ultrafiltration (SCUF) − regulated by gravity or a pump, It generates ultrafiltrate
- Continuous arteriovenous haemo(dia)filtration (CAVH/D) − this approach to CRRT is now obsolete in contemporary practice
- Continuous venovenous haemofiltration (CVVHF) − a pump is required to generate the hydrostatic pressure. Ultra-filtrate is produced and fluid replacement is carefully monitored
- Continuous venovenous haemodialysis (CVVHD) − dialysate fluid is added to the haemofilter and a pump is incorporated to facilitate the process of convection with the use of dialysate
- Continuous venovenous haemodiafiltration (CVVHDF) is a combination of the both the previous modes. − This includes adding dialysate to the haemofilter, whislt the process of convection, ultrafiltration, the use of replacement fluid and the production of ultrafiltrate take place. This approach to CRRT is deemed most effective

This pressure allows plasma water and solutes to move across the membrane to become the filtrate. The drainage from the filtrate compartment ensures a negative pressure on the other side of the membrane. This maintains a pressure gradient.

Proteins and cellular constituents of blood are not able to move across the membrane due to their molecular size. The removal of waste products can only be achieved by removing water with them. The volume of filtrate able to be moved can be over 2 L per hour. In order to maintain cardiovascular stability, fluid must be replaced at the same time.

The indications for starting a form of CRRT are as follows:

- Metabolic acidosis (pH >6.5 and falling)
- Hyperkalaemia (7.6 mmol/L and rising)
- Fluid overload
- Severe uraemic symptoms (e.g., confusion, nausea, vomiting etc.)
- Urea >30 mmol/L and rising, creatinine >300 mmol/L and rising

- Hyperthermia core temperature >39.5°C
- Clinically significant organ oedema
- Drug overdose

All the above indications are a guide, and individual cases may require earlier or later treatment. The overall aims of CRRT are to

- Relieve fluid overload and control volume quickly without inducing volume depletion and hypotension restore and maintain fluid balance
- Remove waste products (e.g., urea and creatinine) efficiently to offer a better chance of survival
- Correct or control metabolic acidosis, serum phosphate levels, protein levels preventing protein malnutrition and so maintain metabolic and electrolyte balance
  - Restore patients suffering from chronic heart disease symptom-free and oedema-free time
  - Provide haemodynamic stability to patients suffering oliguria or anuria due to septic shock

Advantages

- Haemofiltration allows continuous control of
  - waste products
  - fluid balance
- It promotes cardiovascular stability
- It does not require specialist renal staff or equipment
- It can be performed in the ITU, reducing the need for transfer critically ill patients to renal centres

Disadvantages

- Restricts the patient's mobility.
- Constant patient-centred activity can disrupt rest and sleep patterns.
- Anticoagulation must be continuous.
- Removal and administration of large volumes of fluid is nurse intensive and open to potential errors.

Vascular Access

Haemofiltration requires vascular access from a vein. A 'Vas-Cath' is commonly used − a Y-shaped cannula inserted into a large vein:

- Femoral
  - Good blood flow if leg kept straight
  - Difficult to site and expose for observation

- Internal jugular
  - Good blood flow
  - Uncomfortable for patient, difficult to fix to skin
- Subclavian
  - Good blood flow, greater patient mobility
  - Insertion problems, e.g., pneumothorax

One arm of the Y allows blood to be drawn away from the patient and the other allows blood to be pumped back in.

A patient's movement can affect the blood flow.

Terminology Used

- Diffusion — the movement of solutes from a high concentration to a low concentration
- Dialysis — when solutes pass through an artificial membrane the term dialysis is used
- Ultrafiltration — the movement of fluid across a membrane occurs in the presence of a pressure across the membrane. This is due to push and pull processes, known as transmembrane pressure (TMP)
- Convection — the movement of solutes, which occurs with the flow of fluid. When ultrafiltration takes place, substances will be dragged along with it
- Haemodialysis — relies upon diffusion and ultrafiltration. The concentration of waste produced is greater in the blood than in the dialysate — creates equilibrium on both sides
- Haemofiltration — relies upon ultra-filtration and convection, a pressure is created and large amounts of fluid and solutes are forced across the membrane to form filtrate. No dialysate solution — diffusion does not occur
- Transmembrane pressure — blood channel flow/pressure
- Ultrafiltrate — this is the fluid removed generated by the process of ultrafiltration and convection. The fluid balance is determined by the difference between the replacement fluid administered and the ultrafiltrate.

Normal Values

Water and electrolytes need to be replaced to reduce loss:

- Albumin — 35–50 g/L
- Phosphate — 0.73–1.45 mmol/L
- Urea — 2.5–6.7 mmol/L
- Creatinine — 60–150 μmol/L
- Magnesium — 0.75–1.05 mmol/L
- Platelets — 150–400 × 109/L

Factors that Affect Haemofiltration

- Blood flow rate — access needles/tubing/patient blood pressure (BP)
- TMP — the pressure of the blood through the plate and the pressure exerted by the pump/flow of filtrate
- The membrane across the filter
- The patient's blood
  - Haematocrit — increased viscosity, reduced blood flow, reduced TMP
  - Protocrit — protein concentration

Critical Care Nurse's Role

- Continuous ECG and BP monitoring are essential to detect signs of hypovolaemia
- Monitoring of
  - Potassium levels to maintain K^1 between 4.0 and 4.5 mmol/L
  - Six to eight hourly checks of U&Es for creatinine and urea levels
  - Temperature as hypothermia can occur — fluids may need to be warmed
  - Six to eight hourly blood clotting, adjustments of anticoagulant therapy may be necessary
- Replacement fluid — crystalloid to maintain adequate BP
- Vascular access — femoral, artery, vein, catheters or shunts
- Anticoagulation — prevents clotting of filter, different dose regimens
- Prostacyclin 1–12 ng/kg/min — usually used if heparin is contraindicated. Up to 20 ng/kg/min can be used.
  - Side-effects: vasodilatation, reduced BP, nausea and abdominal pain
  - Combined with low-dose heparin
- Fluid balance/documentation — various methods
- Infection control — one-third of renal patients' prognosis is reduced due to infection
- Neurological deficit
- Haemofiltration is continuous; nurse's attention is focused around the patient continuously; steps need to be taken to allow the patient adequate sleep and rest periods
- Psychological care is essential, e.g., communication, information about what is happening etc.
- Ultrafiltrate — waste products — safe disposal of bodily fluids is practiced as per local policy

Plasmapheresis

Plasmapheresis or plasma exchange is the process of removing autoantibodies from the bloodstream mechanically using a process similar to that used in CRRT treatment. The procedure became known as plasmapheresis or plasma exchange meaning plasma separation. It is performed at many major medical centres and critical care units across the country.

In autoimmune diseases, the immune system attacks the body's own tissues and the main attack mechanisms are antibodies and proteins that circulate in the bloodstream until they meet and bind with the target tissue. Once attached, they impair tissue functions and encourage other immune components to respond.

The concept of plasmapheresis is to remove antibodies from the bloodstream, thereby preventing them from attacking tissues. It is important to note that plasmapheresis does not directly affect the immune system's ability to make more antibodies and therefore may only offer temporary benefit. Plasmapheresis is therefore most beneficial in acute, self-limiting disorders.

Specific filters are required especially for plasmapheresis.

Today, plasmapheresis is widely accepted for the treatment of autoimmune diseases such as

- Myasthenia gravis
- Guillain-Barré syndrome
- Lambert-Eaton syndrome
- Chronic demyelinating polyneuropathy
- Goodpasture's syndrome
- Pemphigus
- Rapidly progressive glomerulonephritis
- Systemic lupus erythematosus
- Thrombotic thrombocytopenia
- Immunoproliferative diseases
- Multiple myeloma
- Waldenström's macroglobulinaemia
- Poisoning
  - Sickle cell disease

Some of these conditions become more severe in symptoms, and the availability of plasmapheresis could rapidly improve the patient's life. Its effectiveness in other conditions, such as meningococcal septicaemia, sepsis, Reye's syndrome, multiple sclerosis, polymyositis and dermatomyositis, is not as well recognized or established within the medical arena.

The Plasmapheresis Process

Plasmapheresis is a blood purification procedure. It is a process in which plasma, the fluid element of the blood, is removed from blood cells by a device known as a cell separator. The separator works either by spinning the blood at high speed to separate the cells from the fluid or by passing the blood through a membrane with minute pores that only plasma can pass through. The cells are returned to the person undergoing treatment, while the plasma, which contains the antibodies, is discarded and replaced with other fluids.

Plasmapheresis treatment:

- Requires insertion of a venous catheter, either in a limb or central vein, which allows higher flow rates and is more convenient for repeat procedures — complications, especially bacterial infection.
- Takes several hours and can also be undertaken on an outpatient basis, this is dependent on the patient's underlying disease and overall condition.
- It can be uncomfortable but is normally not painful.
- The number of treatments needed varies greatly depending on the particular disease and the person's general condition.
- An average course of plasma exchanges is 6—10 treatments over 2—10 weeks.
- Treatments vary according to clinician's preference; in some centres, treatments are performed once a week, while in others more than one treatment per week is performed.
- Consists of the removal of blood, separation of blood cells from plasma and return of these blood cells to the body's circulation, diluted with fresh plasma or a substitute.
- Because of concerns over viral infection and allergic reaction, fresh plasma is not routinely used. Instead, the most common substitute is saline solution with sterilized human albumin protein.
- During the course of a single session, 2—3 L of plasma are removed and replaced.

Plasmapheresis procedures available:

- Discontinuous flow centrifugation — only one venous catheter line is required, approximately 300 mL of blood is removed at a time and centrifuged to separate plasma from blood cells.
- Continuous flow centrifugation — two venous lines are used, requires slightly less blood volume to be out of the body at any one time.
- Plasma filtration — two venous lines are used, plasma is filtered using standard haemodialysis or haemofiltration equipment, discarded and replaced by an equal volume of replacement fluid, requires less than 100 mL of blood to be outside the body at one time.

Replacement Fluid

- This is when replacement fluid is given intravenously post plasmapheresis. What fluid is given is dependent on the centre involved.

- Some critical care environments give a plasma substitute, e.g., partial crystalloid replacement or 5% albumin.
- The only indication to replace plasma loss with all Fresh frozen plasma (FFP) is when plasmapheresis has been undertaken to replace missing plasma factors.

Risks Associated with Plasmapheresis

- Hypotension is the most common problem associated with plasmapheresis, which can be connected to episodes of faintness, dizziness, blurred vision, coldness and sweating or abdominal cramps.
- There is also circulatory instability in that there are intravascular volume changes and removal of circulating catecholamines and hypocalcaemia during plasmapheresis.
- Patients with clotting disorders may not be suitable candidates for plasmapheresis because anticoagulation therapy is required for plasmapheresis treatment.
- Bleeding can occur because of the anticoagulant given during the procedure to prevent the blood from clotting.
- Some of these medications can cause other adverse reactions, e.g., tingling around the mouth or in the limbs, muscle cramps or a metallic taste in the mouth. If left untreated, these reactions can lead to an irregular heartbeat or seizures.
- Can cause bleeding in that during the exchange there is removal of coagulation factors.
- An allergic reaction to the reinfusion of human plasma solutions used to replace the plasma can prove to be life-threatening. This type of anaphylactic reaction usually begins with itching, fever, chills, wheezing or a rash. In such a case, the plasma exchange must be stopped and the person treated with IV medications.
- Excessive suppression of the immune system can temporarily occur, as plasmapheresis removes all of the immune system antibodies used to fight infection and as such is not selective. In time, the body can replenish its supply of needed antibodies, but some physicians give these intravenously after each plasmapheresis treatment.
- Care must be taken in relation to asepsis and infection control strategies when treating this group of patients so not to increase their susceptibility to infections. Bacterial infection is a real risk, especially when a central venous catheter is used. Infection can be further precipitated by the fact that plasmapheresis can reduce plasma opsonization.
- Medication dosages need careful observation and adjustment in people being treated with plasmapheresis because some drugs can be removed from the blood or changed by the procedure.

Improvement in Condition

This can sometimes be evident within days, especially in myasthenia gravis. In other autoimmune conditions, especially where there is extensive tissue damage, improvement is much slower but can still be noticeable within weeks.

Effects of plasmapheresis commonly last up to several months, although longer lasting effects are possible.

Transplantation

Transplants are one of the most miraculous achievements of modern medicine. They involve the donation of tissue or organs from one person to another and enable people to take on a new lease of life in the United Kingdom every year.

Types of Transplants:

- Autograft — tissue from one to oneself — skin grafts or coronary artery bypass grafts
- Allografts — organ or tissue between the same species, most human tissue and organ transplant are allografts
- Isografts — organ or tissue between identical twins — although identical allografts the transplant does not trigger an immune response
- Split transplants — an organ for transplant usually the liver can be split between two recipients, an adult to children
- Domino transplants — lungs and heart are transplanted but only the lungs are needed, e.g., cystic fibrosis, the heart is then transplanted into someone else

Transplants are the best possible treatment for most people with organ failure.

Kidney transplants are the most commonly performed. Transplants of the heart, liver and lungs are also regularly carried out. As medicine advances, other vital organs including the pancreas and small bowel are also being used in transplants. Tissue such as corneas, heart valves, skin and bone can also be donated.

The increasing effectiveness of transplantation means that many more patients can be considered for treatment in this way. But there is a serious shortage of donors. For some people, this means waiting, sometimes for years, and undergoing difficult and stressful treatment. For all too many, it means they will die before a suitable organ becomes available.

Organs that can be Transplanted:

Chest

- Kidney
- Heart
- Heart and lung

Abdomen

- Liver
- Lungs
- Pancreas
- Intestine
- Stomach
- Testes

Tissues, cells and fluids

- Hand
- Cornea
- Skin
- Islets of Langerhans
- Bone marrow
- Heart valves
- Bone

Donors are Either Living or Dead

- A live donor donates renewable tissue, cell or fluid or organ, such as kidney, partial liver, lung lobe.
- Deceased donor has been declared brain-dead and the organ(s) are excised for transplantation.

Transplant Rejection

- Minutes to hours after the transplant and the organ has to be removed
- Days, weeks or months after transplant, usually mediated by specific
- T-cell immunity, which attack the transplant organ
- Month to years after the transplant, commonly observed in lung transplants

Symptoms of Rejection:

- Pain at the site of transplant
- Feeling generally unwell
- Flu-like symptoms
- High temperature/fever
- Changes in weight
- Swelling
- Reduction in urine output

Intra-Aortic Balloon Pump

The intra-aortic balloon pump (IABP) provides support for the left ventricle by assisting a failing heart. It does this by mechanically displacing blood within the aorta lowering the systolic BP and raising the diastolic BP. This invasive technique gives support to the heart during such crises as:

- Impending myocardial infarction or myocardial infarction
- Left ventricular failure or insufficiency
- Inability to be removed from cardiopulmonary bypass following open heart surgery
- Cardiogenic shock
- Severe angina with intractable ventricular arrhythmias
- Unstable angina
- Severe ischaemic changes on the 12-lead ECG

By providing extra oxygen and nutrients in the blood to the threatened heart muscle and reducing the needs for oxygen by decreasing the work of the heart, the balloon pump allows time for surgical and medical interventions and for the body's own healing powers to restore the heart to life-sustaining function. The catheter is inserted into the femoral artery and passed up into the descending thoracic aorta so that the tip of the catheter lies just below the subclavian artery.

The IABP helps a patient who has suffered an insult or injury to the myocardium in two ways:

1. It increases blood flow to the coronary arteries, thereby increasing oxygen supply to the myocardium.
2. It decreases the workload of the heart by lowering pressure in the aorta.

Coronary artery blood flow is increased when the IABP inflates and displaces a 30–40 mL volume of blood. The workload of the heart is decreased when the left ventricle ejects blood into the aorta where a previously inflated balloon has just deflated. The balloon should be deflated throughout the length of systole and inflated during diastole.

Balloon Deflation

- Occurs during ventricular systole
- Lowers the systolic pressure the ventricle has to generate, decreasing the demand for oxygen by the myocardial muscle
- Decreases afterload of the ventricle and systolic pressure

Balloon Inflation

- Occurs during diastolic to eject blood into the coronary, hepatic, renal, femoral arteries
- Slows down heart rate
- Increases diastolic BP to allow more time for gas exchange in the capillaries and filling of the chambers of the heart

Complications

- Vessel damage — trauma of the aorta, iliac and femoral arteries during IABP insertion. As the catheter is advanced, it may dislodge arteriosclerotic plaques anywhere along the way.
- Peripheral emboli — most frequently encountered problem, any foreign body in the bloodstream enhances clot formation around it.
- Decreased circulation to the leg — common in critical care patients with small femoral arteries or arteries narrowed by atherosclerotic disease. The leg muscles and peripheral nerves are most sensitive to anoxia, and paralysis and numbness quickly develop.

Problems with the IABP

- Early inflation of the IABP will interfere with aortic valve closure and possibly cause regurgitation in the left ventricle.
- Late inflation of the IABP will not maximize the effect of IABP.
- Late deflation of the IABP will interfere with the onset of the next systole.
- Early deflation of the IABP will not maximize the effects of IABP therapy.
- Leaking of the balloon — if this is suspected then the pump should be turned off.

Dressings to the insertion sites must be changed aseptically.

Special care Considerations

- IABP insertion is an invasive procedure performed by trained healthcare professional. This can either be performed within a theatre setting, cardiac laboratory or CCU/ICU setting.
- If the patient is awake, they should be informed of the procedure, the results that might be obtained/expected, information regarding quality of life and full knowledge of the course of the treatment and the disease process.
- If the patient is asleep, the attending medical staff must, when appropriate, inform the patient's next of kin of the procedure, the results that might be obtained/expected, give information regarding their quality of life and full knowledge of the course of treatment and disease process.
- The area of skin is prepared and draped with sterile towels and a local anaesthetic is administered.
- The IABP catheter is inserted percutaneously through the femoral artery route after the initial guide wire is inserted. Following predilation, the IABP catheter can be advanced over the guide wire, through the subcutaneous tissue and into the arterial system. Following insertion, an X-ray

should be taken to ensure proper positioning in the descending thoracic aorta distal to the left subclavian artery. Ideally, the tip of the IABP should be 2–3 cm below the left subclavian artery and the proximal portion of the membrane should be above the renal arteries in the femorally inserted balloon.

- Once the position of the IABP has been confirmed by the medical staff, IABP therapy may commence.
- The inflation and deflation phase settings are set by the medical staff.
- Regular observations must be carried out to detect early signs of shock, infection.
- Antithrombotic therapy will commence and regular monitoring of blood coagulpathy must be carried out.
- Patients will require assistance to move and gain comfortable position and they will also require assistance with hygiene needs.
- Appropriate pain assessment, analgesia and psychological support must be provided.

Mechanical Circulatory Support

The purpose of mechanical circulatory support by using a ventricular assist device (VAD) is to either supplement the left ventricle when it is not performing well or to completely replace left ventricular function. A VAD will increase the amount of blood that flows out from the left ventricle through the systemic circulation and back to the right side of the heart. The reasoning behind mechanical circulatory support is as a

- Bridge to transplantation
- Bridge to recovery
- Permanent basis 'destination therapy'

Indications for Ventricular Assist Device Therapy

- Escalating inotropic support
- Used to bridge recovery in myocarditis
- Coronary syndromes
- Congenital disorders
- Cardiomyopathy where the treatment is used as a bridge to transplantation
- Post cardiotomy where it is difficult to wean the cardiopulmonary bypass post surgery

Patient Care Receiving Ventricular Assist Device Therapy

- Respiratory management – wean from ventilatory support
- Haemodynamic monitoring – this includes: heart rate (HR), arterial blood pressure (ABP), central venous pressure (CVP), pulmonary artery pressure (PAP), cardiac output (CO)

- Monitoring of VAD values/function
- Monitor renal monitoring − urine output, renal function
- Close monitoring of fluid management − input and output
- Monitor abdominal function − risk of reduced gut motility, nutritional problems
- Drug management − weaning of inotropic support, anticoagulation therapy
- Reduced mobilization − passive and active leg exercises, cardiac rehabilitation programme
- Haematological monitoring − coagulation, full blood count (FBC)
- Infection control management − care of IV access, use of antibiotic therapy, use of appropriate dressing to minimize infection risk, hand washing
- Psychological management − use of multi-disciplinary team (MDT) in promoting rehabilitation and social care and minimizing any worries regarding finances

Complications of Ventricular Assist Device Therapy

- Air emboli intraoperatively
- Haemorrhage
- Neurological damage due to thromboembolic complications
- Impaired renal function
- Right-sided heart failure
- Infection from entry site of VAD access
- Reduced gut motility, nausea and vomiting
- Mechanical failure
- Psychosocial issues related to VAD therapy

Extracorporeal Membrane Oxygenation

This was the first form of extra-corporeal gas exchange to be used, but has proved less successful in the treatment of adults than in the treatment of neonates. Extracorporeal membrane oxygenation (ECMO) works on the principle of giving the lungs a chance to rest and heal by taking over the supply of oxygen and the removal of carbon dioxide from the lungs. Thus, ECMO oxygenates the blood outside the body.

ECMO consists of an extracorporeal veno-arterial circulation with high blood flows being circulated via a gas exchange membrane, this ensures that the majority of the body's gas exchange requirements are achieved and maintained so that there is a preservation of life. A main disadvantage of ECMO is that it requires the insertion of large-bore cannulae and high corporeal blood flows. This combination predisposes patients to a potentially high risk of cell damage, infection and blood disorders.

The main aim of ECMO is to supply the body with oxygen by pumping blood from a major vein, oxygenating it, and then returning it to a major artery.

Carbon dioxide is removed as a result. ECMO can deliver nearly all of the body's oxygen supply at rest; to achieve this, very large flows of blood are needed through the extracorporeal circuit, usually 50% or more of cardiac output.

Indications and Criteria for Extracorporeal Membrane Oxygenation

- Failure to sustain adequate gas exchange, despite maximum critical care support
- Rapid failure of ventilatory support despite FiO_2 (fraction of inspired oxygen) 1.0
- Slow failure of ventilatory support despite a recognized period of critical care management

Extracorporeal Membrane Oxygenation Contraindications

- Chronic lung disease, which includes any major organ, e.g., emphysema.
- Lung failure >7 days − Acute respiratory distress syndrome (ARDS)
- Burns >40% body surface
- Other organ failure(s), including lung failure

Extracorporeal CO₂ Removal

Extracorporeal CO_2 removal ($ECCO_2R$) is an extracorporeal veno-venous circulatory device, which allows for the clearance of CO_2 via a gas exchange membrane. It involves reducing the level of carbon dioxide in the blood to reduce the risk of lung injury with mechanical ventilation.

Low blood flows are adopted so that partial oxygenation support is achieved. Low-frequency positive-pressure ventilation is typically used with $ECCO_2R$ with the adoption of continuous oxygenation delivery throughout inspiration and expiration. The lungs are held in expiration with high positive end expiratory pressure (PEEP) levels (20−25 cm H_2O), limited peak airway pressures (35−40 cm H_2O), with a continuous fresh gas supply. Therefore, the lungs are rested so that recovery from any pulmonary problems may occur.

NICE guidelines (2016) recommend that clinicians wishing to use $ECCO_2R$ should

- Inform the clinical governance leads in their trusts
- Ensure the patient, carers, families understand the uncertain nature of the procedure, risks and provide written information
- Audit and review clinical outcomes

Nitric Oxide

Exogenous application of nitric oxide in the form of inhaled gas has been shown to be effective in relaxing smooth muscle to dilate blood vessels causing pulmonary vasodilatation. It can be used in

- Neonates with persistent pulmonary hypertension.
- Children with congenital heart disease.
- Adults with ARDS or severe asthma.

Despite the promising results with nitric oxide treatment, this has not demonstrated any improvement in patient survival.

3.3 CARING FOR A CRITICAL CARE PATIENT

The Unconscious Patient

Consciousness is an awareness of yourself and your surrounding environment. There are three properties of consciousness, which are affected by the disease process. These are

- Arousal or wakefulness mechanisms and intact cognitive functions
- Alertness or awareness
- Appropriate voluntary motor activity

  These processes require an intact

- Ascending reticular activating system contained within the brainstem (pons, midbrain) and diencephalon, vital to controlling respiration, cardiac rhythms and necessary for essential functions such as swallowing
- Cerebral cortex

  Any interruption along the pathway or disturbance in normal functioning results in a loss of consciousness or a transition from alert to comatose state.
  The causes of unconsciousness are endless and the recovery period would depend on the cause. The common causes of unconsciousness are

- Poison or drug overdose
- Post surgery or cardiac arrest
- Infections — meningitis, encephalitis, sepsis
- Neurological disorders, e.g., seizures, epilepsy, stroke, tumour
- Metabolic disorders, e.g., renal failure
- Trauma — head injury
- Organ failure — respiratory, liver, renal, heart
- Hypothermia, hypoglycaemia, hepatic encephalopathy

The critical care nurse should be aware of the cause of the patient's unconscious state and be observant for any deterioration in the patient's overall condition. Unconscious patients require total nursing care, as the patient's physical state will be dependent on the critical care nurse.

The key factors of caring for an unconscious patient are

- Establish and maintain a clear and patent airway — endotracheal tube (ETT), laryngeal mask airway (LMA), laryngeal airway
- Position patient to minimize aspiration
- Ensure emergency equipment is working and nearby
- Assess the patient's level of consciousness using the Glasgow coma scale (GCS) and record findings
- Record and evaluate patient's vital signs, temperature, pulse, respiratory and heart rate
- Administer oxygen, oxygen saturation monitoring/capnography, undertake arterial blood gases (ABGs)
- Deliver prescribed medication
- Maintain accurate fluid balance chart, IV fluids and urinary output, may require catheterisation; nutrition may require nasogastric tube
- Record 12-lead ECG
- Perform essential nursing care as appropriate to patient's condition, e.g., mouth and eye care
- Regular repositioning of patient as condition allows to promote pulmonary function
- Passive movements of limbs to reduce venous stasis

The skills required:

- Gentleness
- Patience
- Perseverance
- Understanding
- Involvement of the multi-disciplinary team

Immediate nursing care:

- To prevent deterioration of the patent's condition
- Care should be supportive and directed towards preventing complications and damage that may interfere with maximum rehabilitation
- To perform observations and interventions
- Physical nursing care:
  - Positioning — should not occur at 2-hourly intervals as there will be a continued increase in intracranial pressure
  - Airway maintenance, GCS, temperature, pulse, respiratory rate, blood pressure, and monitoring of urine output
  - Oxygen administration
  - Administration of fluids and nutrition
  - Eye care, mouth care, pressure area care, wound management
  - Administration of medications

- Observe reactions:
  - Depression
  - Inappropriate behaviour
  - Understanding and interpretation
  - Speech/swallowing difficulties
- Psychological care:
  - Sleep, sleep deprivation
  - Sensory overload, deprivation
  - Communication
  - Family plays a major role in facilitating the patient to regain functioning and independence

The care of the unconscious patient is geared towards the preservation of life and the avoidance of further complications. In addition to physiological effects, consideration must also be given to the patient's psychological state and the effects of coma on the patient, e.g., isolation, sleep and sensory deprivation and overload.

Pain

Pain is one of the main symptoms that cause people to seek treatment. Pain is synonymous with many conditions observed in critical care. Good pain control (90%; WHO, 1996) can be achieved with well-planned and executed pain management. However, there is a high incidence of patients needlessly experiencing moderate to severe levels of pain while in hospital. The standards of pain management in practice clearly need to be improved.

Pain Pathways

Pain is a sensation that is difficult to measure objectively. It

- Is a sensation that is evoked by the excitation of nerve cells in the brain
- Alerts individuals to damaging forces in the around the body
- Is associated with emotion more than any other sensation, e.g., anxiety, fear, alarm
- Prevents sleep
- Activates the reticular activating system in the brain

Characteristics of Pain

- Sharp, burning, crushing, throbbing
- The character and location of pain depends on
  - The type and situation of the receptors stimulated

- The pathways through which they are transmitted
- Their ultimate destination within the brain

Pain is innervated by autonomic and somatic nerve fibres and arises if there is

- Local ischaemia – angina
- Chemical damage – leakage of enzymes in the pancreas
- Spasm of smooth muscle – colic
- Over distension of a hollow organ – bladder
- Irritation of the peritoneum, pleura or pericardium
- Stimulation of the inflammatory immune response and release of mediators

  Pain related concepts

- Pain threshold – the lease experience of pain, which a subject can recognise
- Pain tolerance level – the greatest level of pain, which a subject is prepared to tolerate
- Hyperalgesia – pain amplification associated with a mild stimulus
- Dependency – experience of side effects with withdrawal of drug following constant exposure
- Addiction – behavioural problem due to compulsive use despite destructive consequences

Classifications of Pain

Pain Reception – Nociceptors

Several million bare sensory nerve endings weave through all tissues and organs of the body, except the brain. Respond to noxious stimuli (those that are damaging to normal tissue) – nociceptors. Injured tissue releases chemicals such as bradykinins, histamine and prostaglandins. ATP released by damaged cells also stimulates pain receptors. Nociceptors are located on A delta and C nerve fibres (Table 3.5); examples include

- Back and neck pain
- Musculoskeletal pain
- Headache
- Osteoarthritic pain
- Rheumatoid arthritic pain
- Postsurgical and trauma pain.

Pain Reception – Neuropathic

Neuropathic pain is caused by a functional or anatomical abnormality of the peripheral or central nervous system. Damaged nerves lead to pathophysiological

TABLE 3.5 Nociceptors and fibres.

Visceral pain – a delta fibres	Deep somatic pain - C fibres
Small myelinated axons 1–4 µm in diameter Conduct at a speed of 6–30 m per second Stimulates receptors in organs of the thorax or abdomen This is fast pain, which presents as • Sharp/dull ache • Piercing • Electric/electric shock • Needle in the skin • Tends to get better • Duration predictable and limited • Has meaning and purpose • Can be localised • Acute type pain	Small unmyelinated 0.1–1 µm in diameter Conduct at a speed of 0.5–2.0 m per second Deep skin layers, muscles or joints Long lasting This is slow pain, which presents as • Burning/aching/itching • Throbbing/nauseous • Associated with tissue destruction • Duration unpredictable • Tends to get worse • No meaning/obscure • Cannot be localised • Chronic type pain

changes resulting in a distortion or amplification of naturally generated signals. Usually described as burning or shooting pains; examples include

- Phantom limb pain
- Neuralgia
- Fibromyalgia
- Peripheral neuropathy
- Complex regional pain syndrome (previously known as reflex sympathetic dystrophy)

Under Management of Pain

Healthcare professionals:

- Poor knowledge of pain management
- Inappropriate attitudes (pain is inevitable due to condition)
- Poor clinical skills (assessing pain)
- Inappropriate beliefs regarding the management of pain (fears of addiction and tolerance to opiates)
- Lack of appreciation of the nonphysical manifestations of pain

Individual patients:

- Low expectations of pain and management and a belief that pain is inevitable
- Inappropriate beliefs regarding pain management strategies (fear of addiction and tolerance
- Beliefs that side effects of medication are inevitable (sedation)

The presence of pain can interfere with obtaining accurate and reliable measurements, which can mask signs of deterioration and lead to false inaccurate readings. Therefore, pain needs to be assessed early. Regular assessment of pain contributes to the quality of communication between nurse and patient and can be a contributory factor in ensuring effective pain relief therapies.

Prior to effective treatment of pain, accurate assessment is essential. Because of the subjective nature of pain, only patients can measure their own pain accurately and so critical care nurses should provide tools to help them assess and communicate their pain; assessment tools can be invaluable in aiding improvement in pain management.

Hygiene Requirements of Critical Care Patients

Patients cared for within a critical care setting, particularly those who are sedated or unconscious, are unable to care for their personal hygiene. As a result, it falls upon the bedside nurse to meet their individual needs. Critical care patients have specific hygiene needs due to the very nature of their often sedated or unconscious state.

General Hygiene

There is some evidence that washing critical care patients at night rather than in the morning is beneficial. However, there are a number of factors, which need to be taken into account before deciding what time is suitable for the patient to be washed. Whatever time is chosen to wash the patient, it must be remembered that regular mouth care, eye care and pressure area care must be performed.

The events leading to washing the patient may be influenced by factors such as whether the patient is sedated. If the patient is not sedated then it is for the bedside nurse to negotiate with the patient when the best time may be. Night-time washes are often encouraged in ICU because it ensures that a patient's energy is conserved for morning activities such as ventilatory weaning, extubation and physiotherapy. Early night-time washes are beneficial as they facilitate long periods of uninterrupted rest to counteract the effects of sleep deprivation and sensory overload.

Always think about the appropriateness of the wash and the effect it will have on your patient's rest and sleep pattern.

All patients on the critical care receive prophylaxis or treatment to try and control the spread of MRSA on the unit. This includes using a special wash for all non-colonised patients and chlorhexidine wash for those who are colonized. It is very important that all chlorhexidine is washed off the patient's skin after they have been treated; if it is not it can cause severe skin reactions.

Mouth Care on a Ventilated Patient

Critical care patients are vulnerable to problems associated with their mouths, which are a well-known complication of ventilation. Care of the mouth is the scientific care of teeth and mouth. The aim of oral care is to

- Keep the mucosa clean, soft, moist and intact to prevent infection
- Keep lips clean, soft, moist and intact to prevent excessive dryness and cracking
- The promotion and maintenance of patient comfort by alleviating pain and discomfort
- The prevention of dental plaque formation and colonisation of bacteria
- The reduction of problems associated with dry mouth and the early identification of problems that may require medical treatment

Drug therapies such as steroids may increase the pathogenicity of these organisms, leading to local and systemic infections. Oral complications can lead to pain, ulcers, infection, bone and dentition changes and bleeding and functional disorders affecting verbal and non-verbal communication, chewing and swallowing, taste and respiration. Therefore, mouth care is an important element of critical care nursing care. See assessment tool for mouth care guidance (Table 3.6).

The oral cavity harbours many varieties of bacteria, which do not normally pose any problems; immunosuppression and systemic treatment such as cytotoxic, antifungal, radiation therapy and steroids may increase the pathogenicity of these organisms leading to local infection. Oral complications can lead to pain, ulcers, infection, bone and dentition changes and bleeding. Functional disorders affect verbal and non-verbal communication, chewing and swallowing, taste and respiration can also occur. Therefore, mouth care is an important part of nursing care practice.

Eye Care

Eye care of patients within critical care is paramount in preventing eye damage and infection. Normal protective mechanisms like blinking and tear production are often impaired in patients who are receiving sedative drugs or are

TABLE 3.6 Oral hygiene assessment tool.

Category	Scores (*if score 1 or 2 for any category please arrange for a hygienist or dentist to assess the patient)			Category scores
	0 = healthy	1 = changes*	2 = unhealthy*	
Lips	Soft, pink and moist	Dry, chapped, red at the edges	Swelling, ulcerated or bleeding	
Tongue	Pink, moist, rough	Coated, red, swollen, fissured	Patches of red or white, swollen, ulcerated	
Gums and surrounding tissue	Pint, moist, smooth, no bleeding or receding gums	Dry, red, swollen, ulcer or sore area, check under dentures	Swollen, bleeding, ulcers, white or red patches, check under dentures	
Saliva	Normal production, watery	Dry, little saliva flow, patient complaining of a dry mouth	Tissues parched and red, little/no saliva production, saliva is thick, patient says they have a dry mouth	
Teeth: Patients' own	Free from tooth decay, no broken or chipped teeth,	1–3 decayed or broken teeth, some roots showing	4+ decayed or broken teeth, roots showing	
Dentures	Intact no broken or damaged areas, fit well, worn daily	1 broken area, painful, worn 1–2 hours throughout the day	1+ broke area, non-fitting dentures need adhesive, lost or not worn	
Oral hygiene	Clean no food debris, no tartar build up in mouth or on dentures	Contains food particles, tartar, plaque in 1–2 areas or on dentures	Contains food particles, tartar, plaque in nearly all areas of the mouth and on dentures	
Pain	No pain expressed by the patient, no behavioural signs	Patient is expressing pain (pain assessment required), behavioural signs, e.g., not eating	Physical signs of pain, e.g., swelling of gums, cheeks, ulcers; verbal and behavioural signs pulling at face, aggression	

Tick this box if the patient has been referred to a hygienist or dentist after oral assessment. □
Modified from Chalmers, J.M., Spencer, A.J., Carter, K.D., King, P.L., Wright, C., 2009. Caring for oral health in Australian residential care. Dental statistics and research series no. 48. Cat. no. DEN 193. AIHW, Canberra.

unconscious. In an unconscious patient, the blink reflex is lost and the eyes are not flushed or cleaned. Eye care is essential for an unconscious patient:

1. Maintain healthy eyes
2. To prevent infection
3. To promote patient comfort

It is important to note that eye infections in this vulnerable group can result in permanent damage to the eye, e.g., loss of vision. Red, inflamed or oedematous eyes will result in patients becoming distressed and agitated and they may be experiencing pain. In turn, this is also upsetting for their relatives and visitors to critical care.

Therefore, a good assessment and delivery of eye care is an important part of nursing care. Eye care involves

- Examining your patient's eyes regularly. If the patient is conscious and able to interact make sure that you get their permission and explain what you are doing.
- If the patient's eyes are clean and they have an intact blink reflex then it is acceptable to leave them and reassess every few hours.
- Look for any discharge or cloudiness, ulceration or scratching of the cornea and assess the blink reflex (this may be absent in sedated patients). Note any differences between the eyes or changes from any previous documented assessments.
- If there is evidence of red eye, cloudiness, ulceration or discharge, report this immediately so that an appropriate medical referral can be made.
- If the eyes appear to need cleaning (they may be 'crusty' or have a discharge) clean the eye with sterile water. Wipe from the inner part of the eye (closest to the nose) to the outer part to remove any discharge or 'crust'. Use a new piece of gauze for each pass and treat the upper lid before the lower. Always wash your hands before beginning this procedure and when moving from cleaning one eye to the other. Always treat a clean eye before one that appears to have a problem.
- If the patient's eyes appear dry, speak to the medical staff about the use of appropriate drops or ointment.

Unconscious patient's eyes must be inspected, cleaned and hydrated regularly to prevent complications.

Eye Care Procedure

- The equipment required is two gallipots (one for the left eye and one for the right eye), sterile gauze and water.
- *Cleaning.* Use each piece of gauze once only, clean from the inside out.
- It should be undertaken at least four times daily for patients without any problem.
- *Observation.* Every 2-hourly, look for redness, discharge or corneal clouding; in these instances, eye care should be increased.
- *Eye drops.* Artificial tears (hypromellose, Viscotears); these are not routinely used but prescribed if corneal wetting is inadequate. There should be two bottles of eye drops one for each eye and clearly labelled L and R.
- *Antibiotics.* May be needed if the eye(s) are red or discharge is present, a conjunctival swab may be required to be sent for microscopy, culture and sensitivity (MC&S).
- *Geliperm.* This may be used to keep the eye closed, as it will not cause trauma or irritation, reduces tear evaporation, prevents infection and keeps eyelids closed and its transparency allows constant observation.

Risk factors for ventilated patients:

- Exposure to keratopathy — caused by incomplete lid closure.
- Dry eyes — drug- or exposure-induced.
- Infection — mostly pathogens from the respiratory tract (*Pseudomonas* and pneumococcus).
- Ventilator eye — conjunctival chemosis (oedema) caused by intermittent positive pressure ventilation (IPPV) and PEEP.

Wound Care

A wound can be due to a surgical procedure, insertion of drain, e.g., chest drain, or device, e.g., IV-line, trauma or formation of a pressure ulcer.

Structure of the Skin

The skin is one of the largest organs of the body and it occupies a surface area of approximately 2 square metres (Guyton and Hall, 2016). It can be divided into two main parts:

The epidermis is composed of mainly stratified squamous epithelial tissue and four major types of cell:

- Keratinocytes
- Melanocytes
- Langerhans cells
- Granstein cells

The dermis is composed of primarily connective tissue containing collagenous and elastic fibres. Other structures found in the surrounding regions are

- Blood supply
- Lymph vessels
- Sensory nerve endings
- Sweat glands and ducts
- Hair, root and follicles
- Sebaceous glands
- Arrectores pilorum

Functions of the Skin

When intact, the skin essentially forms a barrier between the external and internal environments of the body. Its main functions are

- *Protection* – against invasion by foreign and bacterial matter
- *Perception of stimuli* – enables constant monitoring of the external environment
- *Absorption* – allows certain topical compounds, such as drugs, to be absorbed
- *Synthesis of vitamin D* – synthesized by the body as a result of direct exposure to ultraviolet radiation
- *Maintenance of body temperature* – through metabolic processes, the body is continuously producing heat. This is primarily dissipated via the skin, facilitated by three processes:
  - *Radiation* – the ability of the body to give off its heat to another object of lower temperature
  - *Conduction* – the transfer of heat from the body to a cooler object in contact with it
  - *Convection* – the movement of warm air molecules away from the body
- *Water balance* – approximately 500 mL of fluid is lost each day, 'insensible loss', through evaporation

Healing Process

The healing process includes three classifications of healing:

- Healing by *primary intention* – the skin edges are brought together with the aid of suture or skin staples (surgical wounds) or Steri-Strips (minor trauma).
- Healing by *secondary intention* – the skin edges are deliberately not brought together. This is done in order to promote granulation tissue from the base of the wound. Common practice in chronic wounds.
- Healing by *tertiary intention* – a previously sutured wound that has dehisced and has been resutured.

Phases of Healing

There are three phases of wound healing which are continuous, overlapping and merging with the next:

- *The inflammatory phase* — the formation of a blood clot, loosely uniting the wound edges and stimulating the inflammatory response and leading to the characteristic appearance of a wound, e.g., swelling, heat, redness and pain, facilitating healing and repair (0—3 days).
- *The regenerative phase* — the tissue starts to fill and granulation tissue starts the process of wound contraction. The signs of inflammation start to subside, but the wound may be raised in relation to surrounding tissues (0—24 days).
- *The maturation phase* — the process of re-epithelialization begins. The scab should now drop off, as the epidermis is restored to its natural thickness (21 months up to 2 years).

Wound Management

Management for patients with wounds can be both challenging and time consuming, as treatments can be both complex and diverse.

Wound Drainage

This is an abnormal opening in the skin that produces exudates or drainage, which may be caused by disease, trauma or surgery. All drainage should be accurately measured and recorded on the fluid balance chart. Colour, consistency as well as odour and drug therapy must also be noted in the nursing care plan.

Common types of wound or surgical drains are

- *Corrugated strips of rubber*, e.g., Yeats drain — used primarily to drain exudates from fat layers, subcutaneous tissues and occasionally the peritoneal cavity. They guide exudates onto a surface dressing, can be messy and affect normal skin. Application of stoma bag to collect drainage is often used to prevent skin irritation and minimize mess.
- *Tubes and catheter type drains*, e.g., Robinson drain — are the most effective type of drain and can be connected to a closed drainage bag system.
- *Suction drainage systems* — these may involve a closed suction system; ideal for removal of blood and serous fluid, e.g., Redivac drains or under water sealed drains for thoracic surgery.

Ensure that all drains are secured properly so that they are not accidentally dislodged.

Wound Dressing Materials

In order to undertake appropriate and effective wound, drainage and IV line site management strategies, knowledge and understanding of the skin structure and the normal wound healing process is vital. In addition, the ICU nurse should be able to recognize the various stages of wound healing and assess the wound using a recognized and tested assessment tool. Important factors that should be taken into account when choosing a wound dressing are

Best dressing — the ideal dressing should ensure that the wound remains

- Moist with exudates but not saturated
- Free from clinical infection and excessive slough
- Free from toxic chemical particles or fibres released from dressing
- Kept at an optimum temperature for healing to take place
- Not exposed to unnecessary disturbance or wound dressing changes
- Kept at an optimum pH level

Classification of Wound Dressings

Nurses are often restricted to use what is available. However, with the wide range of dressings available, there must be similar alternatives. Wound dressings are classified by their primary functions.

Film membranes are

- Permeable to water vapour and oxygen
- Impermeable to water and microorganisms
- Provide a warm and moist environment
- Comfortable and convenient as they provide a direct observation

Alginates are used to fill cavities and sinuses. They are useful around drainage sites, as they absorb exudates and serous fluid and can easily be removed by irrigation methods.

Foams absorb exudate, which then evaporates into the cells of the dressing and is lost as water vapour. They are also non-adherent.

Hydrogels swell when wet and can retain significant proportions of water within their structure. Their role is to

- Rehydrate wounds
- Debride and clean
- Be painless when applying and removing
- Be soothing

Hydrocolloids. This type of dressing withdraws warm fluid to form a gel that produces a moist environment on the wound surface in order to facilitate healing.

Additional Wound Therapies

Not all wound dressing materials are suited to all wound types, in particular, wounds that are non-healing or copiously draining wounds. However, an alternative method is available in such wounds, the vacuum assisted wound closure system (VAC). This system is often considered when conventional methods have been ineffective.

The VAC system offers

- A closed, noninvasive, active therapy system.
- Negative pressure, which increases the effectiveness of the local wound circulation.
- Active removal of excessive exudates, reducing oedema and haematoma formation.
- Assists with the control of wound leakage.
- Promotes angiogenesis.

Pressure Ulcers

The formation of a pressure ulcer is a complication within a critical care setting and is a real concern among practitioners. A pressure ulcer once formed becomes an open wound and wound management interventions apply.

Pressure ulcers are injuries to the skin and underlying tissue, primarily caused by prolonged pressure on the skin surface. They can occur in critical care patients due to long periods of time confined to bed. Pressure ulcers are common in bony parts of the body, e.g., back of the head, base of the spine, hips, elbows, heels. They can develop over a long period of time or in just a few hours.

Prevention

- Pressure area risk assessment and early application of special mattress or bed
- Regular changing of the patients position
- Checking of the skin integrity to determine early recognition
- Ensure the critical care patient is obtaining nutrition

Grading and symptoms of pressure ulcers:

Grade 1 — discolouration of the skin — red, dark purple or blue patches, usually non-blanching when pressed
Grade 2 — a blister or open wound appears — loss of dermis
Grade 3 — the wound reaches the deeper layers of the skin — full thickness loss
Grade 4 — a very deep wound that can reach muscle and bone

Patients who are at risk of developing pressure ulcers:

- Patients of age 70 years or older
- Bedridden, unable to mobilise, e.g., paralysis, surgery, pain

- Obesity
- Urinary and/or bowel incontinence
- Malnutrition
- Medical conditions − diabetes, peripheral vascular disease, heart or kidney failure, MS
- Polypharmacy

Measures that facilitate the healing of pressure ulcers:

- May require regular cleaning of the wound, a special dressing to facilitate the healing process, removal of damaged tissue
- Ensure the patient is turned regularly from side to side
- Manage nutrition and ensure sufficient calories EF or PN
- The use of specially designed mattresses and/or support surfaces

Specialist Support Surfaces

Pressure ulcer formation is a complication within a critical care setting is a real concern among practitioners. Specialist beds are available within the critical setting that prevent pressure by evenly distributing the patient's body weight over their bony prominences whilst giving bodily support. Specialist beds are designed to constantly change areas of pressure by keeping the patient in continual motion against the bed surface. Certain types of beds facilitate turning while maintaining body alignment and by using specialist beds the problems of

- Shearing
- Friction
- Pressure points being squashed against conventional surfaces can be addressed

In using specialist beds in the care of the critically ill attempts are being made to reduce the pressure exerted on pressure points and thus decrease capillary occlusion pressures. It is important to note that in the majority of critical care patients frequent turning and repositioning alone suffice.

Factors influencing decision for specialist bed:

- Cardiovascular instability, e.g., extreme episodes of hypotension on turning
- Respiratory instability, e.g., extreme episodes of desaturation on turning
- Decreased skin integrity, e.g., severe burns
- Malnourishment
- Receiving vasconstrictive drug therapy
- Extreme weight, e.g., too thin or obese
- Invasive equipment preventing adequate turning, e.g., ECMO, LVAD, RVAD

Despite the advent of pressure relieving aids and specialist mattresses and beds, it remains the case that an immobile patient that is not regularly turned can develop pressure ulcers in time.

Indications for Kinetic Therapy or Continuous Lateral to Lateral Rotational Therapy

Kinetic or lateral to lateral rotational therapy (rotational therapy) treatment is generally indicated for high-risk patients within a critical care setting who are vulnerable to respiratory-associated complications due to immobility and/or prolonged ventilation.

Furthermore, rotational therapy should be considered in all mechanically ventilated patients who are at a high risk of developing pulmonary-related complications. These are

- Increased pulmonary shunt
- Atelectasis
- Pneumonia or lower respiratory pneumonia
- ARDS

  Criteria to discontinue rotational therapy/lateral to lateral rotation:

- Stable and satisfactory improvement in oxygenation
- Patient extubated
- Patient is able to sit out of bed
- 'Do not resuscitate' order

Positioning

Repositioning of unconscious and conscious patients within a critical care setting is a fundamental and essential care element that critical care nurses undertake on a regular basis. It is important to stress the need to correctly position and reposition patients frequently as their physical condition allows.

The major effect of unconsciousness is on patient's body movement. With this decreased movement, an unconscious patient becomes vulnerable to skin breakdown due to problems associated with pressure, moisture, shearing forces and diminished sensation. However, this is not to say that conscious patients are not also at risk of the complications of immobility, e.g., pressure sores and respiratory complications.

The patient should be turned from side to side in the lateral or semi-prone position at least every 2 hours, unless contraindicated. The reason for regular repositioning is so that there is a change to the distribution of ventilation and blood flow through the lungs and mobilization of secretions. This will also have an enhanced effect on the cardiopulmonary system in that changing ventilation and perfusion of the lungs through gravitational effects enhances oxygen transportation.

Log Rolling

The 'log roll' technique is used when there are concerns about the stability of the spinal column and that damage may be caused by the traditional turning manoeuvre. This technique is a labour-intensive process and requires numerous individuals: one to support the head and two on either side of the patient. A modified 'log rolling' technique is also used when nursing patients prone; like log rolling, it is a labour-intensive process and requires experienced staff to prevent further complications, e.g., extubation.

Procedure

- The individual at the head end of the bed should be a qualified nurse or doctor experienced in log rolling and airway management.
- The other four individuals will manage the torso, arms and legs.
- When everyone is in position and ready for the manoeuvre, the leader will indicate when turning is to take place.

In terms of priority of care, the golden rule is to prevent episodes of prolonged pressure. With current technology, numerous preventative tools that can help identify and offer solutions to prevent further complications.

Prone Positioning in Critical Care

Positioning of the critical care patient is a fundamental and essential care element that the bedside nurse undertakes on a daily basis. It is important to stress the need to correctly position and reposition patients frequently in order to decrease the development of pressure sores and reduce respiratory complications.

The use of the prone position within critical care has been used to optimize gaseous exchange in the respiratory compromised patient (Fig. 3.1). Traditionally the use of the prone position was not used often because of

- Fears of healthcare practitioners about performing manoeuvre
- Risk of dislodging infusion lines
- Anxieties surrounding the movement of the neck
- Fears of placing patient's face in an inaccessible position
- Inadequate nursing ratios to manoeuvre patient
- Manual handling issues

Factors that Determine Prone Position

- Problems with patient oxygenation
- Unable to access patient's airway

- Unable to provide adequate hygiene
- Skin care issues
- Increase in facial oedema
- Increase pressure to patient's pressure points
- Requirement to use muscle relaxant to manoeuvre patient and keep them nursed prone
- Nursing ratio

Complication of Prone Position

- Causes hypotension due to inferior vena cava compression
- Risk of nerve compression
- Risk of crush injuries
- Increased risk of venous stasis
- Airway security compromised
- Diaphragmatic limitations due to patient's prone position
- Increased risk of dislodging access lines
- Increased risk of retinal damage
- Increased risk of mucosal breakdown
- Increased risk of unplanned extubation

Contraindications

- Shock
- Acute bleeding
- Multiple trauma patients
- Spinal instability
- Pregnancy (second/third trimester)
- Raised intracranial pressure
- Recent abdominal surgery
- Recent stoma formation
- Unstable thorax/open chest
- Seizures

Procedure

See Fig. 3.1.

The prone position should only be undertaken by practitioners who are familiar with the manoeuvre to minimise complications.

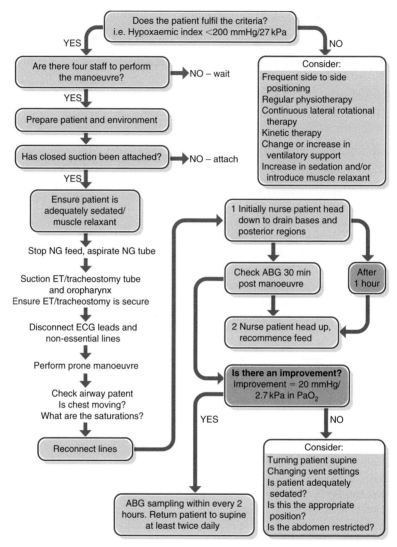

FIGURE 3.1 Moving patient into the prone position. Recommendations for practice: guidelines for moving the patient into the prone position. *ABGs*, five arterial blood gases; *ECG*, electrocardiogram; *ET*, endotracheal; *NG*, nasogastric.

Early Mobilization

Early and progressive mobilization is an important aspect of caring for critical care patients. Mobilization is an extension of the physiological principles of turning and repositioning patients who are confined to their bed.

Reasons for early mobilization:

- Encourages ventilation
- Increases perfusion
- Promotes mobilization of secretions
- Promotes oxygenation
- Decreases venous pooling
- Improves functional residual capacity (FRC)
- Improves patient's psychological state

When and how critical care patients are mobilized is decided on an individual basis in conjunction with the critical care nurse, doctor, physiotherapist and patient. With the advent of specialist chairs and hoists, patients are often mobilized at an early stage. If the physiological condition allows, ventilatory weaning has commenced and sedation has been reduced, there is no reason why a patient cannot be stood up, sat in a chair, encouraged to wiggle their toes and contract calf muscles.

3.4 INTUBATION AND VENTILATION

Physiology

Type 1 Respiratory Failure

- Respiratory alkalosis − normal homeostatic mechanisms and response to an initial increase in CO_2
- Oxygenation is maintained due to increased respiratory rate and depth of breathing, with hypocapnia generally requires supplementary oxygen
- Pulmonary oedema/chest infections/asthma may cause hypoxia but less likely to affect CO_2 removal

Type 2 Respiratory Failure

- Respiratory acidosis − not maintaining homeostasis ventilatory failure with hypoxia combined with hypercapnia
- Indicates homeostastic mechanisms are no longer responding − ventilation required
- Respiratory rate >30/min, cyanosis/tachycardia >110/min, peak flow <33%
- May require additional ventilatory support due to possible exhaustion and hypoventilation

Noninvasive Ventilation

Noninvasive ventilation (NIV) is the delivery of mechanical ventilation, which uses a technique that does not require artificial ventilation, e.g., ETT or TT. Artificial ventilation is invasive and creates complications and is generally confined to specialist areas (Butler, 2005). However, NIV creates fewer complications and is increasingly being used as an effective treatment on acute/specialist wards to provide support for patients with chronic respiratory failure. This includes critical care.

Critical care nurses need the knowledge and skills to care safely for patients receiving NIV.

Conditions where NIV may be considered:

- Acute respiratory failure – hypercapnic respiratory failure (RF)
- Chronic obstructive pulmonary disease – these prevent the use of mechanical ventilation. NIV is a cost effective, successful treatment
- Asthma – not conclusive, literature is controversial, more studies needed
- Acute cardiogenic pulmonary oedema – effective treatment with evidence of quick recovery
- Palliative care – to relieve suffering at the end of life
- Cystic fibrosis
- Upper airway obstruction

Domiciliary NIV:

- Prevents breathlessness in patients not admitted to hospital
- Enables patients with ventilatory failure to have a good quality of life

Breathing involves muscular work and consumes O_2 – at rest, 1%–3% of total body O_2 consumption. If more used for respiratory muscles less for heart and brain aggravating tissue hypoxia. In respiratory failure management, one goal is to reduce the work of breathing and improve tissue O_2 supply.

Terminology includes

- Noninvasive positive pressure ventilation (NIPPV)
- Trademark names such as NIPPY and bi-level positive airway pressure (BiPAP)
- Nasal ventilation
- BTS (2016) guidelines use NIV to describe all types of noninvasive ventilatory support, including continuous positive airway pressure (CPAP)
- The guidelines refer to bilevel systems as bilevel NIV

Plans should include preparations for early intubation if this type of ventilation fails.

The advantages:

- Allows intermittent application
- Reduces the need for sedation

- Does not inhibit speech, swallowing, expectoration, or the need for artificial feeding
- Reverses atelectasis and prevents infectious complications such as pneumonia
- Improves tidal volume/oxygenation/reduces work of breathing
- Reduces pulmonary oedema
- Improves cardiac function, a reduction in afterload

The disadvantages:

- It is slower at improving gaseous exchange abnormalities
- Can lead to gastric distension
- The facemask needs to be tightly fastened; if not, air can leak around leading to reduction in effectiveness
- Uncomfortable mask, necrosis of facial skin
- Eye irritation
- Continuous or accidental removal of the mask can lead to transient hypoxia
- Lack of access to suctioning of secretions, aspiration can occur

Bi-level NIV

This can give pressure support and CPAP combined or alone. It provides a continuous flow of oxygen and air, which enters the patients airways determined on the amount of negative pressure created by the patient on inspiration. This is determined by the respiratory support required by the patient inspired positive airway pressure (IPAP) and expired positive airway pressure (EPAP).

Relatively simple and easy to use, generally uses room air with supplementary oxygen.

Alternates between

- IPAP
  - Increasing breath size
  - Clears CO_2 and reduces patients work of breathing
  - Inspiration higher level airway pressure
- EPAP
  - Expiration low level prevents atelectasis
  - Expands collapsed alveoli improves gas exchange

Modes available:

- Spontaneous (S): no backup if the patient becomes apnoeic
- Spontaneous timed (ST): patient controls breathing rate and pattern, but times backup if apnoea occurs
- Timed (T): breaths delivered at set times where patients are unable to initiate a breath but maintain own airway
- CPAP: may be available on some machines but can be delivered by setting IPAP to the same level as EPAP

Ventilation should work in synchrony with the patient by recognizing

- Patient breathes in (trigger to IPAP).
- Patient breathes out (trigger to EPAP).
- Triggering and cycling should be recognized automatically as breathing patterns change.
- Matched to patient effort to ensure comfort.
- Sensitive triggers require smooth bore ventilator tubing to prevent turbulence triggering the ventilator.
- Low-resistance filter should be used between tubing and the machine.

Continuous Positive Airway Pressure

CPAP is when the alveoli remain open at the end of expiration, leaving a greater surface area for gaseous exchange to take place. CPAP has been available for many years but is being replaced with Bilevel, as it is not often tolerated well. Different types:

- High flow produces higher and more effective pressures
- Low-flow systems produce small volumes of air or oxygen
- Some systems use self-contained circuits or equipment
- Use flow generators further item need to be added

CPAP circuit:

- A flow generator will required additional items to attach, such as tubing and valves which generate positive end expiratory pressure (PEEP).
- Uses high or low flow air (bacterial filter needed).
- Can be attached to O_2 (range from 35% to 95%) supply can quickly drain cylinders.
- Pressure relief valve − a closed circuit is used except for an exit valve.
- Humidifier − prevent drying of the airways thermostat regulated.
- Mask nasal or full face masks with a seal.
- Exit valve − traps the last part of each breath in the airways.

Disadvantages of Continuous Positive Airway Pressure

- Discomfort of the face mask and not being able to fully breathe out
- Pressure ulcers − tight fitted masks
- Hypercapnia − ABGs
- Reduced lung compliance − reduced by prolonged CPAP
- Cardiovascular instability − reduces venous return and central venous pressure
- Gastric distension − air is swallowed
- Noise − irritating and impairs sleep
- Non-compliance − uncomfortable/stress

Inform the patient that this method of oxygen delivery is noisy and may be quite claustrophobic.

Assessment of Patients with CPAP and Bilevel NIV

- Chest wall movements
- Coordination of respiratory effort with the ventilator
- Accessory muscle recruitment
- General observations/measurements: TPR, BP and CVP
- ABG analysis – samples from an arterial line not safe on a general ward as there are issues with management of the line and interpretation
- FEV1 (forced expiratory volume in one second)
- Mental state
- Patient comfort

Continued Evaluation of Patient's Condition

- Maintenance of airway
- Suctioning forms a significant part in maintaining a patient's airway indications:
  - Ineffective cough
  - Depressed level of consciousness
  - Thick, tenacious mucus
  - Impaired respiratory function

  Types of suctioning:

- Suctioning using catheter and gloves.
- Using catheter in sleeve.
- In-line closed suctioning system.

  Areas of contention:

- The instigation of normal saline to initiate a cough reflex and
- The removal of the NIV to undertake suctioning, as CPAP is immediately lost and will take a while to re-inflate.

  Areas to consider:

- Suctioning can be a frightening experience for the patient, explain the process clearly.
- Size of the catheter.

- Pressure used between 80 and 120 mmHg – too low will be ineffective – too high can cause:
  - Atelectasis
  - Hypoxaemia
  - Airway collapse
  - Ulceration
- Pre-oxygenation and duration of suctioning (no longer than 10–15 seconds).
- Equipment, preparation, procedure, documentation.

Continuous Positive Airway Pressure Versus Bilevel Noninvasive Ventilation

Due to smaller starting pressures for bilevel NIV (4 cm H_2O) than CPAP (5 cm H_2O), there is less reduction in cardiac output. Bilevel NIV is more comfortable and quieter than CPAP. CPAP reverses pulmonary oedema more rapidly, although bilevel NIV provides better systemic perfusion. Bilevel NIV provides better long-term physiological effects.

A high proportion of hospitals offer NIV as a treatment choice. The National Institute of Health and Care Excellence (NICE) (2018a,b) recommends that NIV should ideally be used in high-dependency settings, where there are appropriately trained nurses and usually one nurse for every two patients. However, this is not always the case, as NIV is being used on general wards. All wards using NIV should have 24-hour nurse-led support services, e.g., outreach services. The use of NIV requires ongoing investment in equipment, staff development and support.

Maintenance of Airway

Patients are often admitted to critical care with a compromised airway that leaves them at risk from hypoventilation or aspiration of gastric contents. Therefore, a number of methods are adopted to protect a compromised airway. Assisted ventilation is a term used to refer to various methods of invasive ventilation that are used in critical care.

Patients in critical care often have trouble protecting their own airway, and signs of respiratory distress will be apparent (Table 3.7). This can be because of

- Decreased level of consciousness
- Muscle or neurological impairment of the swallow or gag reflex
- Effects of drugs that they have been given or have taken
- Acute airway obstruction
- Need for high levels of inspired oxygen

Always ensure that you have an airway at the bedside in case of accidental extubation.

TABLE 3.7 Respiratory distress parameters.

Physiological	Psychological	Visual
• Increased HR • Decreased HR • Decreased BP • Increased BP • Increased RR • Decreased RR • Dysrhythmias	• Dyspnoea • Panic • Pain • Fatigue	• Increased use of accessory muscles • Increased intercostal retractions • Increased flaring of nostrils • Erratic breathing pattern • ABGs (arterial blood gases) deteriorating

If a critical care patient is unable to protect their own airway, three methods are commonly used to control their airway.

Endotracheal Tubes

Endotracheal tubes (ETTs) are used in managing a patient's airway in critical care. This is a device with an inflatable cuff that is inserted into the patient's trachea via their mouth or nose. It passes through the larynx and the cuff is then inflated with air to seal the trachea. This is to protect the lungs from aspiration; it does not hold the ETT in place. The ETT is secured in place with ties (either a special holder or ETT tape) and a note taken of the length of the ETT at the patient's lips. This is important because tracheal tubes can move and slip further down, entering the right main bronchus so that the left lung is not ventilated. They can also slip upward, passing back through the larynx, which means that the patient can no longer be ventilated through them.

ETT can be passed with in the nose or mouth, which requires direction with Magill forceps to enter the glottis. Confirmation of correct placement of the tube is essential using ABGs.

Endotracheal intubation allows for spontaneous and positive-pressure ventilation. Indications for intubation are

- Acute airway obstruction
- Facilitation of tracheal suctioning
- Protection of the airway in those without protective cough reflexes
- Respiratory failure/arrest requiring ventilatory support and high inspired concentrations of oxygen

Ensure that emergency equipment is checked at the beginning of each shift and is accessible in the event of an unexpected emergency.

Cuffed and Uncuffed Tubes

Uncuffed ETTs are routinely used in young children. It has been traditionally believed that only uncuffed ETTs should be used for intubation in children younger than 8, or even 10, years of age. However, recent literature suggests that the advantages of using uncuffed ETTs in children may be just another myth within the realms of paediatric anaesthesia.

An uncuffed ETT allows a larger internal diameter tube to be used in practice. A larger internal tube minimizes airflow resistance and therefore reduces the work of breathing, in the spontaneously breathing patient. However, this advantage is not applicable in ventilated patients, for whom ventilator settings can be adjusted to provide optimal airflow and decrease resistance.

The advantages of cuffed ETT include

- Protects the airway in presence of copious secretions
- Establishes seal necessary for ventilatory support
- Avoidance of repeated laryngoscopy
- Use of low fresh gas flow
- Reduction of the concentration of anaesthetics gases detectable in the operating room

However, it is important to note that a longer duration of intubation and poorly fitted ETT are increased risk factors for mucosal damage, regardless of whether the ETT is cuffed or uncuffed. A properly sized, positioned and inflated modern (low-pressure, high-volume) cuffed ETT can offer many advantages over an uncuffed ETT. These include

- Greater ease of intubation.
- Better control of air leakage.
- Lower delivery rate and better control of flow of anaesthetic gases.
- Decreased risk of aspiration and infection.

Complications During Intubation

- Trauma/cardiovascular response to laryngoscopy and intubation
- Hypoxia
- Aspiration
- Oesophageal intubation

Complications after insertion:

- Blockage
- Dislodgement
- Damage to larynx
- Complications of mechanical ventilation

Oesophageal Tracheal Airways

These are supraglottic airways that keep the patient's airway open during anaesthesia or unconsciousness. These are an effective alternative to ETT. They are easy and quick to insert and may be inserted blindly. These tubes isolate the lungs from the oesophagus and so prevent aspiration during surgery and unconsciousness.

There is a range of these types of airways available:

- Laryngeal mask airway (LMA)
- iGel supraglottic airway
- Extraglottic airway device (EAD)
- Oesophageal tracheal combitube (ETC)

Tracheostomy

A tracheostomy is a surgical or percutaneous opening into the anterior wall of the trachea. They are inserted through an incision the front of the neck directly into the patient's trachea below the larynx. This procedure is usually performed on the ICU, but occasionally the patient may need to be taken to theatre. The opening is maintained by a tracheostomy tube and facilitates ventilation. Like ETTs, tracheostomy tubes have a cuff to protect from aspiration and are tied into place to make them secure. It comprises of

- A curved tracheotomy tube conforming to the neck anatomy, which is presented in many different sizes
- An inner cannula which can be removed and cleaned frequently to ensure patency of the tube
- A cuff which is of high volume and low pressure that helps to prevent the occluding of capillary blood flow in the trachea

Tracheostomies are usually inserted into patients after they have had an ETT in situ for several days. Tracheostomies are more comfortable for the patient and have fewer long-term effects on the mouth and trachea than a tracheal tube.

Indications

- Upper airway obstruction
- Prolonged artificial ventilation
- Inability to maintain an airway independently
- Removal bronchial secretions
- Upper airway surgery
- Laryngectomy

Advantages of Tracheotomy

- Improved control in long-term ventilated patients
- Secure airway control

- Reduced direct laryngeal injury
- Aids weaning process
- Nursing care aided with easy access to mouth
- Can commence oral feeding
- Speech is aided with fenestrated tube
- Aids patient mobility
- Reduced ICU stay
- Promotes psychological care

Disadvantages of Tracheostomy

- Haemorrhage — posttracheostomy formation or due to erosion of innom-
  inate artery
- Infection around stoma site
- Airway obstruction
- Tube displacement
- Surgical emphysema
- Tracheal stenosis
- Pneumothorax
- Atelectasis
- Tracheo-oesophageal fistula
- Apnoea, bradycardia or hypotension due to vagal nerve stimulation
- Tracheal mucosal injury
- Perioperative complication, e.g., laryngeal nerve injury; nursing care of the
  patient with tracheostomy
- Always have appropriate emergency equipment at the bedside
  - Suctioning facilities
  - Suction catheters of appropriate size and a yankauer sucker
  - Non–re-breathing circuit and/or adult bag-valve-mask with reservoir
    and tubing
  - Oxygen
  - Spare tracheostomy tubes of the same type (one of the same size and
    one size smaller)
  - Tracheal dilators

Always ensure that you have a similar-sized tracheostomy tube and one size smaller by the patient's bedside in the event that it becomes dislodged.

- Maintenance of tracheostomy tube
- Humidification
- Check cuff pressures regularly

- Regular physiotherapy
- Care of the stoma
  - Infection control
  - Regular dressings to clear oozing out of the stoma site — this is a two-person technique to prevent dislodging of the tracheostomy
  - Cleaning of the inner cannulae
  - Oral hygiene
  - Cuff management

Preventing Complications

Complications of a tracheostomy can be prevented or minimized through meticulous nursing care and assessment.

Wound care of a Tracheostomy

Attention to the tracheostomy wound can lessen the severity of infection, and therefore it should be treated as a surgical wound. The wound may be cleaned and covered with a pre-cut tracheostomy dressing to absorb drainage and to keep the neck plate from injuring the neck tissue. This dressing should be changed whenever it becomes soiled.

Send a culture swab if you believe there may be an infection.

Accidental Removal of a Tracheostomy This is a complication that can present as a life-threatening situation. To lessen the chance of such an occurrence, it is essential that tracheostomy ties be secured in a knot not a bow at a tension, allowing one finger to slip between the ties and the neck. It is recommended that a replacement tube of the same size and type and a pair of tracheal dilators be kept at the patient's bedside at all times, in case of extubation. The tracheal opening should be held open with the dilators until the replacement tube can be inserted.

Mucous Plug Formation The complication of mucous plug formation can be avoided if adequate humidification is provided. A mucous plug that obstructs the airway occurs largely as a result of

- Retained secretions
- Inadequate humidification
- Inadequate mobilization of secretions
- Lack of a properly fitted inner cannula

Special Care Considerations Probably the greatest fear of the tracheotomy patient is the inability to speak or call for help when necessary. All measures must be incorporated to facilitate communication. Writing boards and cards should be available for the patient at the bedside and placed within easy reach. The following suggestions may be useful when communicating with tracheotomy patients:

1. Allow ample time for the patient to respond because writing takes longer than speaking.
2. Speak in a normal tone. Although the patient cannot talk, she/he can hear (often there is a tendency to speak too loudly).
3. Avoid asking two questions at once. Again, allow extra time to respond in writing.
4. Encourage use of the paper, writing pad, slate, to ensure privacy of the communication; what is written should be destroyed or erased.

Because tracheostomies and ETT bypass the normal upper airway structures, they leave the patient unable to humidify the air they breathe and compromise their ability to cough and clear secretions. Therefore, humidification and suctioning are essential.

Percutaneous Tracheal Cannulation

Sometimes referred to as a mini-tracheotomy, this is used for the treatment of sputum retention. A mini-tracheotomy is performed with a small-bore tracheotomy tube without a cuff and provides a permanent access to the trachea for suction, while preserving glottic function.

Humidification

Humidification is essential when airway adjuncts are required. This is to ensure a normal respiratory environment, which uses water vapour to moisten the air as it enters the upper airways and lungs.

Either a heat moisture exchanger (HME) or a wet circuit normally provides humidification. An HME is a special filter that traps moisture that the patient exhales and then returns it to them with the next inhalation. In this way, it is very similar to the normal way that the nose humidifies air. HMEs, although they function well enough, are usually only used for short-term humidification. They need to be checked regularly to ensure that excessive moisture is not building up in them. They also need to be changed at least once every 24 hours. A wet circuit humidifier uses a hot plate to heat sterile water, and the vapour then saturates the gas that the patient breathes in. Water bath humidifiers are more efficient than HMEs and can be left in place for longer. Most patients in ICU will receive their humidification via a wet circuit.

When a patient breathes through an ETT or tracheotomy, air is not warmed, moisturized or filtered. Therefore, additional humidity is required, to keep the patient's secretions thin and mobilized as thick, crusty secretions can result in infection.

Mobilizing Secretions

Regular physiotherapy aids the mobilization of secretions. Also important is the turning of patients frequently as well as encouraging deep breathing to prevent pulmonary complications. Depending on the activity level of the patient transferring or assisting him/her to a chair should also be encouraged.

Suctioning

In order to clear secretions from a patient's chest critical care nurses commonly suction using either a sterile catheter or a catheter enclosed in a plastic sheath that is attached to the tracheal tube or tracheostomy permanently. This catheter is passed down the tracheal tube or via the tracheostomy, and suction is then applied to remove secretions.

Suctioning should not be carried out routinely; it should only be performed when there is an indication to do so. This is because the procedure is not risk free; the action of passing the catheter can damage the trachea and the partial occlusion of the airway can lead to complications such as hypoxia, bradycardia or, in extreme circumstances, cardiac arrest. These can be avoided by the use of correct technique and pre-oxygenating the patient prior to suctioning to prevent hypoxia. There are guidelines available for the suctioning of patients and you should take the time to familiarize yourself with these.

Patients with ETTs or tracheostomies often have problems adequately clearing their secretions. This may be because they have an inadequate cough, but even if they can cough, the closed circuit formed by the ventilation circuit attached to their tube prevents them from expectorating. Suctioning is needed when the cough becomes ineffective or secretions too thick for the patient to cough out easily. An inability to expectorate secretions is a common problem for patients with a tracheotomy, and suctioning forms a significant part in maintaining a patient's airway. If the clinical signs of the patient indicate suctioning, the correct catheter size must be at the bedside to minimize trauma to the tracheal mucosa.

The Size and Suction Pressure

- The size of the catheter should be approximately one half the internal diameter of the tracheotomy tube.
- The pressure used for suctioning is important: if the pressure is too low, suctioning will be ineffective; if too high it can cause

- Atelectasis
- Hypoxaemia
- Airway collapse
- Ulceration
- A higher negative pressure does not directly relate to the quantity of mucus extracted. Therefore, suctioning pressure of between 80 and 120 mmHg should be used.

Pre-oxygenation

- In some patients it may be necessary to pre-oxygenate with 100% oxygen using a ventilation bag prior to suctioning.
- This compensates for the oxygen removed from the trachea and bronchi during suctioning and prevents hypoxaemia.
- The procedure should be explained to the patient since suctioning can have a frightening effect. A clear explanation with reassurance decreases the patient's fears.

Suctioning of the upper airway may also be indicated if secretions or vomit are evident or suspected. Patients with a tracheotomy might find it difficult to swallow their saliva at all or adequately. Suctioning in this instance must be applied with care to avoid damage to mucosal surfaces.

Mechanical Ventilation

This is when a machine is used to ventilate the lungs, moving air in and out in several different ways. There are many modes of ventilation, and all different critical care units will have their own combinations or preferences.

Intermittent Positive Pressure Ventilation

IPPV is a method used for mechanical ventilation (the other method, negative pressure, is not discussed here).

Volume Control and Pressure Control

These are two methods that are used to control the way in which gas is delivered to a patient requiring ventilatory support.

In *VC ventilation*, a *tidal volume* is preset and the ventilator delivers that volume with each breath. This ensures the patient always receives the desired amount of volume from the machine. However, the pressures that the machine uses to deliver the breath are not controlled and can therefore reach extremely high levels. High airway pressures can lead to damage to the lungs (barotrauma) and other complications such as pneumothorax.

A way of avoiding the potential problems associated with VC ventilation is to use pressure to control the size of the breath that the patient receives.

By using a PC mode, the ventilator delivers a fixed inflation pressure, so tidal volume varies with lung compliance and airways resistance. This is the preferred mode in most patients with acute lung injury/ARDS. Usually the patient needs to be sedated, and sometimes requires the use of a muscle relaxant. This mode of ventilation allows the clinician to have control over the level of pressure delivered to the patient during ventilation and so prevents barotrauma. A disadvantage of PC ventilation is that it does not guarantee the patient receives an adequate tidal volume, and this can sometimes lead to carbon dioxide retention (hypercarbia) due to under-ventilation.

High-frequency Jet Ventilation

High-frequency jet ventilation (HFJV) is a mode of ventilation that delivers a high-pressure jet of gas, which recruits further fresh gas and is directed by jet towards the lungs. Together with the high gas flow rates additional humidification is required, and this is typically nebulized with the HFJV.

HFJV delivers respiratory rates of 100–300 L/min and in doing so ensures 20 L/min minute volumes. CO_2 elimination is usually more efficient than conventional IPPV, as it lowers peak airway pressures without a reduction in auto PEEP or mean airway pressures. Furthermore, oxygenation itself is dependent on mean airway pressures.

Although not fully understood, the method of gas exchange involves an aggressive gas mixing and convection. Superficial oxygenation readings often fall upon commencing HFJV, though they improve over time.

Indications for High-frequency Jet Ventilation

Bronchopleural fistula is the only proven indication for HFJV, but it has been utilized in assisting with the weaning from mechanical ventilation as the open circuit allows for spontaneous breaths to be taken without the difficulties associated with traditional ventilators. Often a reduction in driving pressure and increase in respiratory rate can facilitate the weaning process. HFJV also ensures adequate ventilation if the patient does not breathe adequately and plays a role in avoiding barotrauma even though high tidal volumes are used.

Establishing High-frequency Jet Ventilation

- A jet must be provided via a modified ETT or catheter mount.
- Entrainment gas is provided via a T-piece.
- Tidal volume cannot be set directly but by setting a combination of jet size, I:E ratio, driving pressure and respiratory rate.
- As the respiratory rate increases, so may the $PaCO_2$ as an increasing PEEP increases the effective physiological dead space.
- The I:E ratio is normally set between 1:3 and 1:2.

- Tidal volumes are determined by a combination of airway pressure and I:E ratio.
- In order to improve oxygenation, external PEEP may also be added to increase the mean airway pressure.

Combined HFJV and Conventional IPPV

Using a combination of HFJV and IPPV may be useful in ARDS or acute lung injuries where HFJV alone is insufficient in providing adequate gas exchange. Guide to ABG interpretation and HFJV manipulation:

- Increase in PaO_2
  - Increase FiO_2
  - Increase I:E ratio
  - Increase driving pressure
  - Add external PEEP
  - Consider the reduction of respiratory rate
- Decrease in $PaCO_2$
  - Increase driving pressure and
  - Decrease respiratory rate.

High-frequency Oscillation

High-frequency oscillation (HFO) can either be applied externally or via an ETT. In ETT delivery techniques, HFO is delivered in high respiratory rates and the gradual decrease of driving pressures. In HFO, the FRC increases as more alveoli are recruited and oxygenation is improved. Once this is achieved, the airway pressure can be decreased, often without any significant deterioration in oxygenation.

This method can be quite noisy, so it is important to inform patient and visitors.

High-frequency Oscillatory Ventilation

If a patient with ALI/ARDS is failing to improve/oxygenate using conventional methods of ventilation, then high-frequency oscillatory ventilation (HFOV) is one of the added therapeutic options available to this group of patients.

For an excellent summary of HFOV in ARDS see *British Journal of Anaesthesia* (2004), 93:322–324.

Ventilation Support

- Controlled or mandatory ventilation, whereby the ventilator delivers all the breaths regardless of the patient's efforts, the machine completely determines the respiratory rate and tidal volume. The intrathoracic pressure seen in normal inspiration no longer occurs; the pressure within the thorax never falls below atmospheric.
- Spontaneous, whereby the ventilator responds to the patient's efforts to breathe, but does not do anything if the patient does not trigger the breath.
- A mixture of the two, where the ventilator delivers breaths but allows the patient to breathe spontaneously between mandatory breaths or the machine senses when the patient fails to breathe and then delivers mandatory breaths.
- The most common settings are synchronized intermittent mandatory ventilation (SIMV) and pressure support (PS).

Intermittent Mandatory Ventilation

The patient breathes spontaneously while the ventilator delivers a prescribed tidal volume at specified intervals, allowing the patient to self-ventilate between cycles.

Synchronized Intermittent Mandatory Ventilation

In SIMV, a preset minute volume is delivered, but it is still possible for the patient to take further breaths through the ventilator; these additional breaths may be supported by pressure support.

Pressure support (PS) is a spontaneous mode in which the patient's breath is supported by a preset pressure once the ventilator has been triggered. As the patient becomes more alert and able to breathe more effectively, the level of support to each breath can be gradually reduced, which works effectively as a weaning tool.

Positive End Expiratory Pressure

This ensures that airway pressure is maintained above atmospheric at the end of expiration. The increased positive expiratory pressure may range from 3 to 60 cm H_2O and produces a continuous positive distending pressure within the airways and alveoli. PEEP improves arterial blood oxygenation by preventing alveolar collapse during the expiratory of ventilation or re-expanding previously collapsed alveoli. This effect maintains or increases the overall FRC, thereby improving the overall diffusion capacity of the lungs.

Continuous Positive Airway Pressure

CPAP is the same as PEEP, but the patient is self-ventilating. It is a spontaneous mode of ventilation that requires the patient to have an intact respiratory drive and the muscle strength to breathe adequately. It is a method of assisting ventilation by providing a continuous pressure in the respiratory system and preventing airway collapse. This makes breathing easier (less effort is required to take an inspiration) and helps to maximize the ventilation of the lungs. It is normally delivered via a high flow oxygen system, but some ventilators are also capable of performing it.

Ventilator Terminology

There are a number of terms and abbreviations that are associated with assisted ventilation.

- Minute volume − The amount of gas (in litres) that a patient breathes in (inspired minute volume) or out (expired minute volume) in a minute. It is calculated by multiplying the respiratory rate by the tidal volume.
- Tidal volume − The amount of gas (in millilitres) in a single inspired or expired breath.
- Peak airway pressure − The highest pressure reached during an inspiration.
- Mean airway pressure − The mean pressure in the airway during a breath.
- PEEP − The pressure maintained in the airway at the end of expiration. It is usually set through the ventilator and helps to keep alveoli open, improving gas exchange.
- FiO_2 − The amount of oxygen a patient is receiving. Written as a decimal where 0.21 is 21% and 1.0 is 100%.
- SIMV − A mandatory mode of ventilation where the machine synchronizes itself to any spontaneous breathing effort the patient may make. It is often combined with *PS*.
- PS − A method of assisting the patient to take a larger breath when they are breathing spontaneously through a ventilator. Often used when 'weaning' patients from ventilation.
- Assisted spontaneous breathing (ASB) − Another name for pressure support.
- Pressure control (PC) − A type of ventilation where a pressure limit is set for each breath delivered by the machine. The pressures in the patient's airway thus determine the size of each breath.
- VC − A type of ventilation where the size of the breath is preset and the machine delivers it regardless of the pressure in the patient's airway.
- Biphasic airway pressure (BiPAP) − A specific mode of PC ventilation where the machine alternates between a high pressure and a low pressure. The patient can breathe in and out at any point but if the patient does not breathe the cycling of pressures provides ventilation.

Ventilator Observations

All patients receiving ventilatory support require the documentation and acquisition of specific observations. The type and degree of documentation is dependent on their mode of ventilation. However, regardless of the mode, there are certain common observations that will usually be recorded.

For mechanically ventilated patients these will include

- Mode — This determines what other observations will be recorded. It is also important to note the mode because different modes are used depending on the general physical state of the patient.
- Respiratory rate (RR) — This indicates how well a patient is coping with breathing spontaneously (*tachypnoea*, RR. 30/min, and *bradypnoea*, RR, 8/min, are both indicators of problems).
- FiO_2 — This tells us how much oxygen the patient is receiving. This reading is used in conjunction with *ABGs* to interpret the effectiveness of ventilation.
- Airway pressures — *Low* airway pressures may indicate leaks in the ventilation circuit. *High* airway pressures can indicate a blockage in the tubing, sputum retention or an overall deterioration in the condition of the patient's lungs.
- Tidal volumes — This indicates the volume of each breath, e.g., a small tidal volume can indicate blockages in the system, leaks or a deteriorating respiratory function.
- Minute volumes — A minute volume can indicate over- (too high) or under-ventilation (too low) as well as problems with the circuit and changes in the patient's condition.

As well as regular observations, ventilator observations should be documented every time there is a significant change so that trends are evident to the critical care team.

Each individual observation outlined above is an important indicator about how well the patient is being ventilated.

Troubleshooting Ventilation Problems

In a case where you, as the bedside nurse, suspect a respiratory function or ventilation problem with the patient you are caring for then you must always seek expert help from a senior member of the critical care team.

In order to assist with the troubleshooting of potential airway/ventilation problems then remember the mnemonic DOPE:

- Displacement — Check to make sure that the patient has not become disconnected from the ventilator and that the ventilator tubing has not become detached from the machine. Check to make sure that the patient's *tracheal tube, tracheostomy tube* or facemask has not become displaced from where it should be. A displaced tracheal or tracheostomy tube is an emergency that must be dealt with immediately by a suitably trained person.

- Obstruction — Check that there is no obstruction in the system. Obstructions can be caused by external sources such as pressure on the ventilation tubing or the patient biting on their tracheal tube. They can also be caused by internal problems such as sputum plugs and bronchospasm.
- Pneumothorax — A pneumothorax occurs when air is able to enter the pleural cavity. This can cause the lung on the affected side to collapse pushing the chest contents out of position. The most dangerous type of pneumothorax, the tension pneumothorax, can prove fatal. The signs of a tension pneumothorax in a ventilated patient include increased airway pressures, reduced minute volume and unequal chest wall movement.
- Equipment problems — Although problems with equipment are uncommon they can and do occur. It is important then to know the equipment you are using and to have emergency equipment available that can be used to ventilate the patient if the primary machine fails.

In an emergency situation place the patient onto a rebreathing 'waters' bag until you seek assistance and rectify the problem; this will ensure adequate oxygenation.

Complications of Ventilator Management

- Upper airways damage
- Infection
- Mechanical malfunction
- Haemodynamic alterations
- Central nervous system disturbances
- Fluid retention
  - Gastrointestinal disturbances
  - Gastric distension
- Acute ulceration of the gastric and bowel mucosa
- Oxygen toxicity — due to persistent high concentration of oxygen
- Absorption atelectasis
- Pulmonary barotrauma
- Intubation of the right main bronchus
- Psychological trauma
- Miscellaneous:
  - Complication encountered with suctioning
  - Complications related to manually ventilating the patient
  - Inadequate warming and humidification of the inspired air

Weaning from a Ventilator

Weaning is the systematic removal of ventilatory support and return of the patient to spontaneous breathing. The weaning process commences the moment the patient is placed on mechanical ventilation. The process consists of

- Correcting the cause of respiratory failure
- Maintenance of muscle strength, i.e., diaphragm
- Maintenance of nutritional intake
- Psychological preparation

All the above processes are equally important in ensuring the successful preparation and extubation of the ventilated patient.

Short-term Weaning

Before any weaning is initiated the patient must be prepared. This includes

- Commence weaning morning or early afternoon, not during night as patient will be tired
- Ensure all sedation etc. has been stopped
- Explain the extubation procedure to patient
- Suction airway
- Ensure continuous monitoring in situ
- Sit patient upright to maximize chest expansion
- Place patient on spontaneous mode, e.g., T-piece
- Stay with and reassure patient at all times
- Monitor all respiratory parameters
- Obtain ABG following 20–30 minutes of spontaneous breathing
- Evaluate ABGs, if normal for patient, extubate onto facemask

Long-term Weaning

Following a long period of ventilation, it is fair to say that weaning is far more prolonged and complex. However, despite this the weaning process follows a similar format to that of short-term weaning. The process itself is more involved in that the whole critical care team will become involved. Once the plan has been formulated, the patient and family are involved in the weaning process. They are informed of the difficulties that may arise and in doing so preparing both the patient and family in the prolonged journey to extubation. It is important to ensure the patient and family are reassured as periods of prolonged weaning can affect the patient's psychological status and thus have an effect on successful and progressive weaning.

Before weaning commences the following process is recommended:

- Initially wean during the day only
- Ensure that all sedation etc. has been stopped

- Explain the weaning process to patient
- Suction airway
- Sit patient upright to maximize chest expansion
- Choose appropriate weaning mode and adhere to this, e.g., PS
- Monitor physiological parameters
- Monitor and record ABGs
- Reassure and remain with patient during this initial phase
- Once set period of weaning has been achieved place patient back onto original ventilation mode
- Reassure patient
- Explain the next phase of weaning to patient

There are generally three phases of weaning.

Pre-weaning Phase

- The decision to wean is made
- The measurable patient data and prior clinical experience of care provides are used when making the decision

Considerations of physiological and psychological readiness for weaning; this includes

- Original disorder treated, reversed if possible
- No evidence of infection, normal temp, no evidence of sepsis or chest infection
- Respiratory status — no respiratory failure, the ability of ventilatory muscles to generate force needed, available energy — no muscle fatigue, ABGs, considerations of secretions and type, breathing spontaneously, coughs, gag reflex, chest X-ray, breath sounds, abdominal distension, measure of tidal volume, oxygen <40%, no PEEP
- Cardiovascular stable — consideration of increased heart rate affecting cardiac workload and oxygen consumption, ECG and arrhythmias, cardiac output not too high, systemic vascular resistance — sepsis, BP >80 or <180
- Haemodynamic status — anaemia as reduced oxygen carrying capacity, blood results, e.g., urea and creatinine within normal limits
- Neurological status — level of consciousness, fully aware of being weaned, consideration of sedation and analgesia
- Adequate levels of pain control — may need analgesia — pain assessment needed so as not to affect breathing
- Metabolic status — calorie intake, blood glucose level maintained, protein levels, too much feeding will increase carbon dioxide levels
- Renal function satisfactory — potassium normal, magnesium or phosphorus can increase muscle weakness, fluid balance, check weight

- Psychological readiness — patient prepared for weaning, expected to feel during procedure, reduce fear and anxiety, shortness of breath may indicate possible failure to wean and extubate. Assurances of a nurse at all times, establish a means of communication. No sleep deprivation and adequate sleep

Weaning Phase

- There is generally no preference to support a preference for using any of the weaning methods and this is generally not a significant issue if the patient has been ventilated for less than 3 days.
    - It is also important to note that successful weaning should commence once the patient is respiratory stable and is receiving an oxygen delivery of >40%.
    - Respiratory assessment during weaning.
        - The patient should be continuously monitored for oxygen saturation, with a regular clinical assessment and review of respiratory parameters.
        - ABGs should be taken after a period of 20–30 minutes as an indicator of spontaneous respiratory function.

    Some of the forms of ventilation above can be used to wean:

- T-piece — advantage is that it tests patient's ability to breathe and allows periods of work and rest, increasing respiratory muscle strength. Disadvantage is the patient may become tired, stressful using oxygen reserves, shortness of breath and afraid when removed from the ventilator; increases dead space and carbon dioxide respiratory drive.
- Intermittent mandatory ventilation (IMV) — this is the most common method; more gradual than T-piece; advantage is that it reduces the need for sedation, reduces barotrauma, and reduces problems with venous return. Disadvantage patient has to get into a rhythm 'mixed up' and increases energy expenditure.
- SIMV — similar to IMV but the disadvantage is removed as the machine synchronizes to the patient, negative pressure valves increase the pressure required, assess for respiratory muscle fatigue when reduced SIMV especially <6 breaths.
- PSV — this is where the introduction of PSV has come in, started at 15–25 cm H_2O above PEEP, spontaneous breathing and inspiratory pressure support 30 cm H_2O patient can be ventilated and reduced gradually, used with SIMV.
- MMV — patient receives a pre-set MV despite variable spontaneous breathing; ensures patient reaches MV prescribed whether they do it by themselves or by the ventilator machine. This method is good if the patient is conscious.

The merits of each of method must match the specific patient situation. Factors associated with failed weaning stage.

- Respiratory muscle fatigue
- Inadequate respiratory drive
- Inadequate cardiac function, e.g., failure
- Uncooperative and confused patient

Factors associated with successful weaning stage.

- P/F ratio >200 mmHg/27.5 kPa
- Haemodynamically stable
- Minute volume <12 L/min
- *Vital capacity >10 mL/kg* Extubation phase

A pre-extubation assessment is required for each patient, which is based on whether an individual patient is ready for extubation. A factor that may affect success and time frame of an extubation are whether the patient has been ventilated on a short-term or long-term basis. Both categories require different weaning strategies. Weaning should commence after an adequate explanation has been delivered to the patient. A spontaneous mode of breathing should be commenced as early as possible as to allow for a reduction in sedative drug delivery, maintenance and promotion of respiratory muscle function. Short-term ventilated patients normally only require a short trial of 20–30 minutes before extubation, but long-term ventilated patients may require weeks of preparation before extubation is successful.

Some questions that arise from this phase:

- What are the indicators of successful weaning that allow the airway to be removed?
- How long does the patient need to be spontaneously breathing before it can be removed, suggested − 2–6 hours ET, 18–48 tracheotomy?

Weaning is suggested to encompass the three phases identified above. When the weaning phase is unsuccessful, patients do not progress to the extubation phase and weaning failure occurs.

Reasons for failure to wean:

- Haemodynamic instability
- Fever, sepsis
- Metabolic abnormalities
- COPD/bronchospasm
- Neurological impairment
- Sleep deprivation
- Psychological reasons − uncooperative
- Disorders of the diaphragm
- Muscle fatigue

Always have your re-intubation equipment at the bedside.

Indications for Re-intubation

- Uncoordinated respiratory function
- Exhaustion
- Agitated
- Clammy
- Decreased peripheral oxygenation

Acid-Base Balance

General Principles of Acid-base Balance

The primary function of the respiratory system is to supply an adequate amount of oxygen (O_2) to tissues and remove carbon dioxide (CO_2). The kidneys will excrete any excess acids or alkali. The respiratory and renal organs together with the buffering effects of blood maintain hydrogen ion (H^+) concentration. H^1 concentration is one of the most important aspects of acid-base homeostasis. When there is an increase in acid production, blood bicarbonate (HCO_3^-), proteins, and phosphate buffer body fluids (Table 3.8). However, there comes a point in the disease process when these buffers can no longer maintain appropriate concentrations of H^+. Patients admitted to or while in critical care can have life-threatening situations such as diabetic ketoacidosis, asthma and severe vomiting, which alter pH balance and exacerbate their problems.

To maintain homeostasis during stress or illness/diseased states there is generally an increase in depth and rate of breathing due to stimulation of the sympathetic nervous system. High alveolar ventilation brings more O_2 into the alveoli, increasing O_2, and rapidly eliminating CO_2 from the lungs (for chemical abbreviations see Table 2.16).

Partial Pressure of Gases

Dalton's law explains the partial pressure of a gas, which is the pressure exerted by a gas within a mixture of gases independent of each gas in the mixture (Marieb, 2017). The partial pressure of each gas is directly proportional to its percentage in the total mixture and in air is determined by atmospheric pressure. Atmospheric pressure is 101 kPa (760 mmHg), 21% of this air is oxygen, and the partial pressure of oxygen (PO_2) in atmospheric air is

$$(21/100) \times 101 = 21.2 \text{ kPa}.$$

TABLE 3.8 The major body buffer systems.

Site	Buffer system	Description
Interstitial fluid (ISF)	Bicarbonate Phosphate and protein	For metabolic acids Not important because concentration is too low
Blood	Bicarbonate Haemoglobin Plasma proteins Phosphate	Important for metabolic acids Important for buffering CO_2 and H^1 Minor buffer Concentration too low
Intracellular fluid	Proteins Phosphates	Important buffer of extracellular H^1 Important buffer
Urine	Phosphate Ammonia	Responsible for most of titratable acidity Important – formation of NH_4^1 and hence excretion of H^1
Bone	Calcium carbonate	In prolonged metabolic acidosis

Within the alveoli the PO_2 is different from air because of enrichment in the air passages (dead space) with CO_2 and water vapour. Alveolar air contains much more CO_2 and water vapour and much less O_2, and so they make a greater contribution to the near-atmospheric pressure in the lungs than they do in air. This is due to

- Gas exchanges occurring in the lungs
- Humidification of air by the conducting passages
- Mixing of gases in the dead space (contains air not involved in gaseous exchange) between the nose and alveoli

In alveoli, PO_2 averages only 13.2 kPa (100 mmHg). Continuous consumption of O_2 and production of CO_2 in the cells means that there is a partial pressure gradient both in the lungs and at the tissue level ensuring diffusion of oxygen into the blood and CO_2 from it.

To calculate mmHg just multiply the kPa by 7.5.

Changes in partial pressures of carbon dioxide (PCO_2) and H^+ are sensed directly by the respiratory centre central chemoreceptors in the medulla (Guyton and Hall, 2016). In contrast, a reduction in PO_2 is monitored by the peripheral chemoreceptors located in the carotid and aortic bodies, which transmit nervous signals to the respiratory centre in the medulla for control of respiration. However, it is the CO_2 'drive' for breathing that dominates in health, although the O_2 'drive' can be significant in some disordered states as an adaptation to chronic evaluations of PCO_2, for example, in chronic obstructive lung conditions.

Metabolic Generation of Acids and Alkali

Each day the body produces acids through normal metabolism, and acid or alkali is ingested in diet. The lungs release or strengthen the bond to acids as necessary and the kidneys also effectively eliminate or reabsorb acids, so there is no impact on whole body acid-base status. If there is an increase in production of acids, the body has a number of buffers outlined in Table 3.8. If there is a reduction in acids or loss of acids the excess bicarbonate (HCO_3^-) is buffered by H^+ to minimize any change in pH.

Normal pH and Hydrogen ion Concentration of Body Fluids

The pH is related to actual H^1 concentration (Guyton and Hall, 2016). A low pH corresponds to a high H^+ concentration and is evidence of an acidosis, and conversely a high pH corresponds to a low H^+ concentration known as an alkalosis. The interrelationships between O_2, H^+, CO_2 and HCO_3^- are central to the understanding of acid-base balance and reflect the physiological importance of the CO_2/HCO_3^- buffer system (see Box 2.3). The CO_2/HCO_3^- buffer system largely takes up the majority of the excess H^+. The $H^1 + HCO_3^2$ converts into H_2CO_3 in the presence of carbonic anhydrase (present in RBCs) and breaks down into CO_2 and water (H_2O) (Box 2.3). The CO_2/HCO_3^- interaction is slow in plasma, but quicker in RBCs due to the presence of carbonic anhydrase.

An Increase in Acids (H^+) in the Body (Acidosis)

There are generally two categories of acid accumulation in the body a respiratory acidosis and a metabolic acidosis, determined if the primary change is either metabolic or respiratory (Table 3.9).

Respiratory Acidosis (Reduction in pH, Increase in PCO_2)

Respiratory acidosis occurs when the respiratory system is unable to eliminate CO_2 produced from cellular metabolism, quickly enough (Richards and Edwards, 2014). An increase in CO_2 increases H^1 ion concentration, and the body's pH starts falling below 7.40. However, normally the body is able to particularly maintain acid-base homeostasis, since the increase in PCO_2 stimulates central chemoreceptors to increase respiratory rate. When PCO_2 can no longer be maintained, e.g., in COPD, the body can still help to maintain pH by the elimination of excess acid in urine, although this is of a slow onset and

TABLE 3.9 Acid-base categories and related conditions.

Acid-base is separated into four categories	The conditions/diseases that lead to acid-base abnormalities
Respiratory acidosis — any disorder that interferes with ventilation (PCO_2. 5.7 kPa; pH, 7.35)	• Any condition that impairs gas exchange or lung ventilation (chronic bronchitis, cystic fibrosis, emphysema, pulmonary oedema) • Rapid, shallow breathing, hypoventilation • Narcotic or barbiturate overdose or injury to brain stem • Airway obstruction • Chest or head injury
Metabolic acidosis (HCO_3^-, 22 mmol/L; pH,7.35)	• Severe diarrhoea causing loss of bicarbonate from the intestine • Circulatory failure/hypovolaemia • Renal disease/failure • Untreated diabetes mellitus • Starvation • Excess alcohol ingestion • High ECF (extracellular fluid) potassium concentrations • Lactic acid production
Respiratory alkalosis (PCO_2, 5.7 kPa; pH. 7.45)	• Direct cause is always hyperventilation (e.g., too much mechanical ventilation, pulmonary lesions) • Brain tumour or injury • Acute anxiety • Early stages of chronic obstructive airways disease • Asthma
Metabolic alkalosis (HCO_3^-. 26 mmol/L; pH >7.40) is the result of excess base bicarbonate ion (HCO_3^-) or decreased hydrogen ion (H^+) concentration, caused by an excessive loss of non-volatile or fixed acids	• Vomiting or gastric suctioning of hydrogen-chloride-containing gastric contents • Selected diuretics • Ingestion of excessive amount of sodium bicarbonate • Constipation • Excess aldosterone (e.g., tumours) • Loss of gastrointestinal hydrochloric acid and potassium (e.g., severe vomiting or gastric suctioning) • Overuse of potassium-wasting diuretics

will not be so effective in, say, acute airway obstruction. An individual can live for many years with conditions such as COPD, partly because of the efficiency of renal compensation.

The Accumulation of Carbon Dioxide in Respiratory Acidosis It is well known that Hb can carry O_2 and CO_2 at the same time, but the presence of one reduces the bonding power of the other, known as the Haldane effect (Richards and Edwards, 2014). The Haldane effect is when CO_2 transported in blood is affected by the partial pressure of O_2 in the blood (Marieb, 2017). The PO_2 in the alveoli normally gives a sufficient pressure (partial pressure) to facilitate CO_2 release from Hb in the alveoli and CO_2 binding in the tissues. The amount of CO_2 transported by Hb in blood is influenced by PO_2. When PO_2 decreases in conditions such as COPD, the CO_2 is less likely to be released from the Hb; consequently, CO_2 levels increase.

In a worsening respiratory acidosis through airway obstruction PO_2 decreases in the alveoli and cannot therefore sufficiently facilitate the release of CO_2 from Hb. A greater proportion of CO_2 remains attached and will eventually lower pH. The deoxygenated Hb carrying an excess of CO_2 is less likely to bind to O_2, thus exacerbating the problem of poor O_2 uptake. In some conditions, administration of oxygen will improve PO_2 and facilitate the removal of the accumulated CO_2 from Hb.

Improved Release of Oxygen in Respiratory Acidosis When there is an increase in CO_2 and H^+, as observed in a respiratory acidosis, e.g., COPD, the blood pH will drop. In an acid environment, less oxygen can be carried by Hb leading to a reduction of oxygen delivery to cells (Marieb, 2017). Conversely, an acid environment in tissues causes Hb to release O_2 more readily to cells and facilitates unloading of O_2. This effect is known as the Bohr effect and is an important adaptation to increased acidity in metabolically active tissues. The increased H^1 binds to Hb in RBCs and alters the structure of the molecule temporarily causing it to release O_2. The Hb molecule therefore gives up its O_2 to tissues under conditions of increased H^+ ion concentration.

Metabolic Acidosis (Reduction in pH and HCO_3^-)

Metabolic acidosis occurs when there is excess acid or reduced HCO_3^- in the body (Richards and Edwards, 2014). Over production or excess H^+ will lead to decreased pH of less than 7.40. This is followed by a reduction in HCO_3^- (used to buffer excess H^1) in an effort to return pH to within the normal range of 7.35−7.45. Body enzymes can only function in a pH range of between 6.80 and 7.80 with reducing pH there is 50% mortality rate at a pH ≤ 6.80.

Compensatory Mechanisms for Respiratory and Metabolic Acidosis When H^1 accumulates in the body, chemical buffers in cells and ECF bind with the excess H^+. As H^+ reaches excessive proportions buffers cannot bind with it and blood pH decreases. The compensation for an accumulation of respiratory or metabolic acids occurs in the lungs and kidneys.

The Role of the Lungs in Compensation. In a respiratory acidosis there is a low/normal PO_2 and a high PCO_2 concentration and a low pH. An increase in CO_2 is observed in all tissues and fluids, including cerebro-spinal fluid (CSF) and in the medulla oblongata. The CO_2 reacts with H_2O to form carbonic acid (H_2CO_3) (quicker in the presence of carbonic anhydrase in RBCs) that dissociates to H^1 and HCO_3^- (Box 2.3). When both CO_2 and H^+ are increased in CSF and tissues, they have a strong stimulatory effect on central chemoreceptors acting on inspiratory and expiratory muscles leading to an increase in the respiratory rate and depth of breathing.

A reduced PO_2 will also contribute to an increase in ventilation since O_2 saturation will decrease. The role of the carotid bodies during a reduced O_2 in lung ailments such as pneumonia, asthma and emphysema is essential and plays a major role in increasing respiration via peripheral chemoreceptors and can increase alveolar ventilation as much as five- to sevenfold (Richards and Edwards, 2014). If the compensation of a deeper and faster respiratory rate is efficient, e.g., in asthma, it may significantly reduce PCO_2 to maintain O_2 levels (Woodrow, 2004). However, the increase in alveolar ventilation may lead to overcompensation and a patient suffering an asthmatic attack may present with a detrimental respiratory alkalosis (Figs 3.2 and 3.3).

In a metabolic acidosis removal of a proportion of the excess H^+ can occur as CO_2, as the equation presented in Box 2.3 is completely reversible. This allows more H^+ to bind with HCO_3^2 to form H_2CO_3 that dissociates to CO_2 and H_2O (Fig. 3.2). Respiration is stimulated due to reduction in pH in CSF stimulating central chemoreceptors, leading to hyperventilation. CO_2 is excreted from the body, and the arterial PCO_2 therefore reduces.

This explains why patients with a metabolic acidosis have a fast respiratory rate, which further increases as acids continue to rise, and can lead to a reduction in PCO_2 to less than is normal in health. A complete compensatory respiratory alkalosis through a reduction in CO_2 is unlikely to completely restore normality because, if it were to do so, the compensatory mechanisms would be eradicated. Therefore, in a metabolic acidosis, respiratory compensation is not sufficient alone.

If PCO_2 cannot be reduced and compensation becomes inefficient, in conditions such as a chest infection or asthma, PCO_2 may eventually start to rise. This may be an indication to instigate additional interventions such as NIPPV (Butler, 2005) or invasive intubation.

The Role of the Kidneys in Compensation. As blood acidity increases, renal compensatory mechanisms act slowly in maintaining pH (Yucha, 2004). In respiratory acidosis excess CO_2 can be converted through the equation in Box 2.3. The retained CO_2 combines with H_2O to form large amounts of H_2CO_3. In the kidneys H_2CO_3 dissociates to release free H^+ and HCO_3^2, and

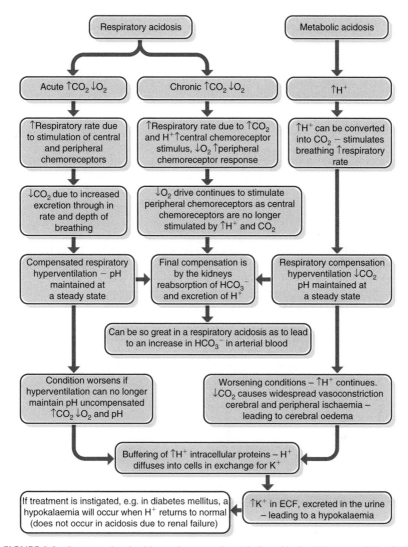

FIGURE 3.2   Processes involved in respiratory and metabolic acidosis. *ECF*, extracellular fluid.

stimulates the kidneys to retain HCO_3^- and sodium ions (Na^+), and excrete H^+. The HCO_3^2 retained is re-circulated and helps to buffer further free H^+.

Similar effects occur in a metabolic acidosis. After about 30 minutes the kidneys start to compensate for the acidosis by secreting excess H^+ secreted in the renal tubule and excreted in the urine as weak acids (Yucha, 2004). For every H^+ secreted into the renal tubule, a sodium and bicarbonate ion are re-absorbed and returned to the blood. The pH is unlikely to be completely

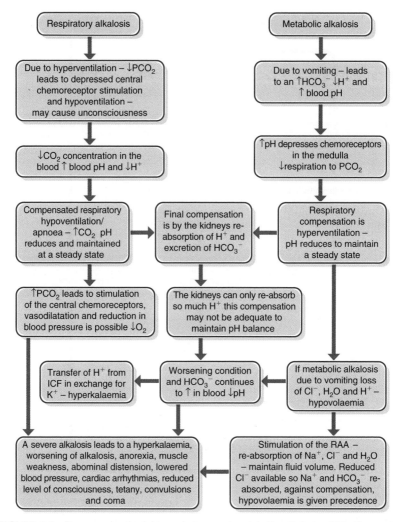

FIGURE 3.3 Processes involved in respiratory and metabolic alkalosis. *RAA*, five renin–angiotensin–aldosterone system.

restored as this would reduce the efficiency of compensatory mechanisms. The CO_2 and HCO_3^2 will be far from their normal values, as a consequence of altered buffering capacity and respiratory compensation.

It takes about 3 days for a patient to have established a steady state of compensation, e.g., a respiratory hyperventilation (Richards and Edwards, 2014). The kidney can only retain so much HCO_3^- with the consequence that the blood contains a higher concentration of HCO_3^- than produced by CO_2 retention alone (Fig. 3.2), hence an improved base excess (BE).

H⁺ Buffer by Intracellular Proteins in Exchange for K⁺. If the concentration of H^+ in ECF rises to a level beyond the compensatory mechanism H^+ moves into cells by simple diffusion to be buffered by intracellular proteins, in exchange for potassium ions (K^+). As cells need to maintain a balanced membrane charge, cells release K^+ into blood in exchange for H^+; this may lead to a high blood K^+ (hyperkalaemia) and characteristic changes in the ECG (peaked T waves and abnormal QRS complexes) may be observed (Richards and Edwards, 2014). However, with normal renal function the majority of excess ECF K^1 will be excreted in urine. If normal ventilation is restored or the acidosis is treated (e.g., in diabetic ketoacidosis it is treated with insulin and glucose) the K^+ will return into the intracellular fluid (ICF) in exchange for H^1 and the patient may then develop a hypokalaemia.

A Decrease or Loss of Acids (H⁺) in the Body (Alkalosis)

There are generally two categories of reduced acids in the body: a respiratory alkalosis and a metabolic alkalosis (Table 3.9). These two conditions stimulate compensatory mechanisms that serve to maintain acid base homeostasis.

Respiratory Alkalosis (Increase in pH, Decrease in PCO₂)

Respiratory alkalosis occurs when the respiratory system eliminates too much CO_2. This reduction of PCO_2 below the range of 4.5−5.6 kPa (30−35 mmHg) causes a reduction in H^1 generation. The decreasing H^+ concentration raises the blood pH above the normal range of 7.45. Any condition that causes hyperventilation can cause a respiratory alkalosis.

If you have an abnormal ABG, always discuss this reading with the person in charge and/ or critical care doctor.

The Processes of Carbon Dioxide Excretion When ventilation is increased above the normal rate excessive amounts of CO_2 are excreted in expired air. In this situation CO_2 is washed out of the body leading to a hypocapnia: the pH rises. A rise in pH is sensed by central chemoreceptors in the medulla and CSF. Both CO_2 and H^+ concentration are reduced resulting in a decrease in ventilation, thus reducing the elimination of CO_2 and reducing pH to within the normal range. ABG analysis will show a lowered PCO_2 and respiratory rate may be decreased in both depth and rate.

The Binding of Hb and O₂ in Alkaline States When there is a decrease in CO_2 and H^+ the pH will rise and consequently more oxygen remains bound to Hb in the tissues (Marieb, 2017). O_2 delivery to cells is therefore reduced as the Hb/O_2 bond is strengthened (the Bohr effect). This will maintain O_2 saturation, but not cellular oxygen delivery. Therefore, the apparent normality of O_2 saturation can be misleading in an alkalosis.

Metabolic Slkalosis (Increase in pH and HCO_3^-)

Metabolic alkalosis (HCO_3^-. 26 mmol/L; pH 7.40) is the result of excess HCO_3^2 or decreased H1 concentration, caused by an excessive loss of non-volatile or fixed acids. Metabolic alkalosis over-excites central and peripheral nervous systems.

Compensatory Mechanisms for Respiratory and Metabolic Alkalosis. When the body HCO_3^- increases in ECF it binds with H^+. As the bicarbonate reaches excessive proportions H^+ cannot bind with it sufficiently to buffer the consequences of pH and blood pH increases. The compensation for a respiratory or metabolic alkalosis occurs in the lungs, kidneys and by the release of H^+ from cells.

The Role of the Lungs in Compensation. In alkaline environments blood H^+ has been lost or there is an excess base HCO_3^-. The unbound excess HCO_3^- elevates blood pH. The arterial blood will show a pH above 7.45, a PCO_2 below 4.5 kPa (35 mmHg) and HCO_3^- above 26 mmol/L. In an alkalosis blood and tissues give up more H^1 as a compensatory response. So as HCO_3^- starts to accumulate in the body H^1 combines with it to form H_2CO_3, this chemical reaction buffers excess.

HCO_3^-.

An increase in blood pH is sensed in the CSF and depresses respiratory centre central chemoreceptors in the medulla. This reduces respiration, CO_2 is retained in an attempt to increase blood PCO_2 and decrease pH. However, this is limited since the reduction in respiratory rate and depth lowers O_2 levels. The reduced CO_2 and H^+ observed in a metabolic alkalosis combine to form two powerful respiratory inhibitory effects on the peripheral chemoreceptors opposing the excitatory effects of a diminished oxygen concentration (Guyton and Hall, 2016). A blood sample taken now will show decreasing HCO_3^- and pH as the body attempts to compensate (Woodrow, 2004).

The Role of the Kidneys in Compensation. After approximately 6 hours the kidneys start to increase excretion of HCO_3^- and reduce the excretion of H^+. This renal compensation returns the plasma H^1 concentration towards normal and urine will be very alkaline with a high pH. To maintain electrochemical balance, excess sodium ions (Na^+) and chloride ions (Cl^-) are excreted along with HCO_3^2. This can lead to a hyponatraemia.

The decreasing pH may in turn cause the respiratory centre chemoreceptors to increase respiratory rate and consequently a compensatory hyperventilation may ensue. If the PCO_2 becomes too low, due to the hyperventilation, this imposes a respiratory alkalosis on top of the metabolic alkalosis and hence metabolic compensation may not be adequate (Yucha, 2004). At this stage the patient could have bradypnoea or Cheyne—Stokes respiration.

A prolonged alkaline environment leads to vasoconstriction, which increases cerebral and peripheral hypoxia (Fig. 3.2). As alkalosis becomes more severe calcium ions increasingly bind to proteins and so hypocalcaemia develops. This increases nerve excitability and muscle contractions. If left untreated an alkalosis can put excess strain on the heart and central nervous system.

Alkalosis in Severe Vomiting. An alkalosis can be seriously exacerbated if there is a severe drop in circulating volume, e.g., in vomiting. In persistent vomiting of gastric contents, electrolytes are no longer available to the body from the alimentary canal to replace those lost in the vomit and in urine (Na^+, Cl^-, HCO_3^-). The principal electrolytes in addition to water lost as a result of vomiting gastric contents are:

- Hydrochloric acid (hydrogen and chloride ions) and
- Sodium chloride (sodium and chloride ions).

The single electrolyte lost in the greatest amounts is Cl^-; as a result the plasma Cl^- concentration falls. A loss of fluid and plasma volume due to vomiting can lead to a hypovolaemic state, which can affect acid—base balance.

Compensation for a hypovolaemia will impose powerful compensatory mechanisms stimulating the kidney to release renin from the juxtaglomerular apparatus stimulating the adrenal gland to release aldosterone. The effect of aldosterone promotes sodium (Na^+) and chloride (Cl^-) reabsorption (and hence water) in the renal tubules to maintain circulating volume in exchange for K^+ and H^+.

The low concentration of chloride in the plasma results in a relatively small filtered load of Cl^- by comparison with Na^1. There are fewer chloride ions to balance the re-absorption of sodium. The body cannot respond by reducing Na^+ re-absorption, which is required to restore circulating volume. The only mechanism available to the kidney is to increase the re-absorption of Na^1 and HCO_3^- and consequently increase the excretion of K^+ and H^+. Vomiting therefore leads to processes of Na^+ and HCO_3^- re-absorption, and K^1 and H^1 loss due to excess Cl^- depletion because of vomiting. This triggers mechanisms that are inappropriate in an existing alkalosis (Fig. 3.2). The retention of electrolytes and fluid during a hypovolaemia takes precedence over acid—base homeostasis.

A cautious IV infusion of isotonic sodium chloride solution at this stage may improve the patient's hypovolaemia. The replacement of the principal ECF electrolytes necessary, e.g., Na^+ and Cl^- will return fluid volume towards normal. It switches the drive from retention of Na^+ and HCO_3^- and excretion of K^+ and H^+ to correction of metabolic alkalosis, e.g., the retention of H^+, Na^+ and Cl^- and excretion of K^+ and HCO_3^-, putting the acid—base problem in order.

H^1 Release from Cells in Exchange for ECF K^+. A decreased H^+ level in ECF causes H^1 to diffuse passively out of cells to buffer excess HCO_3^-. To maintain balance of charge across the cell membrane, ECF K^1 moves into cells. When K^+ cannot be replaced by absorption in the alimentary tract there is a severe depletion of the body's total ECF K^1 content (hypokalaemia), which can ultimately lead to confusion and arrhythmias (Richards and Edwards, 2014).

The primary function of the respiratory system is to supply an adequate amount of oxygen to tissues and remove carbon dioxide. The kidneys will excrete any excess acids or alkali. The respiratory and renal organs together with the blood maintain hydrogen ion concentration. Hydrogen ion concentration is one of the most important aspects of acid—base homeostasis. When there is an increase or decrease in acid production by body tissues, the blood bicarbonate, proteins and phosphate also buffer body fluids. There comes a point in the disease process when these buffers can no longer maintain adequate concentrations of hydrogen ions. Patients admitted to hospital can have life-threatening situations, which alter pH balance.

3.5 TRANSFER OF CRITICAL CARE PATIENTS

Transfer of critical care patients involves not only moving the critically ill patient within the hospital — for example to an imaging department or theatre — but also externally to other hospitals. This may be due to critical care bed shortage within the admitting hospital or need for specialist care and treatment. Prior to transfer of the critically ill patient there are a number of factors to take into consideration.

Always allocate a member of the critical care team to coordinate the transfer.

Important Factors of Safe Transfer

- Patient accompanied by experienced nursing and medical staff
- Appropriate equipment and vehicle are sought and utilized
- Patient fully assessed, stabilized and staff prepared prior to transfer
- All investigations accompany patient on transfer
- All drugs and delivery systems are readily available and prepared for immediate use
- Monitoring systems and battery back up are familiar to accompanying staff
- Continuous monitoring and assessment during transfer
- Knowledge of area transferring patient to. If another hospital, phone ahead and ensure a member of staff waiting at agreed point. For example, a porter waiting in A&E department
- Accurate and concise oral and documental hand over

Organizational and Transfer Decision-Making Factors

A designated consultant is responsible for the decision to transfer the critically ill patient. They should ensure

- Appropriate patient transfer
- Patient can be transferred, risk versus benefits of transfer
- Referring hospital is informed
- Coordination of transfer runs smoothly
- Appropriate staff have been allocated for transfer
- Local policies are adhered to
- Next of kin informed

Specification of Transfer Vehicle

- Ensure good trolley access with appropriate fixing devices
- Good lighting, power points and temperature control
- Sufficient space for attending medical and nursing team
- Sufficient medical gases, electricity and storage space
- Robust surfaces to take into account urgency of transfer, mobilization time, geographical distance of transfer, weather and traffic conditions

Specification of Equipment

- Robust
- Lightweight
- Battery powered
- User friendly
- Audible alarms over unrelated noises during transfer, e.g., sirens
- Illuminated displays

- Emergency equipment available
- Mobile phone for communication

Check with ambulance crew whether they have electricity supply in ambulance.

Accompanying Staff

- An experienced doctor, experienced in resuscitation, airway management, ventilation and organ support with previous transfer experience
- An experienced ICU nurse, operating department practitioner or paramedic experienced in transfer of the critically ill
- Current staffing levels in many hospitals mean that this level of assistant is not always available
- Transferring hospital should provide medical indemnity and personal medical defence cover is also recommended

Always inform accepting hospital before leaving your hospital.

Importance of Patient Preparation

- Stabilization of the critically ill patient prior to transfer is key to minimize the destabilization of the critically ill patient on transfer.
- Is sedation, analgesia and muscle relaxant required?
- Is the patient's oxygenation stable?
- Is the cardiovascular system stable?
- Is IV access adequate?
- Accompaniment of all relevant investigations.
- Full monitoring of patient's vital signs should be in progress prior to transfer.
- Securing airway and IV line management.

Departure Checklist

- Are appropriate equipment and drugs available?
- Sufficient oxygen
- Suction available
- Trolley available
- Ambulance service notified of transfer and patient's condition, nature of transfer
- Bed confirmed at receiving hospital

- Receiving hospital notified
- Medical notes, X-rays and investigations available
- Transfer letter prepared
- Return arrangements known
- Next of kin informed of impending transfer

Transfer of Critically Ill

- Standard of care delivered should be maintained at same level as ICU care
- Continuous monitoring of patient
- Smooth transfer
- Accurate record keeping
- In event of emergency, ambulance to be stopped and/or transport patient to nearest A&E department

Medical and Nursing Hand Over

- Direct communication between referring hospital team and receiving hospital team
- Full hand over of patient's hospital stay alongside and treatments, investigations and results
- Disclosure of next of kin members and contact numbers

Phone next of kin on arrival so that they know their loved one arrived safely

Audit and Training

- Completion of audit documentation
- Completion of any local documentation regarding transfer
- Attend in-house and external training courses regarding safe transfer of critically ill patient

Review of All Transfers by an Allocated Consultant

The clinical conditions possibly eliciting inter-hospital transfer are

- Coma/head injury
- Renal/metabolic failure
- Requirement for computed tomography (CT) scan
- Plastic surgery
- Burns
- Cardiac problems
- Respiratory failure

- Spinal injury
- Major sepsis
- Recipients of transplantation
- Premature babies

Generally, the majority of patients requiring inter-hospital transfer have neurological or respiratory problems requiring further management in a specialist critical care unit. There is an increasing need for inter-hospital transfer of patients requiring liver and cardiac transplant units.

The issue that has led to a decrease in the need for inter-hospital transfer is the development of systems to transmit the images of a CT scan from one hospital to another. This allows the hospital to send the CT images via a phone-line to the specialist neuro-centre where the images can be assessed. The specialist neurologist can then decide whether transport of the patient to the specialist centre is indicated.

When to Transfer?

The importance of the 'golden hour' has been debated, but does the time/outcome equation have any application to the critical care setting? Transfer should occur:

- When the staff of the referring centre feel uncomfortable with the course of the illness injury
- When it is first realized that the patient requires care in a specialist centre. The risks to the patient:
- ETT, IV line dislodgement.
- Lack of appropriate equipment in the transfer vehicle if an unforseen incident occurs en route.
- Break down of the transfer vehicle while transferring patients.
- The vibration of the transport vehicle can cause either hypertension or cardiovascular depression.
- Always ascertain from the ambulance team what equipment etc. they have on board.

The risks of changes in BP can be reduced if the patient is adequately sedated prior to transfer. However, a patient is only ready for transfer after effective resuscitation, after physiological status is stabilized and after mechanical aspects are secured and appropriate equipment is available for transfer.

How should a patient be transferred?

- Ground vehicle transport is most often used.
- Boats are sometimes used to transfer critically ill patients from islands to the mainland.

- The use of aircraft is becoming more widely available in the United Kingdom.
- Helicopters are more frequently used in the transfer of patients over long distances or where traffic would slow the process of ground transport. The helicopter has the benefit of getting to places not accessible to road vehicles and also does not have to contend with the problems of traffic delaying the transfer.

Staff Involved in Transfer

Different areas use different disciplines of staff to accompany patients on transfer:

- Paramedics − ambulance personnel who have undergone further training.
- Specially trained flight nurses − mainly in America.
- Specially trained physicians and nurses, facilitated by ambulance personnel.

There is a pre-transfer checklist, which identifies the need for

- Assessment
- Evaluation
- Stabilization
- Having equipment available for
  - Airway and breathing
  - Cervical spine
  - Circulation
  - Neurological procedures (catheterization, reintubation)
  - Laboratory work (blood gases)
  - Continued medication
  - Safe delivery and documentation

The overall care and responsibility must be the patient's safety during the transport.

Section 4

Common conditions/reasons for admission

Section Outline

This section commences by outlining some of the physiological process of injury and repair that are common to all medical and surgical conditions. In addition, the section details some common conditions that may be observed in critical care and others that may be the reason for admission; others may be complications of interventions/treatments that occurred elsewhere.

4.1 PHYSIOLOGICAL PROCESSES COMMON TO ALL MEDICAL AND SURGICAL CONDITIONS

Principles of Cellular Death/Injury, Repair, and Adaptation

Hypoxic Cellular Death/Injury

When blood flow falls to a critical level below that which is required to maintain tissue viability swelling of the area affected will occur. When the occlusion becomes too great, blood supply is cut off. Eventually the loss of blood flow reaches a level where tissue viability can no longer be maintained (Richards and Edwards, 2014). This damage can occur due to

- Generalized ischaemia
  - Hypovolaemia
  - Hypoxaemia
  - Disseminated intravascular coagulation (DIC)

- Ischaemia of an organ
  - Acute kidney injury (AKI) of the kidney
  - Myocardial infarction (MI)
- Ischaemia of the skin or limb
  - Compression bandages or constrictive devices, such as a tight cast that has been improperly left in place for extended periods of time,
  - Crush or pressure injuries,
  - Pressure ulcers,
  - Swelling of a foot, leg, or arm due to fractures or compartment syndrome,
  - Peripheral vascular disease due to diabetes or heart failure and
  - Inotropic drugs can cause limb and skin ischaemia.

All of these and others can lead to hypoxic injury (Table 4.1), which can affect viability of tissue and its surrounding area. The hypoxic damage may either occur inside the body and be invisible to the naked eye or appear on the surface of the skin. Those areas of hypoxic damage that are invisible are generally due to an MI or AKI leading to heart failure or fluid overload. Hypoxic injury that is visible is due to occlusions of limbs, diabetic foot or pressure ulcers, which may lead to the appearance of offensive unsightly necrotic wounds, which do not heal.

The interrupted supply of oxygenated blood to cells can result in cellular changes, which in turn can stimulate the inflammatory response (IR) (see later). Hypoxia leads to interruption of supply of oxygenated blood to cells, which results in (Fig. 4.1) anaerobic metabolism and cellular membrane disruption.

Anaerobic Metabolism

Nutrients, such as glucose and fatty acids, as well as oxygen, enter the cell across a cell membrane. Hypoxic injury results in an inadequate flow of nutrients and oxygen to cells. As oxygen levels fall in cells, there is a rapid shift from aerobic to anaerobic metabolism. The first phase of glucose breakdown is glycolysis, anaerobic glycolysis (the breakdown of carbohydrates in the absence of oxygen in cells) leads to the accumulation of lactic acid, which reduces the cell's ability to generate cellular energy in the form of adenosine triphosphate (ATP). A reduction in ATP reduces the amount of energy available for cellular work.

The formation of lactic acid diminishes mitochondrial activity, leaving a lack of oxygen available for the third and final phase of glucose breakdown in the mitochondria — the electron transport chain. This event leads to the formation of nitric oxide.

Lactic acid and nitric oxide can rapidly build up in high concentrations in the cell when there is a lack of oxygen for normal metabolic processes. The lactic acid can lower blood pH, and nitric oxide can cause serious

TABLE 4.1 The conditions that lead to death, injury and repair.

Inflammatory response	Hypoxic damage	Oedema
These processes are not mutually exclusive. The inflammatory response can lead to interstitial oedema causing swelling which can cut off blood supply, leading to hypoxic damage and intracellular oedema. Hypoxic damage leading to intracellular oedema can lead to cellular damage and stimulation of the inflammatory response, which will stimulate the release of mediators. In addition, oedema can lead to hypoxia and stimulation of the inflammatory response.		
Trauma Head injury (cerebral oedema) Surgery/anaesthetic Renal/liver disease Pancreatitis Burns Gastrointestinal disorders • ulcers • hernia • irritable bowel syndrome • inflammatory bowel disease • ulcerative colitis Infection/sepsis Pulmonary oedema Drugs Hypertension Heart failure Malnutrition Anaphylaxis Neoplasms Leg ulcers	Hypovolaemia/hypotension Tight compression bandages/casts Compartment syndrome Myocardial infarction/cardiac arrest Shock Heart failure Deep vein thrombosis Pulmonary embolism Acute tubular necrosis Pressure ulcers Cerebral thrombosis or bleed Peripheral vascular disease Neoplasms	Cancer Malnutrition Congestive cardiac failure Fluid overload Left ventricular failure

Modified from Edwards, S.L., 2003b. Cellular pathophysiology Part 2: responses following hypoxia. Professional Nurse 18(11), 636–639.

vasodilatation. The result of anaerobic metabolism is a reduction in the energy available for cell work in the form of ATP, which eventually disrupts the cell membrane.

Cellular Membrane Disruption

The reduction in ATP from anaerobic metabolism leads to electrolyte disturbances. The plasma membrane of a cell relies on sufficient supplies of ATP to maintain a high concentration of sodium in the ECF compartment, and a low concentration in ICF compartments, and to maintain a high concentration of potassium inside the cell and a lower outside. The ATP-dependent sodium/potassium pump in cell membranes maintains the ionic gradients between ECF

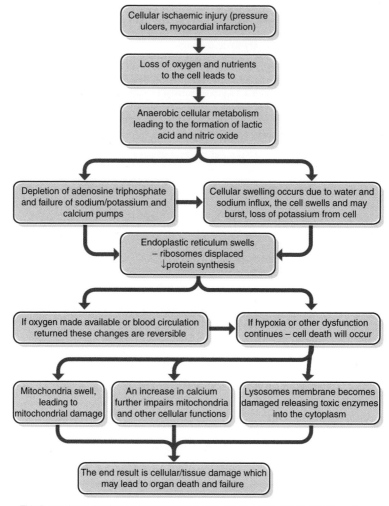

This figure shows that intracellular oedema occurs due to a reduction in ATP; the cell membrane can no longer maintain ionic gradients and sodium and water move into the cell.

FIGURE 4.1 The processes of cellular hypoxia and cell death.

and ICF. A reduced ATP supply to the plasma membrane of cells reduces its ability to maintain the normal ionic gradients of sodium (higher in ECF) and potassium (higher in ICF). The sodium/potassium pumps can no longer function, changing the ionic concentration.

Sodium will accumulate in the cell, drawing water towards it — leading to cellular oedema due to an increase in intracellular osmotic pressure. The cell may burst. Potassium in exchange leaks into the ECF space; the excess potassium is excreted in the urine. At this stage, these processes can be reversed by interventions such as relieving of pressure or administration of oxygen.

It should be noted that the return to normal ionic gradients of the cell might lead to a decrease in ECF serum potassium level.

Physiological Progression

If interventions are not initiated (removal of the occlusion or treatment instigated together with oxygen), intracellular acidosis becomes extreme and cellular dysfunction becomes severe. This leads to further disruption and ICF calcium levels increase. Calcium is present in many cells and is involved in many cellular processes; its concentration accelerates in the cell when stimulated by an electrical impulse (Marieb, 2017). Calcium is prevented from accumulating in the cell by the ATP-dependent calcium pump in the plasma membrane. During hypoxia, the ATP-dependent calcium pump becomes dysfunctional and calcium builds up in cells. Its derangement results in membrane disruption of the mitochondria and structural dysfunction of other organelles in the cell. When calcium accumulates in such large amounts inside cells, it may be the hallmark of irreversible cellular injury and eventually cell death.

An important cell structure within cells that contain destructive enzymes is lysosomes; which break down cell waste (Marieb, 2017). The lysosome membrane is quite stable but becomes fragile when a cell is injured or deprived of oxygen. Lysosomal membrane instability is made worse by the lack of ATP, together with an increase in calcium; cells start to use their own structural phospholipids as a nutrient source. Eventually, lysosome membranes become more permeable and may rupture. This allows the release of lysosome enzymes resulting in self-digestion of the cell. If these processes are permitted to continue, they may finally lead to irreversible cell damage and death.

Tissue Injury: The Formation of Oedema

Oedema is an abnormal collection of fluid in tissues, which can either collect in interstitial or intracellular spaces (Richards and Edwards, 2014). Oedema is a problem of fluid distribution and does not necessarily indicate fluid excess. The causes of oedema are varied (Table 4.1) and include hypoxia (leads to intracellular oedema) (see previous) and the IR (leads to interstitial oedema) (see later).

Interstitial oedema is usually associated with weight gain, swelling and puffiness, tight-fitting clothes and shoes, limited movement of an affected area and symptoms associated with an underlying pathological condition. There are many different types of interstitial oedema, named according to the mechanisms that cause it and localized or generalized. Interstitial oedema is formed in three different ways:

1. Stimulation of the inflammatory immune response (see later).
2. Changes in capillary dynamics due to increased hydrostatic pressure (HP) or decreased plasma oncotic pressure.
3. Lymphatic system obstruction.

Always check albumin levels and/or colloid osmotic pressures in patients with oedema.

Normal Capillary Dynamics

The blood in the capillaries is always under pressure known as the HP, which is determined by the blood pressure (BP). Fluid leaks out of the capillaries all the time into interstitial spaces to allow nutrients to enter cells. However, this leakage of fluid does not affect circulating volume because the movement of fluid in the opposite direction balances it (Fig. 2.2). Counteracting forces determine fluid moving from the plasma to interstitial spaces and vice versa. Fluid moving out of the capillaries and into interstitial spaces is called filtration and fluid moving into capillaries from interstitial spaces is called absorption. Two forces govern movement of fluid across the wall of a capillary.

1 The Hydrostatic Pressure Gradient An HP gradient is the difference between HP of fluid inside the capillary and HP of fluid outside a capillary (filtration). The HP in a capillary varies, because pressure of blood declines continually as blood flows from the arteriolar end of a capillary to the venous end. There is no variation in HP outside a capillary.

Where HP is higher, water tends to move from the side with a higher HP to the lower. A difference in filtration pressure drives water out of capillaries.

The HP inside the capillary declines from 38 mmHg at the arterial end to 16 mmHg at the venous end, and HP outside the capillary is 1 mmHg. Therefore, the HP drops from $38 - 1 = 37$ mmHg at the arterial end to $16 - 1 = 15$ mmHg at the venous end (Fig. 2.2).

2 Colloidal Oncotic Pressure Gradient The colloidal oncotic pressure (COP) is determined by the protein concentration between plasma and ISF because it creates a difference in pressure between the inside and outside of capillaries (absorption). Proteins (plasma proteins) in ECF exert a COP.

The COP gradient is the difference between COP of fluid inside the capillary and COP of fluid outside a capillary. When a COP gradient exists, water tends to flow from the side where COP is higher (osmosis).

Because the concentration of proteins in plasma is higher than the concentration of proteins in ISF, the COP gradient is directed inward and it tends to drive water into capillaries (absorption). The COP of plasma is approximately 25 mmHg, whereas COP of ISF is negligible. Therefore, COP gradient or absorption pressure across a capillary wall is $25 - 0 = 25$ mmHg (Fig. 2.2).

Net Filtration Pressure The direction of water flow across the wall of a capillary is determined by net filtration pressure (NFP), e.g., the difference between HP and COP:

$$NFP = HP - COP$$

When the sign of NFP is positive, HP gradient is greater than the COP gradient, and fluid flows outward (filtration); when NFP is negative, COP gradient is greater than the HP gradient, and fluid flows inward (absorption).

Assuming an HP gradient of 37 mmHg at the arterial end of a capillary and COP gradient of 25 mmHg, the NFP is $37 - 25 = 12$ mmHg, which favours filtration. Assuming HP falls to 15 mmHg at the venous end of a capillary, NFP at the end is $15 - 25 = -10$ mmHg, which favours absorption. Filtration and absorption occur within the same capillary to allow nutrients (glucose) to cross over into cells.

Most of the fluid filtered out of ESF is returned to the circulation, but there is a net deficit of 2 mmHg (Fig. 2.2). It would be assumed that a small amount of fluid remains in interstitial spaces and leads to oedema formation or a reduction in blood volume. This is not the case because about 3 L/day of filtered fluid is picked up from interstitial spaces and returned to the circulation by the lymphatic system.

Changes in Capillary Dynamics

The balance between filtration and absorption can be altered as a result of everyday occurrences (increases and decreases in BP, stress) and as part of the disease process (malnutrition, heart failure). This leads to the formation of oedema due to three different processes.

1 Oedema Formation Due to an Increase in Hydrostatic Pressure Oedema forms when there is an increase in HP either at the arterial end of a capillary or at the venous end. This will raise the pressure of blood in capillaries and cause an increase in the rate of filtration (Marieb, 2017). Using Fig. 2.2, assume that HP in the artery end increases by 5 mmHg from 38 to 43 mmHg and in the venous end from 16 to 21 mmHg, but COP remains the same.

TABLE 4.2 The conditions that lead to changes in hydrostatic pressure and oedema formation.

Condition	Principles	Progression
Liver failure	In liver failure there is a general increase in pressure in the portal venous system and raised pressure in the portal vessels.	This may eventually lead to the formation of ascites.
Heart failure	In heart failure the pressure can rise in either the systemic veins or the pulmonary veins, depending on which side of the heart is affected. Failure of the left ventricle causes pressure to rise in the pulmonary veins and can lead to oedema formation in the lungs as pulmonary oedema.	In right-sided heart failure (complete heart failure) there is an increase in hydrostatic pressure (HP) in the vena cava and other systemic veins. This tends to cause oedema in systemic tissues and oedema will form in the parts of the body that hang down, such as the wrists, ankles and sacrum.
Renal failure	Certain forms of damage to the kidneys interfere with their ability to eliminate excess water and solutes into the urine, which results in the accumulation of excess fluid in the body.	As a consequence, blood volume increases and blood pressure rises throughout the cardiovascular system. The increase in pressure raises capillary HP, which will increase filtration and reduce absorption processes and lead to the formation of oedema.

Therefore, $43 - 1 = 42$, $21 - 1 = 20$, reflects the difference in HP between ECF and ISF. The NFP now equals $42 - 25 = 17$ mmHg at the arterial end and $20 - 25 = -5$ mmHg at the venous end. This leaves a deficit pressure of 12 mmHg leading to an increase in filtration and a reduction in absorption. Large amounts of fluid will collect in interstitial spaces and cause the formation of interstitial oedema in certain conditions, which can lead to poor tissue viability in the affected area (Table 4.2).

2 Oedema Formation Due to a Reduced Colloidal Oncotic Pressure Oedema will also form when there is a reduction in plasma proteins in ECF. Therefore, any condition that will lead to a reduction in plasma proteins will promote changes in capillary absorption. Using Fig. 2.2, assume that COP on the arterial side was to reduce by 5 mmHg from 25 to 20 mmHg, and the same level of reduction of 5 mmHg is reflected at the venous end.

TABLE 4.3 The conditions that lead to changes in colloidal oncotic pressure (COP) and the formation of oedema.

Condition	Principles	Progression
Renal disease	Damage to the kidneys can cause an increase elimination of plasma proteins in the urine (nephrotic syndrome).	This loss of protein triggers a reduction in capillary absorption because of the drop in plasma COP.
Malnutrition	Starvation will reduce the amount of protein available to form plasma proteins. During malnutrition, there are insufficient amounts of proteins being digested through the gastrointestinal tract.	If the malnourished state is allowed to continue the proteins stored in the body are broken down and utilized as a source of energy, by the liver, to maintain cellular and organ function. This leads to reduced amounts of proteins in the plasma inadequate to produce effective plasma COP.

Modified from Edwards, S.L., 2003a. Cellular pathophysiology Part 1: changes following tissue injury. Professional Nurse 18(10), 562–565.

The HP in the ECF capillary is 38 and in ISF is 1 mmHg, therefore $38 - 1 = 37$ mmHg and $16 - 1 = 15$ mmHg, meaning that arterial HP becomes 37 mmHg and venous HP becomes 15 mmHg. Consequently, $37 - 20 = 17$ mmHg at the arterial end and $15 - 20 = -5$ mmHg at the venous end. This leaves a net deficit of 12 mmHg and an increase in filtration but a reduction in absorption leading to an accumulation of fluid in interstitial spaces. This occurs in a number of conditions, leading to poor healing, and tissue viability may be affected (Table 4.3).

3 Oedema Formation Due to Blocked Lymphatic System A cancer growth can form in many tissue types within the body. The tumour can grow to a size that blocks or occludes lymphatic drainage from tissue sites. This will lead to an accumulation of fluid in the interstitial fluid space. The lymphatic vessels and their thin-walled venules offer relatively little mechanical resistance to pressure from cancer (McCance and Huether, 2018).

Other lymphatic vessels supplying the area can normally drain small collections of interstitial fluid away. Large accumulations can cause clinical manifestations related to their volume and the rate at which they accumulate. Lymphatic blockage from any cause can result in drainage of the contents of lymphatic vessels into the pleural space leading to the formation of a pleural effusion (McCance and Huether, 2018). This can cause considerable impairment of pulmonary function.

Tissue Repair: Activation of the Inflammatory Response

Cellular damage, e.g., leg ulcers, surgical procedures, and trauma (Table 4.1), causes stimulation of the inflammatory response (IR) that ends with repair to damaged cells and tissues (Richards and Edwards, 2014). Activation of the IR is part of the innate immune system and represents a major physiological event in the body (Fig. 4.2). Following the damage, tissues release mediators, the most important of which are

- Histamine
- Kinins
- Prostaglandins
- Complement
- Cytokines (monokines and lymphokines)

The list of these chemical mediators is immense and rapidly growing. The mediators are released at the site of injury by the endothelium and will enhance the activity of the body's own nonspecific and specific immune responses. Release of these mediators is to

- protect the body from invading microorganisms,
- limit the extent of blood loss and injury and
- promote rapid healing of involved tissues

The mediators act as a signalling system (chemotaxis) to attract nutrients, fluids, clotting factors, neutrophils and macrophages to damaged sites. The arrival of macrophages in an area of damaged tissue is central to acute inflammation control, but macrophages can remain at sites of prolonged or chronic inflammation. The mediators cause a localized increase in

- Capillary permeability leading to pain and swelling
- Vasodilatation to increase blood supply leading to heat and redness

The endothelium is a major contributor to activation of the IR. It is not just an inert barrier between flowing blood and the substructure of blood vessels and tissue, but an active metabolic organ responsible for coagulation. Coagulation always accompanies inflammation, to prevent excessive blood loss and to isolate the injured site. A victim of an acute tissue injury or a patient with a wound that will not heal or is infected, varicose or pressure ulcers could potentially release inflammatory mediators that circulate in the bloodstream and could alter endothelial integrity elsewhere. This may incite coagulation abnormalities whereby there is a concomitant activation of coagulation or alterations in the haemostatic balance causing systemic thrombosis or gross haemorrhage known as DIC.

A lack of regulation of the IR can lead to an uncontrolled intravascular inflammation that ultimately harms the body. The mediators become toxic to

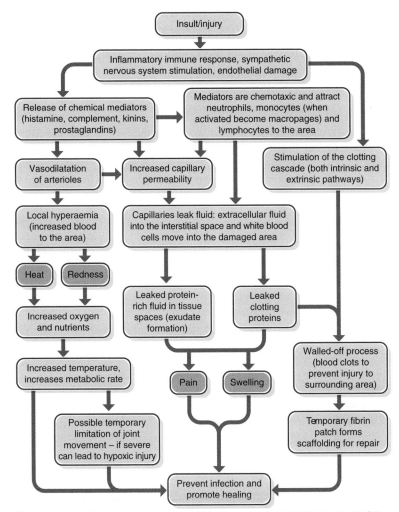

This figure shows that an increase in permeability allows protein-rich fluid to move out of the extracellular fluid compartment, reducing colloidal osmotic pressure; this increases interstitial fluid colloidal osmotic pressure and oedema formation.

FIGURE 4.2 The inflammatory immune response. *Modified from Marieb (2004) with permission.*

other cells, damaging tissues, vessels and organs far away from the initial injury. There are currently no conclusive indicators why some inflammatory processes proceed smoothly to healing while others lead to increase tissue damage. The serious systemic conditions such as multi-system organ failure (MSOF) and systemic inflammatory response syndrome (SIRS) are thought to be caused by over-stimulation of the IR.

Cellular Adaptation

Cells are constantly exposed to changes in their environment. These may occur as a part of normal physiological processes:

- Pattern of food intake may change
- Hormone levels may rise and fall
- May be exposed to extreme temperatures.

If cells were static systems, these changes would affect their function and that of tissues but homeostatic mechanisms allow cells to cope with such stresses.

These mechanisms are also important when cells try to limit damage from injury. Constant injury can lead to the following.

Atrophy

- Decrease or shrinkage in cell size of individual cells with fewer and smaller organelles and less cytoplasm, a decrease in number of cells or both.
- Can affect any organ. Most common in the skeletal muscle, ear and brain.
- Causes include decrease in workload, use, blood supply, nutrition, hormonal secretion and nervous stimulation.

Hypertrophy

- Increase in size of cells and consequently the affected organ.
- Usually due to increased functional demands on a tissue.
- Seen in cells that cannot easily divide, e.g., skeletal and cardiac muscle.
- After removal of one kidney, the other adapts by increasing in size.

Hyperplasia

- Increase in the number of cells resulting from increased cell division.
- May occur as a response to injury. May occur with hypertrophy if the cell is able to synthesize DNA. Can occur in the liver and kidneys.
- Compensatory hyperplasia enables some organs to regenerate. It occurs in the liver. After removal of up to 70% of the liver, regeneration can occur in 2 weeks.
- Nerve, skeletal muscle, myocardial cells and lens cells of the eye cannot regenerate.
- Callus or thickening of the skin is an example of hyperplasia.
- Increased cell mass through hypertrophy or hyperplasia can be physiological:
  - Thyroid increases in pregnancy due to TSH (hyperplasia).
  - Skeletal muscle fibres increase in size (hypertrophy) in response to exercise.

- May occur in response to disease states:
  - Low serum calcium means the parathyroids increase in size.
  - Narrow aortic valve leads to enlargement of muscle cells in the left ventricle.
  - Obstruction of colon leads to increased size of smooth muscle cells proximal to the obstruction.
- Following removal of stimulus to hyperplasia or hypertrophy, the tissue reverts to normal.

Dysplasia

- Abnormal changes in size, shape and organization of cells.
- Related to hyperplasia and may be called atypical hyperplasia.
- Frequently seen in the epithelial cells of the cervix and respiratory tract.
- May be associated with neoplastic growths.

Metaplasia

- The reversible replacement of one cell type by another, sometimes less differentiated cell type.
- Most commonly occurs in epithelial tissues.
- Ciliated columnar epithelial cells of the respiratory tract may become replaced by stratified squamous epithelial cells in the bronchial lining.
- Can be reversed if the stimulus is removed (usually cigarette smoking).
- Metaplasia is not considered to be actual cancer but can be viewed as a premalignant condition that required immediate investigation.

Effect of Treatments on Physiological Processes

The interventions used to treat the insult/injury can lead to further stimulation of the physiological processes identified above. Some of the interventions used such as the following, may prevent these processes from causing serious damage and/or complications:

- Blood transfusions, colloids and crystalloids used to maintain circulating volume, preventing hypoxia to cells.
- Oxygen therapy incorporated to maintain oxygen concentrations to meet the increased demand and prevent anaerobic metabolism and acidosis from developing.
- Enteral feeding may be instigated to maintain levels of nutrients and to aid the healing process.

Instigation of these treatments early may stem the inflammatory immune response (IIR) and neuroendocrine activation and prevent further endothelial damage.

However, surgery and anaesthesia may be required to stabilize bleeding or repair damage. Fasting practices in hospital may lead to starvation. Drug therapies such as antibiotics, steroids and continued stress may lead to immunosuppression. All of these may add further insult and injury to an already compromised patient and further stimulate the physiological processes identified previously.

Blood Transfusions

Blood transfusion is required for the following reasons:

- To replace blood lost during an operation or after an accident
- Used to treat anaemia — iron, vitamin B_{12} or folate
- Medical conditions that require blood transfusions include
  - Haemophilia — affects the ability of blood to clot
  - Sickle cell anaemia, thalassaemia — disruption to the normal production or RBC
  - Leukaemia — RBC is produced at a reduced rate
  - Malaria — RBC are destroyed
  - Renal failure — reduction in production of erythropoietin by the kidneys

Blood transfusions have been implicated in immunosuppression and alterations in the IIR. The changes that occur in stored blood (Box 3.1) may affect an injured patient's progress and precipitate the development of adult respiratory distress syndrome (ARDS), SIRS and DIC and play a part in the development of multiple system organ failure (MSOF).

Various changes occur in blood as a result of its removal from the body. These changes begin within 24 hours of storage and continue throughout the entire 21 days, after which blood is considered outdated. These changes are many and varied and have implications for the patient suffering from injury. Despite blood transfusions being valuable, there are many complications associated with them, e.g., pulmonary damage, metabolic toxicity, blood group incompatibilities and transfusion reactions, all of which can participate in the over-stimulation of the IIR system.

It is important to ensure safety is maintained at the bedside prior to and during blood transfusions to avoid any potential fatal transfusion errors. The following checks should take place:

- The blood has no leaks, discolouration or signs of damage.
- The patient has consented, where appropriate, to the transfusion and information provided.
- Confirm the patient identification by asking them to state their full name and date of birth, which should match the patient wristband; if unable to confirm, then identification can be obtained from the next of kin or equivalent.

- Check the unit of blood against the documentation provided:
  - Patient ID
  - Blood unit number
  - Blood group of the patient and compatibility
  - Check if blood warmer is required
  - Are there any other specific requirements
- Perform regular observations before, during and after the blood transfusion.

Crystalloids and Colloids

In an attempt to reduce blood transfusions, other regimens to maintain circulating volume in times of an insult have been devised, e.g., colloid (gelofusine) and crystalloid (0.9% normal saline) therapies. The use of colloids is to restore plasma volume and improve or maintain oxygen transport and nutrients that are needed for the maintenance and restoration of cellular function. By administering plasma expanders, there is an improvement in oxygen availability, oxygen consumption, circulating volume, haemodynamic status and tissue perfusion.

The result of using crystalloid solutions during or following an insult is that sodium leaks into the surrounding cells and carries with it extracellular water. The use of a salt solution is required to restore extracellular fluid volume. However, between two and four times the amount of crystalloid is required, giving rise to possible risk of oedema and/or haemodilution, and therefore remains controversial.

The need for fluid at this time is to re-perfuse tissues/organs following the loss due to the stimulation of the IIR that causes an increase in permeability and the movement of fluid into the interstitial space. However, fluid therapy after the initial insult may not result in a return to normal functioning but may instead initiate post-ischaemic reperfusion injury. This refers to the continued decrease in blood flow to an area despite normal BP and oxygenation. The damage to the cell can cause severe membrane damage, leading to a worsening oedema, vasospasm, intracellular and mitochondrial calcium shifts and organ failure.

It is thought that an influx of calcium into the cell occurs during resuscitation and consequent reperfusion, not during the ischaemic period. The mechanism by which the calcium content of cells is regulated is then dysfunctional because of a lack of ATP. Intracellular calcium is an important signalling system responsible for activation of phospholipases and proteases, and its derangement results in membrane disruption. As a result, toxic calcium accumulates in the mitochondria, causing structural derangements of the organelles, and may be the hallmark of irreversible cellular injury and eventual cell death.

Surgery/Anaesthesia

Patients undergoing surgical procedures may have impaired immunological activity due to increased stimulation of the sympathetic nervous system due to stress and the increased activity of cortisol. A surgical procedure is accompanied by anaesthesia, trauma to the body, possible blood transfusion and an overall stress response. These effects may further stimulate the neuroendocrine response, which, as previously highlighted, may contribute to shock, ARDS, SIRS, DIC and MSOF if stimulation is prolonged.

Surgery is reported to have implications in reducing cytokine release, which is responsible for the IR. Anaesthesia alone is associated with decreased immuno-responsiveness, with both decreased phagocytosis and lymphocyte proliferation noted. It is difficult to isolate which events cause the alterations to the IIR. Most likely it is the interactions of all of these events that operate synergistically to mediate overall host immunosuppression and thus increase susceptibility to infection. However, when a patient is unable to mount an effective IIR, the likelihood of sepsis or SIRS increases.

Starvation

The recovery from an insult depends upon the consumption and absorption of appropriate amounts of carbohydrates, fats, proteins, minerals and vitamins. Following an insult or injury a patient may not be allowed to consume any nutrition, leading to the start of starvation. During starvation, there is an absence of carbohydrates directly from the gut; the body can utilize carbohydrates stored as glycogen in the liver and skeletal muscles as a source of energy. As a result, glycogen is converted to glucose (glycogenolysis) and released from the liver. This restores blood glucose levels to normal.

It is necessary to commence enteral feeding as soon as possible.

However, despite these mechanisms for supplying blood glucose, they cannot maintain blood glucose levels for very long. Fat stores provide a large energy deposit that may be used for energy. This requires a major body adjustment, as all other body tissues must reduce their oxidation of glucose and switch over to fats as their energy source. As the liver metabolizes fat, ketone bodies are produced in large quantities. These are oxidized by the body into carbon dioxide, water and ATP. As a result of fat utilization as a source of energy, at this stage, hypometabolism occurs so that protein can be spared, and an individual can fast for several weeks, provided water is consumed.

If further injury/insult such as infection or stress occurs, this will result in a hypermetabolic state. Starvation in combination with a hypermetabolic state stimulates neuroendocrine responses and produces a hypo-albuminaemic malnourished state. Carbohydrates, fats and body proteins are broken down in large quantities. In the absence of these energy sources, muscle protein is utilized as a source of energy to maintain cellular functions. Starvation and protein deficiency result in poor immune system function (increasing the risk of infection) and affect the breakdown and removal of damaged tissue from wounds, which leads to poor tissue growth and repair. It is estimated that, once protein stores are depleted to about one-half of their normal level, death results.

Immunosuppression

The patient may be immunosupressed because they are stressed, malnourished, suffering from an insult or injury or receiving drug therapies such as steroids or broad-spectrum antibiotics. The intricacy of the IIR is overwhelming in its complexity, components and interrelationships. Alterations can occur anywhere among the numerous pathways, cells and mediators, leading to disruptions with widespread disorder and confusion throughout body systems.

Interventions to prevent infection or stimulation of inflammation such as hand washing, aseptic technique and nutrition play a major role. These, however, may not be enough to protect the ill patient exposed to alterations in the IIR, resistant environmental pathogens and breakdown of natural defence barriers.

Critical Care Nursing Key Life-saving Interventions

The nursing interventions that relate to the physiological processes that occur following an injury or hypoxia are related to maintaining a normal haemodynamic state and preventing excessive cellular/organ damage and loss of circulating volume. Respiratory failure demands increased and reduced supply of oxygen.

Administration of Oxygen

An imbalance between oxygen supply and tissue demands is fundamental to the nature of the insult. Oxygen supply and demand is maintained in equilibrium as long as supplies of oxygen are available and carbon dioxide is eliminated through ventilation, perfusion, diffusion and cell metabolism. Any alteration of any part of these processes causes impaired gas exchange.

An increase in the demand for oxygen can occur during pulmonary trauma, causing damage to the chest wall and pulmonary contusions. However, an increase in the demand for oxygen may exist when the lungs are not directly injured, as any insult may give rise to an increase demand over supply. As the cells demand more oxygen during injury, compounded by stress, the demand will eventually outweigh supply. This can lead to cellular hypoxia, production of lactic acid and the lowering of blood pH.

In an acid environment, chemoreceptors are stimulated, and consequently oxygen demand is maintained for a short while due to the increase in respiratory rate and depth of breathing. This is an attempt to eliminate the excess acid. The increase in work of breathing can exhaust the patient and increase the demands for oxygen. When the respiratory system becomes overwhelmed, the victim is at risk of pulmonary complications, leading to a supply-demand deficit that gives rise to a reduction in venous oxygen supply and respiratory failure ensues.

The critical care nurse is therefore responsible for administrating humidified oxygen, the continuous frequent monitoring of respiratory rate, depth and pattern of breathing and any signs of change. There are detailed arterial blood gas tests that can be done to determine acid-base balance, but these are not always available in all clinical situations.

Always use humidified oxygen in patients receiving prolonged oxygen therapy.

Prevention of a Low Circulating Volume

Following any tissue injury or damage, the IR is stimulated leading to the release of mediators from the damaged tissue, causing permeability changes leading to movement of fluid into the ISF space and oedema, vasodilatation and coagulation. These processes of inflammation affect the microvasculature, regional circulation and eventually organ function. The vasodilatation in certain areas increases blood flow, the movement of fluid from the circulation due to permeability changes, which causes tissue oedema in the area and contributes to a reduction in normal circulating volume. The stimulation of the clotting cascade may cause blockage of the microvasculature, leading to the development of thrombi, which cause further tissue damage.

The critical care nurse's role is to administer the prescribed fluid regimens for the immediate restoration of an effective circulating blood volume. This may require the use of blood, blood products, a balanced salt and/or water solution, colloid solution or a combination of all solutions.

The Administration of Adequate Nutrition

With the stimulation of the neuroendocrine system, there is a substantial increase in metabolic rate, oxygen consumption and production of carbon dioxide and heat. The increased demand for energy is accomplished at the expense of lean body mass. The loss of lean body mass due to an insult is different from that observed during starvation, which conserves the use of protein stores as a source of energy to the end. A patient with profound injuries will have hyper-metabolism, due to stress, and the release of adrenaline (glycogen stores reduce) and cortisol (fat and protein stores are mobilized) results in the use of mixed fuel sources.

In these instances, energy requirements become amplified. This is needed to supply nutrients and oxygen to active cells, tissues and organs involved in the defence against the results of injury. Inflammation, immune function and tissue repair all require an increase in nutrients to support their function. Therefore, all potential sources of glucose are mobilized as sources of fuel. Proteins and fats are converted into glucose via gluconeogenesis, and glycogen stores are converted via glycogenolysis. The result is a hyperglycaemia.

The release of catecholamines causes decreased deposition of fat stores (lipogenesis) and increased breakdown of fat (lipolysis). The liver converts fatty acids for use as a source of energy. Fats are a more concentrated source of energy than glucose and as such more is broken down than the body can utilize. As a result, fat deposits may accumulate in the liver, leading to signs and symptoms of liver failure, including hyper-bilirubinaemia, elevated levels of liver enzymes, which hepatic encephalopathy. Zinc distributed via the liver becomes deficient, which is associated with impaired wound healing.

If protein continues to be broken down and used for fuel, plasma levels of amino acids reduce. Extracellular fluid proteins are responsible for maintaining COP in the vascular bed; they exert an opposing (reabsorbing) pressure in the capillaries to maintain circulating volume. A decreased level of these proteins, e.g., albumin, results in decreased COP, and hypo-albuminaemia, which causes an accumulation of fluid in the interstitial space, leading to the formation of oedema. Protein loss is accompanied by a loss of potassium, magnesium and phosphate.

The use of all energy sources following an insult causes an exhaustion of energy stores and deprives cells and tissues of nutrients, reducing their ability to produce ATP and to support organ function. There is an increase in cellular metabolism, oxygen consumption, cardiac work and carbon dioxide production. The myocardium becomes depressed leading to cardiac failure.

The loss of energy stores, especially protein depletion, will contribute to morbidity and mortality of patients following an insult. It is therefore imperative to initiate feeding early in critical care patients who are at risk of reducing lean body mass due to injury or insult. The timing and the route of nutritional support can favourably influence the metabolic response to injury.

4.2 NEUROLOGICAL

The brain is a specialized organ that maintains homeostasis in a different way to the rest of the body to ensure that despite a raised intracranial pressure (ICP) cerebral perfusion is maintained to prevent permanent injury or death. This is referred to as autoregulation.

Autoregulation of the Brain

Normal Dynamics

- Brain tissue 80%
- Cerebrospinal fluid (CSF) 10%
- Cerebral blood flow (CBF) 10%

Compensation Mechanisms

- CSF displacement cranial and lumbar
- Reduction CSF production and an increase in CSF reabsorption
- Reduction in CBF venous blood shunted away (can lead to further insult)

Cerebral Blood Flow

- CBF is determined by cerebral perfusion pressure (CPP) and cerebral vascular resistance (CVR). Thus,

$$CBF = CPP/CVR$$

- CVR regulates the arterial BP to maintain CPP above 60–70 mmHg.
- CPP is determined by the mean arterial blood pressure (MABP) minus the intracranial pressure (ICP) and in inversely proportional to CVR.
- Parasympathetic stimulation will decrease heart rate.

A raised ICP can be determined by a rise in BP and a reduction in heart rate.

Brain Trauma

The skull is tough and takes quite a lot of abuse, as the brain is well protected by bone and cushioned by CSF. Many cases of skull fracture depend on age, as the young and the old are vulnerable because their bones and blood vessels are fragile. An accident may result in

- Lacerations to the scalp — damage to the meninges or torn blood vessels — this may result in a bleed and an increase the ICP.
- Fracture of the skull.
  - Linear/simple fracture — two fragments, which remain in apposition.
  - Comminuted — multiple linear fractures, but the fragments are not displaced.

- Compound − communication with outside scalp wound, increased possibility of infection of bone and cranial contents.
- Depressed − fragments are driven inwards, compressing or piercing the meninges or brain as well as the direct injury.

Slight or severe brain injury may or may not be associated with a fracture of the skull. However, brain injury/trauma may lead to

- Intracranial haemorrhage
  - Subdural haematoma − damaged blood vessels on the surface of the brain; blood accumulates over several hours/days, and therefore development of symptoms may be delayed. Occurs on average in 10%−15% of head injuries, generally due to contusion and lacerations.
  - Extradural haematoma − damaged blood vessels inside the skull and occurs in 2% of head injuries. 80% are due to fracture of the skull.
  - Intracerebral haematoma − damaged vessels inside the brain itself. Occurs in 2%−3% of head injuries, generally in the frontal and temporal areas.
  - Epidural haematoma − in the spine.
- Compression of the brain − resulting from a depressed fracture, oedema, haemorrhage; if untreated, will progress into a deepening unconsciousness and a rising ICP.
- Supratentorial herniation − a critical condition associated with brain trauma whereby a portion of the cerebrum herniates through the tentorial hiatus (a space in the base of the brain stem). The rigid skull stops outward expansion, therefore the brain has nowhere to go but down. This leads to compression of the brain stem − brain stem death may ensue.
- Concussion − is a minor head injury, which may cause a brief period of loss of consciousness (less than 30 minutes) or no loss of consciousness due to jarring of the brain and its forceful contact with the rigid skull. As a result, normal brain activity is temporarily interrupted. A concussion is usually spontaneously reversible with no residual damage. The patient may also be dazed, confused, restless and amnesic, complaining of a headache; vomiting may occur in the recovery period.
- Contusion − this is bruising of the brain, which causes rupture of small blood capillaries in the brain in the region that is damaged. The patient may recover but may regress, and it may take several weeks to recover. There may be residual scarring and impaired function.
- Contrecoup injury − this occurs when a stationary object hits the rigid skull, which is stopped instantly. The softer brain rebounds back and forth within the skull.

Always establish from the doctors the range of movement that is allowed for the specific injury, e.g., only to log roll.

Signs and Symptoms

These depend on the nature and severity of tissue damage. May appear immediately or several hours later.

Signs may include

- Cerebral oedema
- Intracranial bleeding
- Ensuing brain compression
- Elevation of ICP

Symptoms may include

- Unconsciousness — either immediately or following a lucid interval
- Headache and dizziness
- Disturbed vision
- Changes in pupillary reactions
- Changes in vital signs
- Disorientation and confusion
- Motor and sensory deficits
- Convulsions
- Speech impairment
- Neck stiffness
- Hyperthermia
- CSF leakage
- 30% of patients have injuries in other parts of the body

Effects of Brain Trauma

- Changes in action potentials
  - Electrical — action potentials become sluggish or are blocked
  - Chemical — neurotransmitters fail to be released at the neuromuscular junction, e.g., acetylcholine
- Changes to hormonal control which as a result fail to initiate a response
  - Failure to activate plasma membrane permeability
  - Reduction in synthesis of proteins or regulatory enzymes — producing building blocks to produce haemoglobin or immunoglobulins of the immune system

- Failure of enzyme activation or deactivation − digestive enzymes
- Reduction in secretary action − reduction in stress response, e.g., adrenaline and noradrenaline
- Stimulation of mitosis − reduction in growth and repair
- Neurological outcomes
  - Epilepsy
  - Transient loss of consciousness
  - Loss of limb movement, weakness, gait
  - Loss of sensation, temperature, touch, pain
  - Changes in sight (partial or complete blindness), hearing (deafness, tinnitus, vertigo), facial (Bell's palsy), lips/jaw movement
  - Incontinence (faecal, urine)
  - Loss of appreciation of size, shape, texture and weight (astereognosis)
  - Loss of cognitive thought, memory, speech, understanding, recognition, interpretation (prosopagnosia), learning ability
  - Aggressive or antisocial behaviour
  - Personality changes, disturbed intellectual ability, disturbances of speech, visual disturbances
  - Hallucinations
  - In addition, the loss of
    - Ability to work
    - Partner
    - Ability to self-care
  - Disturbances of speech
    - Dysarthria
    - Dysphonia/aphonia
  - Disorders of language
    - Dysphasia
  - Impairment of vision/ocular movement
    - Hemianopia
    - Quadrantanopia
    - Diplopia
    - Conjugate deviation of the eyes
  - Persistent vegetative state (PVS) − the body is capable of growth and repair but devoid of thought
  - Locked-in syndrome − efferent pathways are disrupted; patient cannot communicate but is fully conscious and has intact cognitive function
  - Brain stem death − a complete loss of brain stem function

Aims of Care

- Frequent careful observations and monitoring
- Neurological assessment, management of care and interventions
- Prevent complications

- Caring for the unconscious patient
- Rehabilitation
- Caring for the family

Neurological patients require a lot of time and effort to enable them to return to a normal life. This involves initial treatment and interventions, then generally a lengthy period of rehabilitation. When neurological outcomes are the end result, they can be so serious as to affect a person's ability to continue a normal life (Table 4.4). When caring for neurological patients, it is important from the outset to deliver high quality care in an attempt to reduce the devastating effects of these neurological outcomes.

TABLE 4.4 Neurological outcomes.

Neurological outcome	Description
Confusion	• Loss of concentration • Memory impairment • Misinterpretation • Delusions • Reduced intellectual functioning • Anxiety and restlessness • Compulsive behaviour • Reduced alertness • Forgetfulness • Disorientation • Hallucinations
Dysmnesia	• Loss of past memories • Inability to form new memories • Observed in subarachnoid haemorrhage or brain injury, lobectomy, and Alzheimer's
Agnosia	Defect of recognition of objects, both what it is and what it is for – the object may be recognized through other senses, e.g., visual, auditory or touch, language
Dysphasia	• Impairment of comprehension or production of language • Results from dysfunction of the left cerebral hemisphere • Generally involving the middle cerebral artery or a tributary
Alterations in muscle tone	• Hyponia – decreased muscle tone: passive movement occurs with little or no resistance; there is reduced excitability of the neurones; tire easily or are weak • Hypertonia – increased muscle tone passive movement occurs with resistance; spasticity with an increase stretch reflex due to damage of the motor areas in the CNS; rigidity; muscles are firm and tense

TABLE 4.4 Neurological outcomes.—cont'd

Neurological outcome	Description
Alterations in movement	• Hyperkinesia — excessive movements, repetitive movements, compulsions, mannerisms • Hypokinesia — decreased movements, loss of voluntary movements despite preserved consciousness, include the following: • Paresis — partial paralysis, incomplete loss of muscle power • Paralysis — loss of motor function • Akinesia — decrease in voluntary movements, reduced time to do anything • Bradykinesia — slowness of voluntary movements, reduced time it takes to do a movement, all movements are slow, laboured and deliberate and cannot perform more than one movement at a time
Seizures	• Partial — locally, temporal lobe, simple (the patient remains conscious) or complex (loss of consciousness) • Generalized — symmetrical multifocal

Myasthenia Gravis

Myasthenia gravis is a disorder of neuromuscular transmission characterized by

1. Abnormal weakness and fatigue of some or all of the muscle groups
2. Weakness worsening on sustained or repeated exertion, or towards the end of the day, and relieved by rest

This condition is a consequence of an autoimmune destruction of the nicotinic postsynaptic receptors for acetylcholine. Myasthenia gravis is rare, with a prevalence of 40 per million. The tendency for patients with myasthenia gravis to carry certain histocompatibility (HLA) antigens increases the incidence of autoimmune disorders in first-degree relatives, which suggests an immunological basis for the condition.

Aetiology

Antibodies bind to the receptor sites resulting in their destruction. These antibodies are referred to as acetylcholine receptor antibodies (AChR antibodies) and are found in the patient's serum.

The role of the thymus:

- Thymic abnormalities occur in 80% of patients.
- The main function of the thymus is to process T-cell lymphocytes, which participate in immune responses.
- Thymus function is impaired in a large number of disorders, which may be associated with myasthenia gravis, e.g., systemic lupus erythematosus.

Clinical Features

- 90% are adults — peak age of onset is between 20 and 40 years
- The disorder may be selective, involving specific groups of muscles
- Several clinical subdivisions are recognized:
  - Group I — ocular muscles, only 20%
  - Group IIA — mild general weakness, 30%
  - Group IIB — moderate generalized weakness, 30%
  - Group III — acute fulminating, 20%
  - Group IV — severe upon mild or moderate at onset, 20%
- Approximately 40% of group I will eventually become group II. The rest remain purely ocular throughout the illness
- Groups IIB, III and IV develop respiratory muscle involvement
- Bulbar signs and symptoms:
  - Ocular involvement produces ptosis and muscle paresis
  - Weakness of the jaw muscles allows the mouth to hang open
  - Weakness of facial muscles results in expressionless appearance
  - On smiling, buccinator weakness produces a characteristic smile (myasthenic snarl)
  - May result in
    - Dysarthric speech, dysphonic speech
    - Dysphagia
    - Nasal regurgitation of fluids
    - Nasal quality to speech
- Limb and trunk signs and symptoms
  - Weakness of neck muscles may result in rolling of the head
  - Limb muscles tend to be involved proximally
  - Movement against a constant resistance may demonstrate fatigue
  - Limb reflexes are often hyperactive and fatigue on repeated testing
  - Muscle wasting occurs in 15% of cases

Treatment

- Anticholinesterase drugs — interfere with cholinesterase, the enzyme responsible for the breakdown of acetylcholine allowing enhanced receptor stimulation. As a result, more acetylcholine is available to effect neuro-muscular transmission

- Cholinergic overdose (can be masked by atropine) will result in generalized weakness — cholinergic crisis:
  - Muscle fasciculation
  - Increased secretions — sweating
  - Respiratory difficulty
  - Pupillary signs — miosis
- Steroids — prednisolone for those patients who do not respond well to anticholinesterase therapy
- Thymectomy
- Plasmapheresis

Guillain-Barré Syndrome

Sometimes referred to as acute idiopathic postinfectious polyneuropathy. The condition occurs following virus infection but also with other infections, e.g., mycoplasma, gram-negative infection and following surgery or trauma. Some 50% of patients describe an infectious illness in the 4 weeks prior to the onset of neuropathy. It is a cell-mediated immunological reaction directed at peripheral nerves comprising of an acute demyelinating polyradiculopathy. Patients who present with Guillain-Barré syndrome (GBS) often have a history of viral infections and immunizations.

GBS includes a progressive, areflexic motor weakness with its progression manifesting over days and weeks. Patients often present with minor sensory disturbances, and autonomic dysfunction is not unusual. On CSF examination, there is no evident cell count increase, but protein levels typically rise gradually. Another manifestation of GBS is muscle tenderness and back pain. However, other causes of muscle weakness and back pain must be excluded before a diagnosis of GBS is finally made. At the beginning there is

- Loss of feeling
- Then weakness
- Gradual ascent of paraesthesia from the feet, then upper legs, thighs, buttocks and abdomen
- In several cases respiratory and bulbar involvement occurs

Major contributors to mortality and morbidity in patients presenting with GBS are respiratory muscle weakness and autonomic dysfunction, e.g., arrhythmias, hypotension.

Treatment

- Is mainly supportive with management of the paralyzed patient
- Occasionally ventilation and tracheotomy may be required

- There is a mortality rate of 10% survival in all cases; some disability can occur if respiratory failure; some severe or moderate, and in milder cases, outcome is excellent
- IV γ-globulin
- Plasmapheresis, it is important that this treatment is started within 14 days of onset of symptoms for it to be effective
- Steroids are sometimes used but have not been shown to be useful
- Regular chest physiotherapy
- Monitoring of $PaCO_2$ for early signs of respiratory failure
- Continuous cardiovascular monitoring for early detection of autonomic dysfunction
- Nutritional support especially if ileus present from autonomic dysfunction
- Adequate analgesia for muscle pains etc.
- Regular pressure area care
- DVT prophylaxis due to reduced mobility

Spinal Trauma

The spinal cord consists of 31 pairs of nerves:

- Cervical − C1−8
- Thoracic − T1−12
- Lumbar − L1−5
- Sacral − S1−5
- Coccygeal − C0

The higher the injury to the spinal cord, the worse the patient outcome in relation to the ability to move (Table 4.5), depending on the level of the spinal injury or whether the injury is complete or incomplete. There are about 20 spinal cord injuries each week in the United Kingdom, the most common age being 16−35 years.

The causes are

- Motor vehicle accidents, 46%
- Falls, 21%
- Penetrating trauma, 15%
- Sports injuries, 14%
- Diving accidents, less than 2%

Spinal Cord Transection

Refers to severance of the spinal cord and can be complete, partial or slow (Table 4.6). It is important to assess the level and completeness of spinal cord injury, as this allows a prognosis to be made. If the lesion is complete from the

TABLE 4.5 Functioning and potential outcomes by level of spinal cord injury.

Level of injury	Muscle functioning	Outcome
Cervical C4 and above	Loss of all muscle functioning including muscles of respiration. Injuries are usually total because of respiratory failure.	Usually death.
Cervical C5	The phrenic nerve innervating the diaphragm is usually spared. Loss of intercostal muscle functioning often causes respiratory problems.	Quadriplegia with poor pulmonary capacity. High level of dependency for activities of living.
Cervical C6–C8	Muscle movement of the neck. Some chest and arm movement remains. Therefore, some muscles of respiratory continue to function.	Quadriplegia but adequate muscles of the arms and hands are spared. Independence in feeding, some dressing and propelling of wheelchair.
Thoracic spine T1–T3	Neck, shoulder, arms, and hand muscle functioning intact. Loss of muscle functioning from above nipple line and all of trunk and lower extremities.	Considered a quadriplegic if lesion above T3. Much more independence: intact arm function. Needs support in upright position because of loss of trunk muscles.
Thoracic T4 (nipple line), T10 (umbilicus)	More of the chest and trunk muscle functioning remains. All neck and shoulder, arm and hand functioning intact.	Paraplegic - involves only the lower part of the body. Can perform all activities, transfer easily. Achieves mobility with a wheelchair.
Thoracic 11– lumbar 2	Same as above. Muscle function extends to upper thigh.	Bladder control located here and sexual erections. Loss of voluntary bowel and bladder control but can have reflex emptying.
Lumbar 3– sacral 1	Muscle functioning at all of upper body, chest, and most of leg muscles.	Paraplegic with many muscles of mobility intact. Loss of voluntary bladder and bowel control, but can have reflex emptying.
Sacral S2–S4	Same as above but more leg functioning.	The centre for micturition is situated at this level. Destroys the reflex arc to the bladder and bowel. Results in flaccidity and complete loss of bladder and bowel control. Loss of ability to have a reflex erection.

TABLE 4.6 Incomplete/partial spinal cord injury.

Type of injury	Cause of injury	Recovery
Anterior cord syndrome	• The anterior part of the spinal cord is injured by flexion-rotation force causing dislocation or compression fracture of the vertebral body • Anterior spinal artery compression – spinal tracts are damaged by direct trauma and ischaemia	• Results in loss of power • Reduced pain and temperature sensation below the lesion
Central cord syndrome	• Observed in older patients with cervical spondylosis • A hyper-extension injury often from minor trauma compresses spinal cord • Cervical tract serving arms suffers brunt of injury	• Flaccid lower motor neurone weakness of the arms • Relatively strong but spastic upper motor neurone leg function • Sacral sensation and bladder and bowel function are partially spared
Posterior cord syndrome	• Seen in hyper-extension injuries with fractures of the posterior elements of the vertebrae • Contusion of the posterior columns	• Good power, pain and temperature sensation • Profound ataxia due to loss of proprioception makes walking very difficult
Brown-Sequard's syndrome	• Results from stab injuries • Common in lateral mass fractures of the vertebrae • A hemi-section of the spinal cord occurs	• Reduced or absent power • Relatively normal pain and temperature sensation on the side of the injury • The uninjured side has good power • Reduced or absent sensation to pin prick and temperature

outset, that is, there is no sign of spinal cord function below the level of injury, recovery is far less likely than in an incomplete lesion. There are three types:

1. Sudden complete transection, which results in all of the following below the level of injury:
   a. Total paralysis of all skeletal muscles
   b. Loss of all spinal reflexes
   c. Loss of pain, temperature, proprioception and the sensation of pressure and touch
   d. Absence of somatic and visceral sensations

e. Unstable, lowered BP due to loss of vasomotor tone

f. Loss of perspiration, bowel and bladder dysfunction

g. Abnormal, painful and continuous erection (priapism)

2. Partial transection − the patterns of incomplete injury can be viewed in Table 4.6.

3. Slow transection − there is no spinal shock (results from tumours, multiple sclerosis).

Spinal Shock

This is an abrupt cessation of impulses firing from the higher centres, which result in flaccid paralysis below the level of injury. Damage may lead to

- Paralysis
- Paresthesia
- Weakness
- Numbness
- Pain

The main effects of spinal cord injury (Table 4.5):

- Loss of voluntary movement below lesion
- Loss of sensation below lesion
- Potential effects on respiratory system
- Loss of normal control of sympathetic nervous system, affecting most of the body, including
  - Cardiovascular system
  - Loss of ability to regulate temperature below lesion
- Loss of normal bowel function
- Loss of normal bladder function

Meningitis

Viral meningitis is generally aseptic and not usually serious. Bacterial meningitis is septic, has an increased mortality and, if untreated, is almost always fatal (see Table 4.7).

Symptoms

- Severe headache
- Malaise
- Fever, cold hands and feet
- Vomiting
- Photophobia
- Convulsions

TABLE 4.7 Differences and similarities between meningitis and encephalitis.

	Meningitis — inflammation of the meninges	Encephalitis — inflammation of the brain substance
Differences	• Bacterial — serious and can be fatal • Antibiotics — benzylpenicillin, ampicillin, chloramphenicol, gentamicin, cephalosporins • Organisms that cause the inflammation • Epidemics can occur and can be serious in children • Bacterial meningitis is a notifiable infection • Cerebrospinal fluid (CSF) findings — protein and pressure increased, glucose is reduced or absent, turbid or clear (this varies between bacterial and viral meningitis)	• Viral — serious and can be fatal • Antibiotics — aciclovir • Organisms that cause the inflammation in blood and CSF • Epidemics very uncommon • Not a notifiable disease • CSF findings — increased protein and pressure, fluid clear, glucose normal
Similarities	• Clinical features — fever, malaise, anorexia, cerebral dysfunction, altered conscious level, abnormal behaviour, seizures, headaches, nausea/vomiting, tremor, positive Kernig's sign • Diagnosis — lumbar puncture, blood cultures • Differential diagnosis — cerebral abscess, subarachnoid haemorrhage • Antibiotics if tuberculosis (TB) suspected • Treatment — steroids, sedatives, analgesia, isolation, artificial ventilation/care of the unconscious patient	• Clinical features — headaches, neck stiffness, seizures, drowsy, confused leading to unconsciousness, fever, septicaemia, photophobia, positive Kernig's sign, purpuric rash • Diagnosis — lumbar puncture, blood cultures • Differential diagnosis — cerebral abscess, subarachnoid haemorrhage • Antibiotics if TB suspected • Treatment — steroids, sedatives, analgesics, isolation, artificial ventilation/care of the unconscious patient

- Confusion and irritability
- Meningeal irritation:
    - Neck and spinal stiffness
    - Joint and muscle pain
    - Resistance to extending the knee when the thigh is flexed (Kernig's sign)

- Apathy
- Pale, blotchy skin, spots/rash that do not fade under pressure
- Drowsiness, difficult to wake
- Progressing to unconsciousness
- In elderly and immunosuppressed patients, these signs may be absent; mental confusion may be the predominant feature

A patient with fever with spots/rash that do not fade under pressure is a medical emergency.

Differential Diagnosis

- Meningeal irritation can occur without meningitis — may be a feature of other types of severe infection:
  - Subarachnoid haemorrhage
  - Cerebral abscess
  - Encephalitis

Causal Organisms

Meningococcus — dies quickly outside of a body temperature of 37°C. There have been eight strains identified; five strains are carriers rather than cases. Therefore, only three strains are significant: A, B and C.

- A strain almost eradicated.
- B strain is responsible for most infections.
- C is increasing over recent years.

An incubation period of 3 days is usually required, the source is generally human nasopharynx where the bacteria colonises and invades the bloodstream/CNS resulting in meningitis. It easily spreads via infected respiratory secretions. Sometimes there are epidemics. Generally treated with benzylpenicillin. Swelling of the brain is most marked in the parietal, occipital and cerebellar regions.

Haemophilus influenzae — parvobacterium, common in normal respiratory tract, but tends to be more common in children/infants 1 month to 4 years of age. Treatment is with chloramphenicol.

Streptococcus pneumoniae (pneumococcus) — a normal commensal of upper respiratory tract; many types, not all of them infective; generally observed in

- Middle-aged and elderly
- Reduced general health
- Secondary to pneumococcal infection of the lungs, sinuses and middle ear

- Treated with benzylpenicillin
- Infection generally restricted to the anterior lobes

Mycobacterium tuberculosis — 100 cases/year in England and Wales. Treatment generally involves rifampicin, isoniazid, ethambutol and pyrazinamide.

Diagnosis

- History — infectious ear, sinuses or contact.
- CSF examination — appears cloudy, turbid, with an increased white blood cell count, protein and pressure. Glucose is reduced.
- Blood cultures.
- Nose and throat swabs.
- Chest X-ray.

Treatment

- Antibiotics as above
- Steroids
- Sedatives if patient is fitting or agitated
- Isolation if meningococcal is suspected
- Artificial ventilation may be required if unconsciousness results from
  - Encephalopathy
  - Cranial nerve palsy
  - Cerebral infarction or abscess
  - Obstructive hydrocephalus
  - Subdural effusion of sterile or infected nature

Encephalitis

This is inflammation of the brain substance leading to oedema/necrosis or haemorrhage and an increase in ICP and differs from meningitis in a number of ways (Table 4.7).

Causes

- Herpes simplex
- Herpes zoster
- Measles/mumps — can be caused by vaccinations and known as post-vaccination encephalitis
- Viral infection, which is very serious and has a high mortality such as
  - Rubella
  - Arbovirus
  - Polio

- Enterovirus
- Epstein-Barr
- Cytomegalovirus (CMV)
- Bacterial
  - Tuberculosis
  - Syphilis

The most common method of transmission is in the bloodstream; less common is via nerves and can lead to brain damage and cranial nerve damage. The spread of the infection is via the faecal or oral route but can be spread via direct contact with respiratory secretions.

Symptoms

- Sudden or gradual
- Fever
- Malaise
- Anorexia
- Cerebral dysfunction
- Altered level of consciousness
- Abnormal behaviour
- Seizures
- Headaches
- Tremor
- Positive Kernig's sign

Diagnosis

- Lumbar puncture, which will have increased protein and pressure; fluid may be clear
- Stool specimen, which will contain the enterovirus
- Blood serum antibodies
- Computed tomography (CT) scan

Treatment

- Isolate the patient
- Aciclovir
- Steroids may be beneficial

Cerebral Vascular Accident

Interruption of the blood supply to the brain due to

- Any injury to nerve cells and/or pathways to the brain
- Increase of pressure within the cranium

This results in loss of, or reduction in, the function of the part of the brain affected and the organs and tissues supplied by the affected nerves due to

- Ischaemic stroke — caused by blockage(s) cutting off the blood supply to parts of the brain; 85% of all strokes are ischaemic:
  - Thrombosis — more common in elderly associated with underlying disease, occlusion occurs slowly, 50% will experience TIAs (transient ischaemic attacks — attacks of intermittent reduction in supply of oxygen to the brain)
- Atherosclerosis — hardening of the arteries caused by fat deposits forming plaques, rare cause of stroke as collateral circulation may develop
- Embolism — leads to maximum immediate neurological deficit:
  - Clot detached from the heart following an MI or subacute bacterial endocarditis.
- Haemorrhagic stroke — bleeding within the brain and accounts for 15% of all strokes; 1 in 10 patients dies before reaching hospital
  - Abrupt hypertensive episode, often precipitated by activity
  - Rupture of an atherosclerotic vessel
  - Cerebral aneurysm

Incidence

- There are about 100,000 strokes in the United Kingdom each year
- It is the fourth leading cause of death in the developed world and the leading cause of disability
- Incidence rises with age:
  - <65 years 25%
  - 65−75 years 25%
  - 75 years 50%
- 5% of the population older than 65 years will have suffered a stroke or TIA
- More commonly associated with men:
  - 1/3 will die
  - 1/3 will survive with some degree of disability
  - 1/3 will recover
- Estimated cost of stroke to society is £26 billion a year
- Stroke patients occupy 11%−15% of NHS beds and take 5% of NHS budget
- Development of specialist stroke units have been recommended as people are more likely to survive and recover function if admitted promptly to a hospital-based specialist co-ordinated stroke team

Risk Factors and Prevention

Risk factors:

- Smoking
- Hypertension
- Diabetes

- Heart disease — rare
- High-cholesterol diet
- Women taking oral contraceptives increased further if they smoke

  Prevention:

- Decreasing predisposing risk factors such as above by
  - Changing diet
  - Low salt intake
  - Monitoring of and appropriate treatment of conditions, e.g., diabetes, heart disease, TIAs and hypertension

Blood Flow to the Brain

The brain requires 20% of the body's total circulating volume.
  Major arteries:

- Middle cerebral artery
- Carotid artery
- Vertebro-basilar artery
- Anterior cerebral artery
- Posterior cerebral artery

  The brain is supplied with blood by the carotid arteries situated in the neck, which branch off from within the brain into multiple arteries, each of which supplies a specific area.
  The vertebral arteries supply the posterior part and the brain stem — even a brief disruption in blood supply can cause neurological deficit.
  Symptoms of a CVA will vary depending on the area that has been affected, ranging from dysphasia to hemiplegia.

Abnormalities Caused

Middle cerebral artery area:

- Some loss of field of vision occurs with a right hemiparesis
- Lack of awareness of affected side
- Facial numbness
- Weakness in arm more than leg

  Carotid artery area:

- Weakness and hemiplegia on opposite side, numbness, sensory changes, visual disturbances
- Headache or altered level of consciousness

Vertebro-basilar:

- One-sided weakness, numbness around mouth and lips, altered vision in both eyes, double vision, dysphasia
- Ataxia
- Dysphagia
- Loss of memory

Anterior cerebral artery:

- Weakness and numbness especially lower limbs or loss of motor power and coordination
- Incontinence, confusion, personality change

Posterior cerebral arteries:

- Visual disturbances, sensory impairment
- Dyslexia
- Paralysis usually absent

Types of Stroke

Transient ischaemic attack:

- Temporary paralysis lasting 10–15 minutes
- Presenting with speech difficulty or numbness
- Sudden onset; recovery within 24 hours

Reversible ischaemic neurological deficit:

- Resolves within 72 hours

Partial non-progressing stroke:

- Neurological deficit does not develop further into a complete stroke

Progressing stroke/stroke evolving:

- Symptoms fluctuate for 24–76 hours

Complete stroke:

- Once occurred the stroke is considered complete

Symptoms

- Specific changes in brain function will depend upon the location and extent of the damage.
- Symptoms are typically on one side of the body but may be isolated to specific functions and may include:
  - Loss of movement/paralysis or weakness of arms and legs

- Decreased sensation, numbness, tingling, weakness
- Decreased vision
- Language difficulties/dysphasia
- Swallowing difficulties
- Inability to recognize affected side of the body
- Loss of memory and thinking
- Vertigo, loss of coordination
- Personality changes, depression/apathy
- Consciousness changes, sleepy, lethargic, comatose
- Loss of bladder/bowel control
- Dementia, impaired judgement, limited attention span
- Facial paralysis, uncontrollable eye movements, lid droop
- Seizures, unpredictable movements
- Pain and headaches

High Temperatures

There are four general states of increased body temperature (Richards and Edwards, 2014):

Pyrexia (fever)

This involves a condition whereby the thermoregulatory mechanisms remain intact, but the body temperature is maintained at a high level. It generally has an infective aetiology, but there are other non-infectious causes of pyrexia. These include acute MIs, haemolysis (seen in reactions to blood transfusions) and thyrotoxicosis.

The cooling methods used to treat such as, tepid sponging or fanning has been criticized. Such cooling methods are of no use, as they result in

- A compensatory response by the hypothalamus, which will produce heat-generating activities like chills and shivering
- The hypothalamus interpreting the sent information from localized nerve endings in the skin as indicating that body temperature is decreasing, so will further increase set point temperature
- Compromising an unstable patient by depleting their metabolic reserve and can create a new temperature spike that is as high or higher than the original one
- The patient feeling weak, especially during the early stages when the temperature is still rising

Treating a high temperature by cooling and tepid sponging can therefore serve to increase the temperature further and cause the patient discomfort and possible harm. The best way to treat a high temperature is by the use of anti-pyrexia drug therapy.

Hyperpyrexia

This is generally observed in conditions such as septicaemia and bacterial meningitis when the hypothalamus set point temperature is very high, e.g., above 40°C. A temperature between 41°C and 43°C produces nerve damage, coagulation, convulsions and death.

Hyperthermia

This occurs when there is hypothalamic injury, due to neoplasms, surgery, central nervous system problems, and when over-heating overwhelms the heat loss mechanisms — causes cerebral metabolism to increase and the brain has great difficulty keeping up with the increase in carbon dioxide production. It does not respond to anti-pyrexia therapy.

Treatment is difficult as the body fails to activate compensatory cooling mechanisms. This tends to increase cellular metabolism, oxygen consumption and carbon dioxide production.

It is essential the temperature is carefully monitored and cooling methods such as fanning and tepid sponging are instituted, as the hypothalamus will not respond to anti-pyrexia drug therapy, irreversible brain damage and death.

Malignant Hyperthermia

This is a life-threatening inherited disorder that leads to hyper-metabolism involving the skeletal muscles. Certain drugs can lead to a malignant hyper-thermia such as

- Diuretics,
- Antiseizure therapy,
- Analgesics,
- Some common anaesthetics,
- Antiarrhythmics and
- Antibiotics.

Symptoms include

- Muscle rigidity
- Hypoxia, progressive lactic acidosis and excessive production of carbon dioxide
- Increase in heart rate, supraventricular or ventricular arrhythmia
- Abnormally rapid breathing
- Increasing body temperature >38.8°C, a relatively late sign, but may not occur if adequate treatments is started early
- Rhabdomyolysis

A malignant hyperthermia also presents in four other conditions:

- Heat cramps
- Heat exhaustion
- Heat stroke
- Neuroleptic malignant syndrome (NMS)

Heat cramps and heat exhaustion are generally not life-threatening. However, heat stroke, malignant hyperthermia and NMS must be recognized quickly, as, untreated, they may be fatal.

Treatment includes stopping the trigger agent(s) and hyperventilation using intravenous opioids, sedatives and non-depolarizing muscle relaxants (Schneiderbanger et al., 2014). The administration of dantrolene 2 mg/kg, sodium bicarbonate administration for metabolic acidosis, fluid resuscitation and vasopressor drug therapies may be needed to stabilize haemodynamics. Furosemide can help to prevent AKI. If hyperthermia is present internal cooling with cold infusion fluids and external cooling with ice packs.

Hypothermia

A drastic decrease in body temperature is known as hypothermia, is characterized by a marked cooling of core temperature and is defined as a core temperature below 35°C (Richards and Edwards, 2018). Progressive temperature reduction below this level will result in reduced metabolism and risk of cardiac arrest. At 28−30°C, loss of consciousness will ensue. Low temperatures cause compensatory shivering and vasoconstriction, to shunt the blood to vital organs and prevent excess heat loss from skin surfaces, causing metabolic and cardiorespiratory stress to ill patients. Hypothermia can be accidental or therapeutic.

Accidental Hypothermia

This is a temperature below 35°C resulting from sudden immersion in cold water or prolonged exposure to cold environments. Can be associated with alcohol and some sedatives and narcotics, which diminish conscious perception of cold. Healthy subjects who experience hypothermia often survive profound hypothermia with medical support.

Therapeutic Hypothermia

This is used to slow metabolism and preserve ischaemic tissue during surgery. It can also occur through exposure of body cavities to the relatively cool operating room environment, irrigation of body cavities with room temperature solutions, infusion of room temperature intravenous solutions, and inhalation of unwarmed anaesthetic agents. These types of therapeutic hypothermia can extend into the post-operative period.

The nurse needs to be aware of any patients at risk of hypothermia and take notice of how long the patient has been exposed in theatre. Rewarming methods are divided into three groups:

- Passive external rewarming (removal of wet clothes, blankets, warm room)
- Active external rewarming (radiant lights, convection air blankets)
- Active internal rewarming (warmed gases to respiratory tract, warmed intravenous fluids).

The process of rewarming should proceed at no faster than a few degrees per hour. If a patient is rapidly rewarmed oxygen consumption, myocardial demand and vasodilatation increase faster than the heart's ability to compensate and death can occur.

4.3 ENDOCRINE DISORDERS

The endocrine system along with the nervous system is responsible for control and communication within the body. The glands are ductless and secrete their products directly into the blood stream to act upon a target organ that may be far away from the gland itself (Richards and Edwards, 2018).

Diabetes Insipidus

This is a disease of the posterior pituitary gland, which is the size of a pea and secretes many vital hormones, important in the control of other endocrine glands. Known as the 'leader' or 'master' endocrine gland.

Types of Diabetes Insipidus

- Central or neurogenic diabetes insipidus – there is a lack of antidiuretic hormone (ADH) being released into the circulation in response to an osmotic stimulus, e.g., osmoreceptors increase their firing when blood osmolality increases (concentrated/thick).
  - Most often due to a lesion in the hypothalamus or posterior pituitary gland including
    - Tumours
    - Aneurysms
    - Thrombosis
    - Infections
  - There is a total or partial inability to concentrate urine.
  - Total urine output varies between 4 and 12 L per day.
  - Acute onset and dehydration may develop rapidly.
  - Transient usually incomplete central diabetes insipidus is noticed frequently in critical care patients with head injury.

- Dipsogenic or psychogenic diabetes insipidus — is precipitated by excessive intake of water very rare.
- Nephrogenic diabetes insipidus — deficient action of ADH.
- Pregnancy-related diabetes insipidus is also recognized to occur.

Clinical presentation:

- Polyuria — an excessive passage of urine or large production of urine
- Nocturia — voiding during the night
- Thirst — generally the desire for cold drinks
- Inability to replace water may result in signs of hypovolaemia
- Low urine osmolality — urine SG between 1001 and 1005
- High plasma osmolality due to dehydration
- The essential feature is that urine osmolality is inappropriately low compared to plasma osmolality
- Urine volumes over 4–6 L/day or 3 mL/kg over 2 consecutive hours (in neurosurgical patients may point towards diabetes insipidus)

Investigations:

- Random plasma and urine osmolality
- Plasma and urine osmolality relationships
- Blood chemistry — blood glucose, 24-hour urine osmolality and electrolytes, blood and urine electrolytes, urea and creatinine
- ADH test — if tests above are positive then ADH (usually as DDAVP (desmopressin) nasally) is given
- Hypertonic saline — used to evaluate osmoreceptor mechanism
- Magnetic resonance imaging (MRI) scan — assessment of pituitary function

Treatment:

- Replacement therapy with a synthetic ADH:
  - Aqueous vasopressin (arginine) — short-acting agent can be given intramuscularly or subcutaneously
  - DDAVP — long-acting agent, given intranasally
- Oral hydration is often sufficient

Diabetes Mellitus

This is a common condition characterized by a persistently raised blood glucose level due to a deficiency or lack of insulin. An estimated 1.4 million people in the United Kingdom have diabetes (Richards and Edwards, 2018).

The Pancreas

The pancreas releases glucagon, which is synthesized by α-cells of the islets of Langerhans in the pancreas. Glucagon is released in response to a low blood glucose level and inhibited by a high blood glucose level. Glucagon will mobilize the release of glucose into the blood to increase the blood glucose level. Target/effect of glucagon is the

- Liver
  - Glycogenolysis (glycogen to glucose)
  - Gluconeogenesis (synthesis of glucose)
  - Release of glucose into blood
- Adipose (fat) tissue
  - Fat catabolism, release of fatty acids into blood

The pancreas also releases insulin synthesized by the β-cells of the islets of Langerhans in the pancreas. The release of insulin is stimulated by a high blood glucose level and inhibited by a low blood glucose level. Target/effect of insulin is

- All cells except liver, kidney, brain
  - Increased glucose uptake into cells
  - Promotes protein synthesis and fat storage
  - Encourages glucose storage as glycogen in the liver and skeletal muscles
  - Lowers blood glucose levels

A hyposecretion of insulin leads to diabetes mellitus (type 1 or type 2), as glucose is not absorbed into cells and therefore the body cannot utilize glucose, which accumulates in the blood. The kidneys attempt to excrete any excess in urine. A hypersecretion of insulin is generally due to an overdose of insulin and will lead to a hypoglycaemia, which can be life-threatening.

Type 1 Diabetes Mellitus

- Dependent on insulin − without it the patient will die
- Less than 25% of people with diabetes are insulin dependent
- Thought to be an autoimmune disorder − β-cells in the pancreas are targeted by antibodies and eventually totally destroyed
- Some individuals have a genetic predisposition − trigger factor is needed, generally a virus
- Highest incidence around 11−12 years of age but can occur at any age; uncommon over the age of 40 years

Clinical features:

- Polyuria
- Thirst
- Polydipsia

- Weight loss — breakdown of protein and fats as source of energy, emaciation
- Production of excessive ketones — acid and appear in urine
- Lack of energy — cells are starving, loss of muscle mass, weakness

Treatment:

- Insulin therapy — cannot be given orally because gastrointestinal enzymes render it ineffective. May require up to four injections per day (see Section 6).

A hypoglycaemia is a medical emergency, and the patient requires something sweet to eat or drink if conscious; if semi- or unconscious, the patient needs either glycogen or glucagon immediately.

Type 2 Diabetes Mellitus

- There is either insufficient production of insulin or an inability of the body to use the insulin adequately (insulin resistance)
- Patients not dependent on insulin may receive some insulin to help control their diabetes but can live without it
- Different from type 1, as it does not usually happen in the young, may have the disorder for years and not know it
- Symptoms develop much more insidiously; incidence increases with age and as people are living longer, so the disease is getting more common
- Disorder is linked to obesity and can run in families
- Can be controlled by diet alone or by medication such as oral hypo-glycaemic agents, to bring down blood glucose

Diabetic ketoacidosis is a medical emergency and intervention is urgently required.

4.4 RESPIRATORY

Respiratory Trauma

- The most common is closed chest injury from an RTA (road traffic accident) with associated extra-thoracic injuries, all of which may be life-threatening.
- Swift assessment and resuscitation are carried out simultaneously.
- Initial management is directed towards detection and correction of life-threatening effects from the sustained injuries.

Direct Chest Injuries

- Knife wounds
- Injury due to a fall
- RTAs
- Violent incidents (beatings, boxing)
- Inhalation burns
- Blast injury

Effects

Ruptured Aorta

- Determined by
  - Widened mediastinum
  - Left haemothorax
  - Depressed left main bronchus
  - Fractured first rib

Ruptured Diaphragm

- Due to abdominal compression (risen since seat belts made compulsory)
- Risk of gut strangulation
- Left-sided rupture is more common, right being difficult to diagnose due to the presence of the liver

Disruption of Major Airways

- Frequently determined due to
  - respiratory distress
  - subcutaneous emphysema
  - haemoptysis
- In the presence of ruptured bronchus, a pneumothorax is common

Massive Pneumothorax/Haemothorax

- Causes the lung to collapse
- There is a tear in the lung and air and/or blood escapes into the pleural space

Pulmonary Contusion

- Bruising of the lungs
- Avoid over-hydration

Myocardial Contusion

- Common in blunt chest trauma
- May result in arrhythmias — nonspecific T wave changes to pathological Q waves
- Cardiac failure may be evident — generally should be managed as a MI

Oesophageal Perforation

- Due to penetrating injury, occurs rarely with closed chest trauma, the patient develops
  - Retrosternal pain
  - Difficulty in swallowing
  - Haematemesis
  - Cervical emphysema

Systemic Air Embolism

- More common in penetrating injuries — life-threatening
- Uncommon, but is thought to generally be under-diagnosed
- Caused by a bronchopulmonary vein fistula

Cardiac Tamponade

- Suspected in a patient with thoracic trauma with a low BP and raised venous pressure
- Differential diagnoses are
  - Tension pneumothorax
  - Severe heart failure
  - Prolonged and inadequate treatment of shock
- Aspiration of the pericardial sac under ECG (electrocardiography) control

Flail Chest

- Disruption of the normal structure of the chest due to
  - Fracture of three or more adjoining ribs in one or more places
  - Rib fractures with costochondral separation
  - Sternal fractures
- Limits the negative intra-thoracic pressure needed to move air into lungs and paradoxical movement occurs:
  - On inspiration, the intact chest expands; the injured flail segment is depressed.
  - The intrapleural pressures on the unaffected side are greater, displacing the mediastinum towards it.

- This is known as mediastinal flutter, which
  - impairs ventilation;
  - reduces cardiac output and venous return;
  - reduces intrapleural pressure during inspiration;
  - impairs circulating dynamics and venous filling;
  - can be observed by visual inspection of movement of both posterior and anterior breathing patterns;
  - is worsened by pain and
  - ventilator support may be required
- On expiration, the flail segment bulges outward, thus interfering with breathing out
  - The negative pressure on the unaffected side is less than that on the affected side − the mediastinum shifts towards the affected side
  - Ventilation impairment depends on injury or presence of pneumothorax or haemothorax
- Mediastinal shift occurs
  - During inspiration, the increased intrapleural pressures on the unaffected side displaces the mediastinum towards it.
  - During expiration, the negative pressure on the unaffected side is less than that on the affected side, and the mediastinum shifts towards the affected side (mediastinal flutter).
- Changes on inspiration lead to reduced cardiac output

Indirect Injuries (Dealt with Elsewhere in this Section)

- Pulmonary embolism
- Carbon monoxide poisoning
- Hanging
- Obstruction
- Aspiration
- Drowning
- Anaphylaxis and asthma

Unrelated Injuries

Any conditions whereby the demand for oxygen outweighs supply can lead to unrelated trauma to the respiratory system, due to

- Stress
- Major trauma
- Hypovolaemia
- Diabetic ketoacidosis
- MI
- Pancreatitis
- Liver/renal failure
- Hyperpyrexia, hyperthermia, hypothermia

Interventions

- Control any bleeding
- Insertion of an IV cannula
- Basic circulatory resuscitation is initiated
- Administration of oxygen
- Exclude or treat pneumothorax or haemothorax — insertion of a chest drain or 12- or 14-gauge intravenous cannula percutaneously in life-threatening emergencies
- Assessment of extra-thoracic trauma, head, neck and abdominal injuries and significant concealed blood loss must be excluded
- Gastric decompression — risk of regurgitation (vomiting or aspiration)
  - Extremely common in severe cases of chest trauma
- Provide pain relief
  - Will relieve respiratory distress in patients with fractures of the ribs and/ or sternum
- Reconsider endotracheal intubation, ventilation if:
  - Dangerous hypoxaemia and/or hypercarbia
  - Significant head injury
  - Gross flail segment and contusion
  - Respiratory distress

Asthma

Inflammatory condition of the airways mediated by a wide range of stimuli — immunoglobulin (Ig) E, the release of chemical mediators. Thus leading to bronchospasm and an imbalance between:

- Cholinergic (parasympathetic)
- Adrenergic (sympathetic)

Asthma can produce symptoms of all grades varying from very mild to life-threatening. Its danger should never be underestimated, and several people die each year from asthma.

Contributes to difficulty in breathing out, plugging mucous and oedema. Extrinsic asthma:

- Childhood
- Identifiable factors provoke wheezing
- Associated with hay fever and eczema
- Nocturnal cough (only a symptom)

Intrinsic asthma:

- Usally begins in adult life and obstruction is more persistent
- Obvious stimuli other than respiratory tract infection

Acid-base changes occur:

- Respiratory alkalosis − normal physiological processes in the early stages of asthma; homeostasis maintained
  - Dyspnoea − increase in respiratory rate
  - End-tidal CO_2 normal or low
  - Cough/wheezing
- Respiratory acidosis − indicates the patient is no longer able to maintain homeostasis; intubation may be required if:
  - Worsening wheeze
  - Respiratory rate >30/min
  - Cyanosis/tachycardia >110/min
  - Peak flow <33%

Drug therapy:

- Salbutamol and/or ipratropium inhaler/nebulizer regular and on demand
- Inhaled short-acting steroid
- Longer acting β-agonist
- Theophylline in severe cases of status epilepticus
- Prednisolone
- Antibiotics only if asthma attack precipitated by an infective focus

Chronic Obstructive Pulmonary Disease

Chronic bronchitis and emphysema; commonest cause linked to cigarette smoking.

Chronic Bronchitis

- Productive cough for most days of the year for three consecutive months for more than 1 year
- Characterized by excessive mucus production

Emphysema

- Permanent enlargement of the air sacs within lung tissue
- Destruction of pulmonary tissue loss of elastic recoil

Clinical Features

- Develops over many years, rarely before middle age
- Morning cough, little sputum
- Breathlessness on exertion, gradually dyspnoea occurs at rest
- Bronchitis predominates; periodic chest infections occur; cyanosis leading to a blue tinge to the skin
- Emphysema predominates; extreme breathlessness; often not cyanosed but retains excessive carbon dioxide, and colour can appear pink
- Wheeze, use of accessory muscles of respiration
- Extreme anxiety during very breathless periods
- Changes occur to acid-base balance to maintain body pH:
  - Respiratory acidosis (PCO_2 >5.7 kPa; pH < 7.4)
  - Metabolic alkalosis (HCO_3^2 >26 mEq/l; pH > 7.40)

Drug Therapy

- Bronchodilators:
  - Salbutamol
  - Atropine analogues — ipratropium bromide
- Theophylline
- Corticosteroids
  - Oral prednisolone
  - Inhaled steroids
- Antibiotics only if acute exacerbation is due to an infection
- Diuretics if heart involved

Pneumonia

An acute inflammation of the substance of the lungs due to:

- Bacteria
- Chemical causes
- Aspiration of vomit
- Radiotherapy
- Allergic mechanism (asthma)

Common Bacteria

- *Streptococcus pneumoniae*
- *Mycoplasma pneumoniae*
- *Haemophilus influenzae*
- *Staphylococcus aureus*
- *Legionella pneumophila*
- *Mycobacterium tuberculosis.*

Aspiration Pneumonia

Aspiration of gastric contents either solids or liquids can lead to severe illness; can be fatal as gastric acid contents in the lungs is very destructive; aspiration material enters the right lung more readily — wider right bronchus infection; usually an anaerobic organism.

Predisposing Factors

- Recent extubation
- Metabolic coma
- Altered consciousness
- Drug overdose, anaesthesia, epilepsy, CVA, alcoholism
- Dysphagia, oesophageal disease
- Stricture, fistula, hiatus hernia, reflux
- Neurological disorders
- Myasthenia gravis, motor neurone disease
- Nasogastric tubes
- Terminal illness

Management

- Oxygen therapy
- Bronchodilator therapy
- Cardiovascular support
- Bronchoscopy
- Antibiotics
- Corticosteroids
- Mechanical ventilation if condition worsens

Prevention

- Posture — sit the patient up in bed
- Suction
- Cricoid pressure
- Airway protection
- Nasogastric tube
- Antacid therapy, H_2 receptor antagonists and sucralfate
- Metoclopramide

Pneumonia in the Immunocompromised Patient

- Opportunistic infections
- Rapid pneumonias extensive and life-threatening
- Viral, fungal, protozoal or bacterial in origin
- *Pneumocystis jiroveci* (formerly *carinii*) is the commonest

Pulmonary Oedema/Fluid Overload

Fluid in the interstitial and alveolar spaces of the lungs, generally caused by an increase in hydrostatic pressure (HP) within the pulmonary circulation due to:

- Left ventricular failure
- Fluid overload − increased infusions of
  - Crystalloids
  - Colloids
- MI
- Pulmonary hypertension

  Treatment involves the following:

- Morphine is given to reduce anxiety and to cause systemic vasodilation; however, there is a lack of evidence as to its efficacy (Chioncel et al., 2015)
- Diuretics furosemide is considered a first-line therapy for pulmonary oedema
- Vasodilators such as glyceryl trinitrate (GTN)
- Inotropes, if systolic BP and cardiac output reduces, such as dobutamine and dopamine
- Noninvasive or invasive ventilation to improve oxygenation

Pulmonary Embolism

A pulmonary embolism (PE) is an occlusion of pulmonary vascular bed by an embolus or a thrombus, tissue fragments, lipids, fats or an air bubble:

- 90% of PE is the consequence of clots that are initially in the leg veins and the pelvis.
- Half the people diagnosed with pulmonary embolism die within 2 hours of the diagnosis.
- PE is responsible for 10% of hospital death and 80% of the time PEs go undetected.
- Most PE deaths occur within 1 hour of diagnosis.
- PE causes hypoxia, vasoconstriction, pulmonary oedema or decrease in surfactant.

  The effect of the embolism depends on the extent of the pulmonary blood flow obstructed, the size of the affected vessels, nature of the embolism and the secondary effect. The size of the pulmonary artery in which the blood clot is lodged determines the severity of symptoms and prognosis. If the embolus blocks the pulmonary artery and one of its main branches, immediate death may occur. Patient may complain of

- Chest pain
- Sudden pain or shock
- A sudden sharp or abdominal pain if embolism blocks smaller vessels.

A large pulmonary embolus is a medical emergency and can result in sudden death.

The Pathophysiology of Pulmonary Embolism

PE is more common in patients who have had surgery of the lower limbs and trauma patients. When trauma to the blood vessels is inevitable, for example during total hip replacement, blood vessels will constrict to slow down blood flow. With pulmonary infarction an area of the lung will be destroyed through blocking the circulation to the lung cells, leading to death of the tissue. Permanent lung injury does not occur if the infarction is not severe; patient may present symptoms similar to those of pneumonia.

During this process factor Xa is formed, which converts prothrombin II to thrombin. Thrombin will produce a soluble protein, fibrinogen, and this in turn produces an insoluble protein, fibrin. Fibrin releases a meshwork of strands to trap platelets. As these seal the wall of the dead blood vessel, a clot may break loose and travel to the lungs and occlude the circulation before fibrinolysis. As a result of the pulmonary circulation, dyspnoea, chest pain, ventilation/perfusion (V/Q) imbalances, pulmonary infarction and decreased cardiac output may occur.

Diagnosis of Pulmonary Embolism

- Bloods are taken for a D-dimer test.
- Impairment in gas exchange, i.e., partial pressure of oxygen is low, partial pressure of carbon dioxide is normal and pH is normal.
- A computed tomography pulmonary angiogram (CTPA) should be conducted as first line diagnostic if possible.
- PE should be suspected in critical care patients who collapse suddenly 1–2 weeks following surgery.
- If large, PE is a medical emergency – leading to death.
- Clinical features depend on size of embolus:
  - Sharp, knife-like pain in the chest, well localized in a small embolus
  - If large, the pain is more central
  - Shortness of breath
  - Anxiety and distress
  - Haemoptysis
  - Hypotension, tachycardia, pallor
  - Cyanosis (suggests a large embolism)
  - Collapse, cardiac arrest or shock.

Treatments of Pulmonary Embolism

The aim of therapy is to prevent further thrombus formation and embolization.

- The administration of oxygen is required to relieve shortness of breath and to supply oxygen to the affected areas of the lungs.
- Morphine 10 mg may be given to relieve chest pain.
- Low-molecular-weight heparin (LMWH) or fondaparinux is the first line of treatment (NICE, 2012).
- Unfractionated heparin is used for patients with existing renal failure and/or haemodynamic instability.

Care of a Patient with a Pulmonary Embolism

- Involves supportive measures and prevention of heart failure and further emboli formation.
- Observe for: bleeding of the gums and avoid pressure when brushing teeth, excessive or easy skin brusing and unexplained nose bleeds.
- The vital signs the nurse has to look for include when a patient appears to be in shock or having difficulty in breathing and pain.

Pneumothorax

An accumulation of air in the pleural space due to the following:

- Spontaneously in young, tall, thin men
- Trauma
- Asthma, COPD, TB, pneumonia, lung carcinoma
- Cystic fibrosis and any diffuse lung disease
- IPPV, aggressive bagging following intubation
- Insertion of a CVP line

Clinical features:

- No symptoms if small and in a fit young man
- Dyspnoea depends on size, mild to very severe
- Pleuritic pain – sometimes transient
- The patient may suggest that they felt something 'snap' before the onset of pain and dyspnoea
- Decreased breath sounds, respiratory distress
- Agitation, cyanosis, tachycardia
- Reduced respiratory movement on affected side
- Increase or decrease in BP

A tension pneumothorax is a medical emergency. A flap develops and acts as a one-way valve, air is trapped following inspiration. Mediastinal shift — the medial structures become misplaced towards the unaffected side.

- Reduces venous return and cardiac output
- Death may occur very quickly
- 16—18 gauge needle third—fourth inter-coastal space at the mid-clavicular line will relieve pressure

Tension pneumothorax is a medical emergency.

4.5 CARDIOVASCULAR

Hypovolaemia

Hypovolaemia is defined as a diminished circulatory fluid volume. Hypovolaemic shock (see Section 1) is a further decrease in circulatory fluid volume so large the body's metabolic needs cannot be met.

The decline in blood volume decreases venous return and cardiac output (Richards and Edwards, 2018). Numerous compensatory mechanisms are activated when the circulating volume is reduced and the venous return is decreased.

The baroreceptors (in the aorta and carotid sinus) become stretched to a lesser degree, decreasing their rate of discharge, resulting in vasoconstriction. The vasoconstriction will greatly increase the peripheral resistance, maintain arterial BP and return more blood to the heart.

A decreased renal blood flow will result in an enzymatic chain reaction — renin converts angiotensinogen to angiotensin I then to angiotensin II, which stimulates the production of aldosterone, in an attempt to restore extracellular volume, by conserving sodium and water. Angiotensin II stimulates the release of noradrenaline (a powerful α-receptor stimulant) and when circulating in the blood will cause widespread peripheral vasoconstriction, in an added attempt to improve BP and renal blood flow.

However, the continued vasoconstriction in the kidneys may cause the glomerular filtration rate (GFR) to become depressed; as a result, minimal urine is produced. If hypovolaemia is prolonged, AKI can occur leading to renal tubular damage. The continued failure of the kidneys to excrete hydrogen ions causes a metabolic acidosis, with a consequent decrease in the pH. The acidosis results in an impaired cardiovascular response with depression of myocardial function.

To maintain fluid and electrolyte balance, water and electrolytes are in constant motion, between intracellular (about 25 L) and extracellular compartments (divided into interstitial fluid − 12 L, and plasma volume − 3 L). Thus, if concentrations of sodium (the major cation in extracellular fluid) are increased, as is the case when there is a loss of extracellular water, osmoreceptors in the hypothalamus are stimulated. The osmoreceptors increase the production of antidiuretic hormone (ADH), which increases water reabsorption from the kidney's distal tubules and collecting ducts and arouses the sense of thirst.

These protective mechanisms will eventually cease to function, and circulatory failure ensues. If the metabolic acidosis, circulatory failure or volume is not corrected or treatment instigated, death will occur in a short period of time.

The principal aetiologies of hypovolaemic states can be classified as haemorrhage, plasma loss, third-space shifts, bleeding disorders, dehydration and high temperatures.

Hypovolaemia Caused by Haemorrhage − the Loss of Whole Blood

This is the most common cause of hypovolaemia and can if untreated lead to hypovolaemic shock. The greater the duration and severity of haemorrhage, the more pronounced the overall state of hypovolaemic shock. An acute loss of 10% of total blood volume reduces arterial pressure by 7% and cardiac output by 21%; the loss of 20% of the total blood volume reduces arterial pressure by 15% and cardiac output by 41%.

The consequent loss of red cells seen in haemorrhage decreases the oxygen-carrying capacity of the blood and contributes to hypoxia. Hypoxaemia can develop into an acidosis (reduced pH) and together these stimulate the vascular chemoreceptors, specialized areas within the aortic and carotid arteries that are sensitive to concentrations of oxygen and hydrogen ions (pH) in the blood (see Oxygen saturation, below).

Hypovolaemia Caused by Plasma Loss

This is the result of an increase in capillary permeability leading to a shift of plasma fluid from the vascular space into the interstitial space. This type of hypovolaemia occurs most often in individuals with large partial-thickness burns, full-thickness burns, or burns over more than 20%−25% of the total body surface area. The rate and volume of plasma deficit are roughly proportional to the extent of the area burned. Other conditions of plasma loss that produce similar types of plasma deficit are known as third-space fluid shift.

Hypovolaemia Caused by Third-Space Fluid Shifts

Any type of trauma or cell damage (e.g., surgical, MI, head injury), whether it is external and visible or internal and invisible, will automatically trigger an IR. The normal body response will be to send nutrients, fluids, white blood cells and clotting factors to the damaged site to repair tissue, prevent infection and if necessary stem blood loss. Capillaries vasodilate and become more permeable to allow these factors to reach the site of injury, leading to localized swelling and lymphatic blockage.

The permeability causes movement of fluids, allowing water, electrolytes and other particles (such as albumin) into the interstitial spaces, and is known as a third-space fluid shift. When third-space fluid shift occurs, a patient can appear paradoxically 'dry' or hypovolaemic as fluid has moved into the intravascular spaces yet may still have the same or greater quantity of body water. The vasodilation is caused by the release of cell mediators (e.g., histamine, kinins, complement) from the damaged endothelium, and causes a reduction in BP, peripheral vascular resistance and an increase in heart rate, further compounding the appearance of a hypovolaemic state. This relative (rather than true) hypovolaemic state stimulates baroreceptors, volume receptors and osmoreceptors to reabsorb sodium and water to cause vasoconstriction in an effort to restore circulating volume and increase BP.

Hypovolaemia Caused by Bleeding Disorders

Platelet and coagulation disorders can cause or fail to prevent an internal or external haemorrhage. Disorders of platelets are generally visible through the skin as a discoloration known as a purpura, which occurs when there are not enough normal platelets to plug damaged vessels. Disorders of platelets include thrombocytopenia and thrombocytosis and can be caused by drugs, such as anti-inflammatory agents, antimicrobials, antidepressants and adrenergic blocking agents. Coagulation disorders tend to result in more bleeding and are usually caused by a deficiency of one or more clotting factors. These disorders are usually caused by a deficiency in one or more of the clotting factors, an insufficiency of vitamin K, liver disease or DIC.

Hypovolaemia Caused by Dehydration

Dehydration is more commonly seen in the elderly and if prolonged can induce hypovolaemic shock. It may be a consequence of either a primary deficit of water, a primary deficit of salt or both. A primary deficit of water leads to cellular dehydration and circulatory failure. By contrast, a primary deficit of salt leads to a reduced extracellular fluid volume, a reduced blood volume and increasing difficulty in maintaining an adequate circulating volume. For the different types of hypovolaemia due to dehydration, see Table 4.8.

TABLE 4.8 The different types of dehydration.

Isotonic dehydration

This is where there are alterations in both the total body water (TBW) and electrolyte balance. It generally results from reduced fluid intake rather than increased loss but can occur from haemorrhage, severe wound drainage and excessive diaphoresis. The most common cause of reduced fluid intake in clinical practice is the inability of the individual to acquire an adequate amount of fluids. Water dehydration causes weight loss, dryness of skin and mucous membranes, decreased urine output and symptoms of hypovolaemia, such as a rapid heart rate, flattened neck veins and a decrease in blood pressure. In severe cases, hypovolaemic shock can occur. Individuals at risk of dehydration related to water deficit include infants, the elderly and immobilized individuals.

Hypertonic dehydration

This is where there is an increased concentration of extracellular sodium (hypernatraemia) in relation to water. This is associated with fever or respiratory infections, which increase the respiratory rate and enhance water loss from the lungs. Also severe diarrhoea causes water loss in relation to sodium. Insufficient water intake also can cause hypernatraemia, particularly in individuals who are comatose, confused or immobilized. In hypertonic volume depletion, which is excess water loss relative to sodium, the urine specific gravity will be greater than 1.030; the haematocrit, plasma proteins and plasma osmolarity will be elevated above normal.

Hypotonic dehydration

This is where there is a reduction in sodium (hyponatraemia) and an increase in water. This is associated with a reduced intake of sodium, continued diuretic therapy and vomiting. Sodium deficits usually cause a reduction in the plasma osmolarity with movement of water into the cells. This movement will reduce the overall circulating volume and thus give the impression of dehydration.

Dehydration – a deficiency of both salt and water

This is the most appropriate term to indicate both sodium loss and water loss. A deficiency of both salt and water occurs when fluid is lost from the gastrointestinal tract.

Hypovolaemia Due to a High Temperature

The vasodilatation observed during a high temperature can make a patient appear hypovolaemic, as fluid space has increased, yet there is still the same amount of circulating volume. The vasodilatation causes a reduction in BP, peripheral vascular resistance and an increase in heart rate and electrolyte imbalance. Dehydration may result due to fluid loss during sweating and from the lungs due to increased respiratory rate. Dehydration, together with the profuse vasodilatation of blood vessels may serve to add to the 'appearance' of a hypovolaemic state.

Hypovolaemic shock caused by any of the six aetiologies described is indeed a critical state that begins with an adaptive response to illness or injury and may progress to multiple system organ failure.

Assessment of a Patient with Hypovolaemia

Nurses can collect data to determine the circulatory status of a patient, and every nurse is aware of the crucial importance of astute and accurate observation. This starts from the very moment the patient is admitted to a critical care area, as the nurse automatically observes details such as

- Facial colour
  - Pallor
  - Flushed or cyanosed
- Any respiratory difficulty
  - Rapid or shallow breathing
- Cool moist or dehydrated skin
- Ischaemia of the eyelids, lips, gums and tongue
- Facial expressions
- Oedema
- Increased or decreased body weight
- Pulsating neck veins
- Posture and dry mucous membranes
- Observations are made for signs of
  - Anxiety or distress
  - Evidence of confusion, disorientation, apprehension, restlessness, agitation or calm (Milovanovic and Adeleye, 2017).

These observations will direct the nurse's subsequent, more systematic objective approach to data collection.

Mental State in Hypovolaemia

A reduced oxygen supply caused by the loss of red blood cells observed in haemorrhage will stimulate the adrenal medullar to secrete noradrenaline, an alpha-receptor stimulant that causes vasoconstriction of the systemic circulation. The continued reduction in blood flow leads to a reduction in blood supply to the brain's reticular formation (located in the brain stem), whose function it is to modulate sensory awareness and input. These changes may account for the deterioration in mental state often observed in hypovolaemic states, and can present themselves in different ways, e.g., apathy, confusion, restlessness and apprehension.

Restlessness in hypovolaemic patients may serve to increase their depth of respiratory movements and may improve venous return by increasing the intra-thoracic pressure, helping to compensate for the continued reduction in cardiac output from continuous bleeding. However, others are quiet and apathetic, and their senses become dulled, probably as a result of cerebral ischaemia and acidosis. In addition, a reduction in perfusion to the brain stem will affect respiration, BP and heart rate.

A general assessment of the patient's mental state can alert the nurse to impending neurological deterioration. The Glasgow Coma Scale is an example of a specific tool designed to produce a uniform method of determining and recording the activity of the ANS or mental state. It focuses on the evaluation of three parameters: eye opening, motor response and verbal response. The person's best achievement is scored separately for each parameter and the total can range from a maximum score of 15, where a person is fully alert and orientated, to a minimum score of 3, where a person is completely unresponsive.

Supporting the Patient with Hypovolaemia

When considering support for the circulation, there needs to be effective clinical management of bleeding to ensure the rapid establishment and maintenance of fluid volume replacement and the control of haemorrhage. The immediate restoration of an effective circulating blood volume through the use of blood, blood products, a balanced salt solution, colloid solution or all four is needed to minimize, prevent or reverse hypovolaemic states.

The current concepts of fluid resuscitation are complex and full of controversy, and there are constant discussions about whether whole blood (Table 3.1), colloid (Table 3.2) or crystalloid (Table 3.3) therapy should be given. It might be easy to just propose that blood be given for haemorrhage, colloids be given for plasma loss, clotting factors for bleeding disorders and crystalloid for dehydration and third-space fluid shifts. However, this argument, even though rational and logical, is much too simplistic.

Acute Coronary Syndromes

There is a period of time, prior to the development of acute coronary syndromes (ACS), which begins with the build up of

- Fatty streaks appear within the endothelium of the lumen of a coronary artery, which progresses to narrowing of the vessel
- Eventually this may lead and/or rupture leading to the stimulation of the inflammatory immune response
- Attracts platelets and a thrombus can form
- Resulting in angina

Stable Angina

Angina is a pain in the chest, felt as a result of lack of blood supply (ischaemia) to the heart. There is a narrowing of the coronary vessels, due to deposits of atheroma.

- A pain in the chest, felt as a result of lack of blood supply (ischaemia) to the heart.
- There is narrowing of the coronary vessels due to the deposits of atheroma
- The pain of angina can be brought on by exertion, described as mild (tightness, squeezing pain or discomfort) and often confused with heart-burn and the patient ignores it
- Relieved by rest and/or glyceryl trinitrate (GTN) tablets sublingually

  Usually managed by the GP with medication therapy:

- Nitrates GTN, isosorbide mononitrate and isosorbide dinitrate
- β-blockers atenolol to reduce workload of the heart and oxygen demands of the heart
- Calcium antagonists if angina is caused by coronary artery spasm
- Aspirin, lipid-lowering drugs statins e.g., atorvastatin

ACS are degenerative disorders, which occur over time, can be insidious; with symptoms only emerging when the stable angina has progressed. ACS include

- Unstable angina
- ST-segment elevation myocardial infarction (STEMI)
- Non−ST-segment elevation myocardial infarction (NSTEMI)

ACS does not occur without some degree of coronary artery disease (CAD). The plague is rupturing or has eroded, and it is difficult to differentiate between unstable angina and an MI, there, ACS is now used to describe both. Some risk factors such as age, gender and family history cannot be changed; thus, the main focus is on primary prevention:

- Modification of diet and increase exercise
- Hypertension
- Diabetes mellitus
- Smoking
- Obesity
- Menopause
- Stressful lifestyle

Unstable Angina

This may be a sign of an impending heart attack:

- Episodes of pain become more frequent
- Occur without obvious cause and at rest

- Can present with pleuritic pain, indigestion or dyspnoea
- Urgent angiography is required for diagnosis and treatment.
- Chest pain does not respond to usual therapy, e.g., GTN spray and rest and is what usually brings a patient into hospital:
  - The administration of oxygen is only necessary if the patient is presenting with signs of hypoxaemia (Shuvy et al., 2013)
  - Insertion of an IV cannula

Myocardial Infarction

- Myocardial infarction (MI) refers to necrosis of myocardial cells caused by cessation or a severe reduction in the blood supply.
- The condition once occurred is that of irreversible necrosis of a portion of heart muscle due to prolonged ischaemia.
- The prolonged, unrelieved ischaemia results in hypoxia, and as the amount of oxygen to the cardiac cells diminishes cellular death ensues − cardiac cells can withstand ischaemic conditions for about 20 minutes, even though they are metabolically altered and non-functional.
- If oxygen supply is not resumed the death of a segment of heart muscle, i.e., a MI, is the result.

The elderly or diabetic patient may sometimes have a 'silent' MI where no chest pain is experienced.

Coronary Circulation

The site of an infarction depends on which coronary artery is blocked. The tissue beyond the obstruction dies due to lack of oxygen to the tissues, which may become scar tissue, resulting in loss of strength and function of the muscle. There are two major coronary arteries:

1. The left coronary artery (LCA) − has two divisions
   a. Circumflex artery
   b. Left anterior descending artery (LAD)
2. The right coronary artery (RCA) − has branches:
   a. Right marginal branch
   b. Posterior interventricular artery

Near the apex of the heart, the posterior descending artery merges (anastomoses) with the anterior descending artery.

If the circumflex artery or any of its branches are occluded the infarction will cause damage/injury to the

- Lateral wall of the left ventricle
- Anterior wall of the left ventricle
- Anterior part of the septum (anterior MI)
- Abnormal arrhythmias may occur such as atrial fibrillation, atrial flutter

If there is occlusion to the LAD, the infarction will cause damage/injury to the

- Inferior wall of the left ventricle

Occlusion of the RCA will cause injury to the

- Posterior and inferior surface of the left ventricle
- Posterior part of the septum (inferior MI) (Table 4.9)
- Right ventricle, which supplies the nodes of conduction; more serious arrhythmias can occur such as bradyarrhythmias which can lead to a first- or second-degree heart block

Functional Changes

The severity of functional impairment depends on the size of the lesion and the site of infarction. Functional changes may include

- Decrease in the ability of the heart to contract
- Altered left ventricular compliance
- Decreased stroke volume
- Decreased ejection fraction
- Increased left ventricular end diastolic pressure
- Sino-atrial node malfunctions

This may lead to a number of serious complications that may be observed following an MI (Table 4.10).

TABLE 4.9 Infarction sites and artery blocked.

Infarction site of myocardial infarction (MI)	Blocked artery
Anteroseptal/anterior	Left anterior descending (LAD)
Anterolateral/posterior, lateral	Left circumflex
Inferior/posterior	Right coronary

TABLE 4.10 Complications of a myocardial infarction (MI).

Complication	Interventions that may be undertaken
Arrhythmias	Some form of rhythm disturbance occurs in nearly all MI patients, and is likely to occur within the first few hours.
• Ventricular ectopic beats (VEB) • Ventricular fibrillation (VF) and ventricular tachycardia (VT)	Does not generally require any treatment. Requires immediate DC cardioversion.
• Accelerated idioventricular rhythm (AIVR) — common in inferior MI	Slow VT, generally benign and treatment is rarely necessary.
• Atrial fibrillation (AF)	May not require treatment if patient is asymptomatic. IV β-blocker or amiodarone can be used to slow the ventricular rate. Digoxin is the drug of choice if heart failure is present.
• Atrial flutter (AFlutt)	Difficult to treat, as drug therapy is usually ineffective. Most patients will generally revert to sinus rhythm in time. If this does not occur, rapid atrial pacing or synchronized DC cardioversion may be necessary.
• AV nodal and AV re-entry tachycardia (AVNRT and AVRT)	These are uncommon; adenosine is the treatment of choice. Verapamil should be avoided, especially in patients with heart failure.
• Bradyarrhythmias	Temporary pacing is indicated. Atropine, or isoprenaline for immediate treatment, while pacing is being instituted or if pacing facilities are unavailable.
• Complete heart block	Generally, secondary to inferior MI usually recovers within a few days and has a good prognosis, but temporary pacing is required if the ventricular rate is slow. Permanent pacing is rarely necessary.
Cardiac failure	Diuretics and nitrates and inotropic support. Angiotensin-converting enzyme (ACE) inhibitors are recommended for all patients with significant LV dysfunction.
Cardiogenic shock	Mortality is very high — 80%. Definitive proof that expensive strategies improve survival is being researched.
Thromboembolism	Thrombus formation overlying the infarcted myocardium is common 30% of patients. Heparin and warfarin is recommended. Warfarin is generally stopped on discharge, but there is evidence that prognosis is improved when warfarin is continued.
Cardiac dilatation and left ventricular aneurysm formation	Occur in patients with large infarcts, causing stretching and dilatation of the ventricle. ACE inhibitors appear to limit dilatation and help to preserve LV function and prognosis.

TABLE 4.11 Grades of encephalopathy.

Grade	Description
1.	Absent minded, forgetful
2.	Drowsy, night to day reversal
3.	Semi-conscious, rousable (intubate adults at this level)
4.	Comatose
5.	Irreversible brain swelling

Acute Coronary Syndromes Recommended Interventions/ Treatment (NICE, 2014)

NSTEMI or Unstable Angina

- Aspiring and anti-thrombin therapy
- Coronary angiography with percutaneous coronary intervention (PCI) within 72 hours
- Coronary artery bypass grafts (CABG) depending on angiography findings
  - Coronary artery bypass surgery is a procedure by which graft is placed between the aorta and a point in the coronary artery beyond the narrowed or blocked area.
  - A graft is required for each of the main coronary arteries affected.
  - The internal mammary artery is generally used, which is less likely to narrow over time than a vein graft.
  - A heart-lung bypass machine is generally used during the operation; the heart is stopped while the bypass grafting takes place.
  - Coronary artery bypass grafts can take place without the use of a heart-lung bypass machine; this is known as 'beating-heart surgery'.

Acute STEMI

- Fibrinolysis with acute STEMI presenting within 12 hours of onset of symptoms
- Coronary angiography with STEMI presenting more than 12 hours after the onset of symptoms
- If cardiogenic shock is present coronary angiography, with follow-on primary PCI if indicated

Cardiomyopathy

Dilated Cardiomyopathy

Characterized by dilatation and impaired contraction of the left ventricle or both ventricles. It may be

- Idiopathic
- Familial/genetic
- Viral and/immune
- Alcoholic/toxic
- Associated with recognized cardiovascular disease in which the degree of myocardial dysfunction is not explained by the abnormal loading conditions or the extent of ischaemic damage

Clinical Presentation

- Pulmonary congestion and/or low cardiac output
- Exertional symptoms and fatigue for many months or years before diagnosis
- An acute illness or the development of arrhythmia, in particular atrial fibrillation, may precipitate acute decompensation and prompt the individual to seek medical attention
- Family or routine medical screening
- May present with systemic embolism or sudden death
- Nutritional deficiencies and endocrine abnormalities may produce heart failure; therefore, it is important to take a drug history of both prescribed and non-prescribed medications.

Investigations

- Electrocardiogram − T wave changes, septal Q waves, prolongation of atrioventricular (AV) conduction and bundle branch block. Sinus tachycardia and supraventricular arrhythmias are common, in particular atrial fibrillation (AF), non-sustained ventricular tachycardia (NSVT)
- Echocardiogram
- Exercise testing
- Viral serology
- Endomyocardial biopsy

Treatment

- To control symptoms and to prevent disease progression and complications such as progressive heart failure, thromboembolism and sudden death. Diuretics are used to treat congestive symptoms.
- Angiotensin converting enzyme inhibitors − improve dyspnoea and exercise tolerance, reduce hospitalization rates and reduce cardiovascular mortality. They also prevent or slow down disease progression in

asymptomatic patients. Angiotensin II (AII) receptor antagonists may be prescribed in the case of intolerable side effects from ACE therapy, as they have a similar effect.

- β-blockers are prescribed.
- Spironolactone has recently been associated with a 30% reduction in the overall risk of death in patients with an ejection fraction of 35%.
- Anticoagulation may be required in patients with dilated atrial chambers and those with AF.

Non-pharmacological treatment of advanced heart failure:

- Patients with intractable symptoms and end-stage disease may be referred for cardiac transplantation or for left ventricular assist device (as a bridge to transplantation).
- Multi-site ventricular pacing.
- Dual-chamber pacing has been advocated as a method for restoring AV synchrony and improving left ventricular coordination.
- In severe congestive heart failure − bi-ventricular pacing.

Hypertrophic Cardiomyopathy

Characterized by left and/or right ventricular hypertrophy, which is usually asymmetric and involves the interventricular septum:

- The left ventricular volume is normal or reduced.
- Systolic gradients are common.
- Familial disease with autosomal dominant inheritance predominates.
- Arrhythmias and premature sudden death are common.
- The condition appears to be a common genetic malformation of the heart affecting 1 in 500 of the population.

Pathophysiology

Four main abnormalities are found:

- Ventricular hypertrophy
- Rapid contraction of the left ventricle
- Impaired relaxation
- Intracavity systolic gradients

Symptoms

- Patients can present at any age with dyspnoea, chest pain, unexplained syncope, arrhythmia, or sudden death.
- Many patients have none or very minor symptoms and in children and adolescents the diagnosis is often made during family screening.

- Chest pain on exertion occurs in up to 30% of adults, and many complain of atypical pain that is prolonged and occurs at rest and after meals.
- Dyspnoea is common.
- Less common is paroxysmal nocturnal dyspnoea and orthopnoea, which may occur in the presence of apparently mild disease.
- Approximately 15%–25% of patients experience syncope, and 20% complain of presyncope.

Diagnosis

- A detailed family history, especially noting any sudden unexplained deaths.
- May be diagnosed as a result of family screening or as an incidental finding during a medical examination.
- Adults are often asymptomatic so in the majority of patients the physical examination may be unremarkable.
- Once a diagnosis has been given it is vitally important that first-degree relatives of an affected person are offered cardiac evaluation.

Investigations

- ECG is abnormal in the majority of patients and may show evidence of right and left atrial enlargement.
- Echocardiogram is normal.
- 24-hour Holter − 24-hour ambulatory electrocardiographic monitoring − paroxysmal supraventricular arrhythmias occur on Holter monitoring in 30%–50% of patients.
- NSVT occurs in 25% of adults.
- Most episodes are slow and asymptomatic and occur at rest.
- Atrial fibrillation is present in 5% of patients at diagnosis.
- Echocardiogram.
- Exercise testing.
- Cardiopulmonary gas exchange during exercise.
- During upright exercise patients commonly demonstrate an abnormal BP with either a fall in BP or a failure of it to rise; this is a risk factor for sudden death.
- MRI − useful to assess the degree of hypertrophy when the diagnosis with echocardiography remains unclear.

Treatment of Hypertrophic Cardiomyopathy
Non-Obstructive − Medical Treatment

- β-blockers, verapamil and diltiazem are used to treat dyspnoea and chest pain and improve exercise intolerance.
- Diuretics may be used in the short term to treat pulmonary congestion.

- Amiodarone is an effective and widely used drug.
- Patients who experience atrial fibrillation will require anticoagulation to reduce the risk of thrombus formation.

Obstructive HCM – Medical Treatment

- β-blockers are the first line of treatment and the majority of patients will show improvement in symptoms.
- Verapamil should be avoided in obstruction because of possible peripheral vasodilation and haemodynamic collapse.
- Disopyramide is used to treat patients with gradients and is best used in combination as used alone it may accelerate AV node conduction and increase the potential risk of supraventricular arrhythmias.

Obstructive HCM – Surgical Treatment Choices are

- Surgical septal myectomy
- Dual-chamber pacemaker

Genetic Testing

The genotype-phenotype relationship remains unclear. Recent studies have suggested that some mutations may have prognostic significance. A genetic test is not yet available, and research in this area continues.

Arrhythmogenic Right Ventricular Cardiomyopathy

A familial myocardial disease characterized pathologically by right ventricular (RV) myocardial atrophy and fibrofatty replacement. Long-term follow-up data from clinical studies indicate that arrhythmogenic right ventricular cardiomyopathy (ARVC) is a progressive heart muscle disease that, with time, may lead to more diffuse RV involvement and left ventricular (LV) changes and may culminate in heart failure.

Pathological Features

- Diffuse or segmental loss of the myocardium of the right ventricular free wall. It is frequently transmural.
- May be difficult to diagnose as the patient may be asymptomatic until the first presentation with cardiac arrest.
- Diagnosis may be missed and the patient may present in later years with congestive heart failure, with or without ventricular arrhythmia.

Causes

- A familial background has been demonstrated in nearly 50% of cases, with an autosomal dominant pattern of inheritance.
- As yet the involved genes and the molecular defects remain unknown.

- At the present time a genetic test for screening is not currently available.
- In some cases, there is either no evidence of inheritance or there is insufficient information about the individual's family to assess inheritance.
- A further difficulty is that, within a family, features of the disease may be variable and the disease may appear to skip a generation.

Symptoms

- May be asymptomatic or may present with palpitations, syncope, pre-syncope, lethargy, dyspnoea and oedema.
- The severity of symptoms and risk of complications varies greatly between people, and many people never have any serious problems related to their condition.

Diagnosis

- Requires right ventriculogram, electrophysiological studies (EPS), genetic testing, 24-hour monitoring, exercise testing, echocaridogram, surgery or endomyocardial biopsy because the diagnosis may be difficult to establish.
- To fulfil the diagnosis, the patient must demonstrate two major criteria, one major criterion plus two minor criteria or four minor criteria.

Investigations

- A full physical examination and careful family history are recorded.
- Electrocardiogram − T wave inversion and QRS prolongation (0.110 ms) in leads V1−V3, and complete or incomplete right bundle branch block. In 30% of patients a small deflection may be seen at the end of the QRS complex, the so-called epsilon wave, caused by delayed right ventricular activation.
- Signal average electrocardiogram (SAECG) − permits identification of very low amplitude electrical signals believed to emanate from damaged areas of myocardium.
- Echocardiogram − evaluate right and left ventricular size and function, which are important major and minor criteria for the diagnosis.
- VO_2 maximum exercise test − assess peak exercise capacity, maximal oxygen consumption, peak heart rate and stroke volume. BP is also monitored and changes in heart rhythm recorded.
- Right ventricular angiography − assess the areas commonly involved in ARVC such as
  - The infundibulum
  - The anterior right ventricular free wall
  - Inferior wall
  - Sub-tricuspid area
- CT and MRI − scanning enables visualization of anatomical features of the right ventricle and can show tissue characterization and may identify areas of myocardial thinning.

Treatment Options

- Management is tailored to the individual's clinical presentation.
- Pharmacological therapy.
- β-blockers.
- Antiarrhythmic drugs are used; either sotalol or amiodarone (alone or in combination with β-blockers) are the most effective drugs with a relatively low proarrhythmic risk.
- The efficacy of this treatment may be based on reported symptoms, and further evaluation using 24-hour Holter and exercise testing.
- In patients with sustained VT or VF, antiarrhythmic drug treatment guided by programmed ventricular stimulation with serial drug testing is an option.
- Catheter ablation.
- Implantable cardioverter defibrillator − most effective safeguard against arrhythmic sudden death and is the treatment of choice for survivors of cardiac arrest, and those patients with VT.

Restrictive Cardiomyopathy

- The least common of the cardiomyopathies, this is defined as heart muscle disease that results in impaired ventricular filling, with normal or decreased diastolic volume of either or both ventricles.
- Systolic function usually remains normal, or at least early in the disease, and wall thickness may be normal or increased, depending on the under-lying cause.
- Usually results from increased stiffness of the myocardium that causes pressure within the ventricle (or ventricles) to rise precipitously with only small increases in volume.
- As the condition affects either or both ventricles, the patient may present with signs of left or right ventricular failure.
- It is important to distinguish this condition from constrictive pericarditis, which may also present with restrictive physiology but which is often cured surgically.
- May be a primary disorder due to endomyocardial fibrosis.
- Secondary restrictive cardiomyopathy can be due to infiltrative disease such as amyloidosis, postirradiation therapy or storage diseases such as haemochromatosis, glycogen storage disease or Fabry's disease.
- Idiopathic restrictive cardiomyopathy is sometimes familial and seems to be associated with distal skeletal myopathy.

Clinical Presentation

- The underlying cause of restrictive cardiomyopathy may not be obvious on presentation: the patient may present with symptoms similar to those of dilated cardiomyopathy.

- Commonly exercise intolerance is a frequent symptom, as the heart cannot increase cardiac output by tachycardia without compromising ventricular filling.
- Presentation may be sudden cardiac death.
- Other symptoms include dyspnoea, paroxysmal nocturnal dyspnoea, orthopnoea, peripheral oedema, ascites, fatigue and weakness.
- Angina does not occur except in amyloidosis, in which it may be the presenting symptom.
- In advanced cases the patient may present with all the signs of heart failure except cardiomegaly.

Investigations

- ECG − sinus tachycardia, atrial fibrillation and complex ventricular dysrhythmias.
- Echocardiogram − reveals thickened ventricular walls, small ventricular cavities and dilated atria.
- Characteristic feature is a deep and early decline of ventricular pressure at the onset of diastole with a rise to a plateau, and a higher left ventricular end diastolic pressure.
- Chest X-ray − may be normal; cardiomegaly, pleural effusions and pulmonary congestion may be evident in those who have progressed to heart failure.

Treatment

- Palliative and similar to that of dilated cardiomyopathy and heart failure. Medical intervention includes the use of diuretics, ACE inhibitors, anti-arrhythmics and anticoagulant.
- A pacemaker may be used to treat AV conduction block. Cardiac transplantation can be considered in patients with refractory symptoms in idiopathic or familial restrictive cardiomyopathy.

Nursing Considerations in Cardiomyopathy

- Presents the critical care nurse with many challenges; the presentation of cardiomyopathy within a family may range from the asymptomatic patient who requires no treatment to sudden cardiac death and heart failure.
- It is important to remember that nurses will encounter patients who are living with a cardiomyopathy at various stages of disease progression. Understanding the different types of cardiomyopathy, their inheritance patterns and treatment strategies will enable the critical care nurse to offer valuable support and advice.
- Psychological adjustment to a diagnosis of cardiomyopathy may depend on effective communication with clinical staff, and support and understanding from family and friends.

- The Cardiomyopathy Association (CMA) is a patient organization that offers support and advice to sufferers, their families and health professionals on all types of cardiomyopathy.

Heart Failure

Heart failure is when the heart is no longer acting as an efficient pump and cannot respond to the demands made upon it (Richards and Edwards, 2014). The heart is two pumps: the right side and the left side, and either side can fail independently; however as both sides are linked together as one structure, if one side fails the other will eventually follow.

When either one or both sides of the heart fail, its ability to

- Contract efficiently is reduced and it can no longer respond to increase filling pressure by contracting more strongly.
- Is not strong enough to pump blood efficiently around the body and various organs receive insufficient blood supply.
- The kidney activates the renin-angiotensin system and causes salt and water retention and oedema.
- Breathlessness may occur due to oedema of the lung tissue — leading to left ventricular failure and pulmonary oedema. Fluid collects through the lungs into the right side of the heart and backtracks into the systemic circulation causing systemic venous congestion and peripheral oedema.
- The major organs receive oxygen and blood supply at the expense of other organs e.g., muscles, which are starved, and this may lead to fatigue.
- When both sides, e.g., left and right, of the heart fail the condition is not curable. There is a failure of the heart to eject blood efficiently from the ventricles, resulting in elevated intra-cardiac pressures.

Chronic heart failure can be kept under control with the use of drugs.

Left Ventricular Failure

In most cases the left ventricle fails first known as left ventricular failure (LVF). There is damage to, or overload of, the left ventricle, which leads to pulmonary oedema.

The myocardium becomes weak, which impairs the ability of the left side of the heart to pump efficiently.

- With each consequent beat blood (the amount depends on the severity of the weakness) remains in the left ventricle, decreasing the amount of blood pumped out from the left ventricle.
- Nervous stimulation will increase heart rate to maintain cardiac output for a while, but the blood continues to build up in the left ventricle leading to a back flow from the left ventricle into the lungs.

- This will raise the HP in the blood vessels in the lungs leading to pulmonary oedema.

Cardiovascular Causes Include

- Hypertension
- Mitral and aortic valve disease
- Cardiac arrhythmias e.g., atrial fibrillation
- Over transfusion e.g., fluid overload
- MI
- Ischaemic heart disease
- Cardiac arrhythmias, e.g., atrial fibrillation
- Cardiomyopathy.

Non-Cardiovascular Causes Include

- Pregnancy and childbirth
- Thyrotoxicosis
- Hypovolaemia/fluid overload
- Pulmonary embolism
- Sepsis
- Anaemia
- COPD

Clinical Features

- Severe breathlessness
- Moist, wheezy breathing
- Anxiety, feeling of suffocation
- Tachycardia
- Cold, clammy skin
- White, frothy sputum, may be pink in terminal stage
- Chest X-ray shows enlarged heart, diffused density in the lung bases
- 12 lead ECG may show normal sinus rhythm, q waves and left axis deviation

Treatment and Drug Therapy

- Sit the patient up in bed to allow maximum lung expansion
- Administer oxygen as prescribed
- Urgent diuretics are needed to relieve the pulmonary oedema
- Small dose of morphine can relieve panic and anxiety and helps to reduce strain on the heart

Heart Failure

This is when the increased pressure pushes backwards into the pulmonary artery and into the right side of the heart leading to failure of the right side of the heart (Richards and Edwards, 2014).

Heart failure is the most common complication following an MI.

- The stress on the heart from the necrotic muscle reaches a critical level.
- There is impaired contractility of the cardiac muscle and cardiac output declines.
- There is an increase in volume in the right ventricle.
- The right ventricle cannot pump and there is a backlog of blood in the right atrium and then the vena cava.
- The venous system then becomes congested.
- Blood pools in the systemic circulation leading to peripheral oedema.

Clinical Features

- Increased breathlessness
- Due to increased pressure in the systemic veins oedema forms
- Weight increases
- Distended jugular veins, which are visible
- Fall in cardiac output results in salt and water retention by the RAAS system of the kidneys
- Ascites may occur
- All the abdominal organs are engorged with blood and in the liver; this may cause abdominal pain
- Loss of appetite, lethargy and fatigue, muscle weakness
- Mental changes such as irritability, reduced attention span and restlessness

Treatment and Drug Therapy

Generally, the same as LVF with the addition of additional medications (NICE, 2018)

- Diuretics continue
- Digoxin for patients with atrial fibrillation
- ACE inhibitors are recommended
- β-blockers
- Anticoagulants
- Mineralocorticoid receptor antagonists (MRA) added to ACE inhibitors and β-blockers if heart failure worsens
- In the chronic stage ivabradine or sacubitril valsartan
- Treat depression

- Ventricular assisted device (VAD) mechanical circulatory support for advanced heart failure
  - The device once implanted can improve a patient's survival and quality of life (Birati and Jessup, 2015).
  - The VAD can be used to partially or completely support the failing heart. The device works by pumping blood from the left ventricle into the ascending aorta.
  - VADs can be used for
    - Prior heart transplant
    - As a therapy for those heart failure patients where transplant is not an option
    - Patients too sick to undergo transplant surgery to improve physical condition
    - As a bridge for patients who may recover, e.g., due to fluid overload

Implantable Cardioverter Defibrillators

Used for patients who have life-threatening abnormalities of heart rhythm. Implantable cardioverter defibrillators (ICDs) send electrical pulses to regulate abnormal heart rhythms and are used to treat two types of rhythm:

1. Ventricular tachycardia
2. Ventricular fibrillation.

The ICD constantly monitors the heart rhythm; if it senses that a rhythm disturbance is beginning, it can deliver one of the following treatments:

- Pacing − If the cardiac rhythm is not too serious, the ICD delivers a short series of low-voltage electrical impulses which will correct the heartbeat without the need for any further action.
- Cardioversion − If the heartbeat is irregular the ICD can deliver a light electrical shock.
- Defibrillation − If a more serious arrhythmia is sensed the ICD will deliver a bigger electrical shock to the heart in order to stop the abnormal beating and get the heart rhythm back to normal − defibrillation.

There is generally a delay of between 3 and 12 seconds between the ICD detecting an abnormal heart rhythm and delivering the electrical shock.

4.6 RENAL

Renal function can be affected by a variety of disorders, the common cause being infection. Stones or a tumour can obstruct the urinary tract. Renal function can be impaired by disorders of the kidney itself or by many other systemic diseases. Because the kidney filters blood, it is directly linked to every other organ system. Therefore, renal conditions that lead to renal failure can be life-threatening. Two different causes

- Inflammation (Fig. 4.2) − infection, obstruction, tumours
- Reduced blood supply to the kidneys (Fig. 4.1) − hypoxic damage, acute tubular necrosis (ATN), hypovolaemia

Acute Renal Failure

There are considered to be three types of acute renal failure that lead to an AKI all include varying causes (NICE, 2013):

Prerenal Acute Renal Failure

The causes of prerenal acute renal failure are dehydration, heart failure, sepsis and severe blood loss, and if not corrected or treated early can lead to intrinsic damage.

It is also associated with pre-existing conditions such as atherosclerosis, hypertension, and chronic liver disease, diabetes mellitus.

The patient usually suffers from dizziness, dry mouth, low BP, rapid heart rate, thirst and weight loss.

Urine output is usually low.

Postrenal Acute Renal Failure

The causes of postrenal ARF are an acute obstruction that affects the normal flow of urine out of both kidneys. There is a backflow of urine in the nephrons leading to an increase in pressure and causing them to fail.

Urinary Tract Obstruction

Can occur anywhere in the urinary tract:

- Renal or bladder stones formed from calcium loading in the urethra
- Enlarged prostrate
- Trauma
- Tumours
  - Neural lesions interrupt innervation of the bladder
  - Renal cell carcinoma common neoplasm
  - Metastasis to the liver, lung, bone
  - Bladder tumours − high rate of recurrence

Causes a collection of urine behind the obstruction, affecting surrounding organs leading to inflammation and ischaemic atrophy, which is dependent on

- Location with the urinary tract
- Unilateral or bilateral
- Partial or complete − GFR reduced or zero

- Acute or chronic duration — chronic partial obstruction causes compression of kidney structures reducing renal ability
- The underlying cause

The relief of renal obstruction is followed by a variable period of diuresis, with losses of large amounts of urine; this lasts for a few days without symptoms of volume depletion.

Intrinsic Acute Renal Failure

This is acute renal failure that is not caused by prerenal or postrenal factors. Intrinsic renal failure involves structural damage or injury to one or both kidneys. This includes

- Vascular disease
- Acute glomerulonephritis (AGN)
- Renal artery/vein obstruction
- Ischaemia a reduced blood flow to the kidneys ATN
- Toxins such as antibiotics, chemotherapy

Urinary Tract Infection

- Usually caused by bacteria from retrograde movement into urethra and bladder
- Diagnosed by culture of specific organisms
- Counts of 100,000 bacteria/mL of freshly voided urine
- Can occur anywhere along the urinary tract
- Cystitis — inflammation of the bladder, which is the most common site; generally more common in women; common organisms include
    Escherichia coli
    Klebsiella
    Proteus
    Pseudomonas
    Staphylococcus

Pyelonephritis

- Infection of the renal pelvis, acute or chronic (persistent or recurrent)
- Cause is usually bacterial but can be fungal or viral
- Generally spread by ascending organism along the ureters but may occur via the blood stream
- Acute, responds well to 2 weeks of organism-specific antibiotics

Glomerular Disorders

Glomerulonephritis Inflammation of the glomerulus caused by

- Immune responses
- Toxins or drugs
- Vascular disorders
- Systemic diseases

Classification of glomerulonephritis:

- AGN
- Rapidly progressive glomerulonephritis (RPGN)
- Chronic glomerulonephritis

Nephrotic Syndrome Excretion of at least 3.5 g protein in urine per day.

- Hypoproteinaemia, hyperlipidaemia and oedema
- Caused by loss of plasma proteins across the injured glomerular filtration membrane
- Reduced protein leads to oedema

Treatment involves:

- Normal-protein, low-fat diet
- Salt restriction
- Diuretics
- Steroids
- Occasionally albumin replacement

Differentiating Between Prerenal and Intrinsic Factors can be Difficult

In Prerenal

- Urine output is diminished.
- Urinalysis will show normal constituents with a high specific gravity, high osmolality, low urine sodium, urea and creatinine.
- There is no actual damage to the kidney itself so the kidney will respond to therapy.

In Intrinsic

- Urine output may or may not be diminished.
- Urinalysis has a low specific gravity, low osmolality, increased urine sodium, low urine urea and creatinine.
- There is damage to the nephrons, so improvements will not be seen with the correction of the cause.

Classification of Renal Dysfunction

- Renal insufficiency refers to a decline in renal function to about 25% of normal or GFR of 25–30 mL/min
- Renal failure refers to significant loss of renal function
- End-stage renal failure (ESRF) is when less than 10% of renal function remains

Generally, two different types:

- AKI – prerenal, renal, postrenal
- Chronic renal failure

Phases of Acute Renal Failure

- Initiating stage – begins when the kidney is injured renal impairment is evident with an altered BUN and creatinine levels and decreasing urine output
- Oliguric stage – decrease in urine output of less than 400 mL/24 hours, oedema may appear, hyperkalaemia leading to cardiac arrest, metabolic acidosis; if there is less than 100 mL/24 hours this is termed anuria
- Diuretic stage – an increase in urine output and uraemia resolves, loss of massive amounts of fluid through excessive urination, dehydration, hypokalaemia
- Recovery stage – recovery depends on the number of functioning nephrons, if too few can suffer from hyperfiltration and die leading to chronic renal failure

Clinical Features

- Asymptomatic
- Oliguria
- Increasing blood urea
- Nausea and vomiting
- Confusion
- Loss of appetite

(See Table 4.12).

Acute renal failure can cause sudden, life-threatening disturbances in the biochemistry of the blood and is a medical emergency.

TABLE 4.12 Caring for a renal patient.

Symptoms	Investigations	Treatments	Specific nursing care	Complications
• Incontinence	• Past medical history	• Fluid challenge	• Fluid balance chart – +ve and –ve balance	• Renal failure
• Pain	• Urinalysis	• Surgical - removal of tumour or stones, formation of ileoconduit	• TPR, BP, CVP	• Metabolic acidosis
• Haematuria (painless)	• Urine sample for MC&S: gram +ve or gram –ve	• Medical e.g., drugs diuretics, chemotherapy, radiotherapy, anti-hypertensive drugs, dopamine, dobutamine	• Analgesia, pain assessment	• Electrolyte imbalance
• Frequency of micturition	• Central venous pressure monitoring	• Urinary catheterization if appropriate	• Diet e.g., restricted protein, potassium	• Fluid overload
• Proteinuria (generally the first identifiable problem)	• Cystoscopy	• Fluid therapy, fluid restrictions	• Fluid therapy, care of IV lines	• Hyperkalaemia (generally the cause of death in end-stage renal failure)
• Reduced glomerular filtration rate	• Surgical investigative procedures e.g., IVP Urograms (X-ray)	• Blood transfusions	• Care of RRT lines, insertion site, aseptic technique	• ECG changes
• Reduced urine output	• TPR, blood pressure (BP)	• Renal replacement therapy (RRT) e.g., haemofiltration	• Catheter care, hygiene	• Hyperventilation, respiratory complications
• Oliguria	• Ultrasound for kidney stones	• Peritoneal dialysis	• Administration of drugs	• Heart failure (cardiogenic shock)
• Oedema	• Renal biopsy	• Renal dialysis	• Blood results	• Oedema
• Hypertension	• Blood analysis:	• Analgesia	• Cardiac monitor	• Fluid overload
• History of an hypotensive episode, or cardiac problems	↑ BUN (blood urea nitrogen) creatinine	• Antibiotic therapy	• Keep patient informed, provide support for family and friends	• Hypoproteinaemia
• Confusion and disorientation	↑ potassium	• Renal transplantation	• MDT support	• Hypoxia
• Dehydration	↑ calcium levels	• Changes in lifestyle: diet, low potassium and protein	• Inform doctor of any changes	• Hypertension
• Painful/painless micturition	↓ Hb anaemia		• Psychological and social needs	• Anaemia (due to reduced erythropoietin production)
• Anaemia	↓ sodium levels		• Communication	• Infection, sepsis
• Confusion	• Blood glucose		• Changes in lifestyle e.g., loss of control, altered body image, stress	
	• ECG elevated			
	T wave, ↑ heart rate			
	• 24 hour urine collection			
	• Daily weight			

Chronic Renal Failure

The kidney has many important regulatory functions, but renal symptomatic changes do not become apparent until the renal function declines to less than 25% of normal. The causes are prerenal, postrenal and intrinsic.

Clinical Features

- Gastrointestinal tract − anorexia, nausea and vomiting, hiccups
- Skin − itching, uraemic frost
- Blood − anaemia, tendency to bleed
- Bones − inadequate vitamin D, bone pain, pathological fractures
- Cardiovascular system − hypertension, coronary artery disease
- Nervous system − uraemic neuropathy leading to apathy, confusion, irritation, tremors and seizures

Management of Chronic Renal Failure

- Blood and urine analysis − check haemoglobin for anaemia, electrolytes, creatinine and urea, urine testing for protein
- Fluid and electrolyte balance − potassium − ECG changes, sodium, phosphate and calcium balance, fluid and diet intake are strictly controlled, fluid output
- Acidosis − metabolic acidosis begins to develop when GFR decreases by 30%−40%, maintained by respiratory system removal of carbon dioxide

Renal replacement therapy:

- Haemodialysis − intermittent, traumatic to the circulation, reduced BP
- Haemofiltration − continuous, less traumatic to the circulation
- Peritoneal dialysis − intermittent generally at home at night, managed by the patient
- Transplantation − variable success with organ donation, but some improvement with live donations

CRF accounts for the death of a small group of patients. Death can sometimes be easy to predict because dialysis has been discontinued. They can suffer from pain during the last days and this underscores the necessity for medical and nursing staff to be skilled providers of modern palliative care. If the symptoms of ESRF are poorly managed, they lead to misery at the end of life. Knowledge of palliative care in these instances is essential.

The end result of renal failure is generally death (See Table 4.13).

4.7 GASTROINTESTINAL

Patients admitted to critical care may have undergone GI surgery for a number of the conditions identified here or may have developed bleeding due to peptic ulcer, liver failure or cirrhosis. Some conditions are severe and may

TABLE 4.13 The broader issues involved in caring for a renal patient.

Physiological issues	Social issues	Psychological issues	Ethical principles/ issues	Wider issues	Palliative care issues
Inflammation process	Financial	Altered self and	Cost of	The environment of care:	Discussion of
Hypoxic injury:	Job security	body image	treatment	• Ward/unit philosophy e.g., is	issues regarding
• Cardiac respiratory disease	Transport to	How others see	When to stop	children allowed to visit,	dying
• Hypovolaemia/	and from	patient with renal	Do no harm/	holistic care advocated.	Answer questions
hypotensionSystemic diseases:	dialysis	failure	do good	• Care planning nursing	concerning anger:
• Liver failure	The cost	Mental state	Age/family	process, nursing model	'Why me?', 'is
• Sepsis	Is it	Pain – too much	position	• Primary nursing/team nursing	there a God?'
• Peripheral vascular disease	transferable	may affect	Availability of	• CommunicationManagement	Pain control
• SLE (Systemic lupus erythematosus)	to children?	psychological	treatment in	styles	Decisions
Diet/fluid administration	Mobility	reasoning	area and	Family involvement in care	regarding family/
Urinalysis/urine output	Housing	Effects of controlled	funding	and decision-making	family support
Drug therapy e.g., diuretics	conditions	diet and restricted	Autonomy	Government funding for	Living will
Pain management – knowledge of	Depression	fluid intake	Informed	kidney dialysis	Religious needs
how they work, side effects	Welfare	Sexuality	consent	Charity involvement	Talk about issues
Care of IV lines and dialysis access.	benefits	Children	Responsibility		around dying
Functions of the kidneys –	Appropriate	The wife coping	and		where, what if,
observations of change:	referral	help may be	accountability		what to do in the
• Potassium – ECG changes	Multi-	needed	of staff towards		event of
• Oxygen administration	disciplinary	Concerns regarding	patients		Alternative
• Acid base balance – respiratory rate	team	who is going to pay	When to stop		therapies that
• Fluid balance – oedema formation,		the bills	treatment and		might help e.g.,
protein loss		Dialysis leading to	begin		relaxation,
• HypertensionTransplantation issues		life restrictions	palliative care		massage
Fluid restriction		(Maslow)			Effective pain
Blood results		The worry			management
Neuropathy		regarding other			Respite care for
Bone problems		family members			wife if needed
Blood transfusions		Transplant concerns			End of life
		mental state			decision-making
		regarding			
		acceptance of this			

require critical care interventions — e.g., peritonitis, pancreatitis, bleeding oesophageal varices.

Nutrients are required to carry out vital functions to sustain life, to form new body components or to assist in the functioning of various body processes, such as, breathing and physical activity.

The Effects of Stress on the GIT

The majority of patient in critical care suffer from stress and malnutrition, which can lead to complications of the GIT such as ulceration and hypoxia. This compounds to prevent the replenishment of energy sources (direct or indirect) reducing patients' ability to heal and recover.

The Stress Response

- Initiated by the nervous and endocrine systems
- Stress stimulates the SNS, promoting:
  - Suppression of reproduction, growth and thyroid hormones
  - The medulla of the adrenal gland releases catecholamines into the blood stream, adrenaline and noradrenaline
  - It is noradrenalin that has the major effect on the GIT:
    - GIT relaxation
    - Inhibiting GIT activity and absorption
    - May be significant to cause ischaemia to the stomach and duodenal mucosa
- The adrenal cortex is also activated in long-term stress:
  - Release of cortisol, GIT effects of cortisol:
    - Promotes gastric secretion
    - May be enough to cause ulceration of gastric mucosa
  - Effects carbohydrate, protein and fat metabolism resulting in an increase in blood glucose
  - Maximises the action of catecholamines

Conditions of the GIT

Critical care patients can suffer from conditions related directly to the GIT including

Upper GIT disorders
Lower GIT disorders

Symptoms of Gastrointestinal Disease Could Include the Following

- Dysphagia
- Dyspepsia

- Heartburn
- Flatulence
- Haematemesis
- Abdominal pain/acute abdomen
- GI bleeding
- Melaena
- Steatorrhoea
- Loss of weight
- Abdominal pain
- Anorexia
- Diarrhoea and vomiting
- Constipation

Disorders of the Upper GIT

This includes the oesophagus, stomach and duodenum.

Hiatus Hernia

This is a herniation of part of the stomach through the diaphragm.
Common and is one cause of reflux oesophagitis.

Types Sliding hiatus hernia is when the stomach herniates into the thorax when the patient is in the supine position

- Standing causes the stomach to slide back into the abdomen.
- Exacerbated by any factors that increase intra-abdominal pressure such as coughing, bending, straining and pregnancy.
- Management is medical weight reduction, antacids and sleeping in the sitting position.

Rolling or para-oesophageal hernia the fundus of the stomach herniates through the hiatus alongside the oesophagus

- Reflux is less common but there is a danger of congestion, constriction and ulcer formation.
- The hernia may strangulate which is a major complication.
- Diagnosis is by barium studies and endoscopy.

Oesophageal Varices

- These occur secondary to liver disease caused by portal hypertension distended and tortuous veins.
- 70% of patient with cirrhosis will develop varices.
- Bleeding is likely from large varices and in severe liver disease.
- They are frequently the cause of life-threatening haematemesis when they rupture.

- The mortality rate varies between 30% and 60%.
- Recurrent bleeding from varices has a poor prognosis with most patients dying within the year.
- Emergency treatment of bleeding varices:
  - Prompt correction of hypovolaemia.
  - Vasoconstriction therapy − vasopressin or Glypressin may be used.
  - A Sengstaken-Blakemore tube is usually used.

Helicobacter Pylori

- This organism *Helicobacter pylori* is a spirochaete and is known to be involved in gastritis, gastric ulcer (GU) and duodenal ulcer (DU) formation and cancer.
- Is the commonest cause of gastritis.
- Generally occurs in 50% of patients over 50 years of age.
- Mode of transmission is thought to be through water; otherwise it is uncertain.
- Diagnosis is by C urea breath tests, which is very simple but not always accurate, endoscopic mucosal biopsy and culture of the organism is the best way for certain diagnosis.
- Treatment is by triple regimens, as most strains are resistant to single antibiotic therapy:
  - Amoxicillin
  - Metronidazole
  - Omeprazole
- Eradication of the infection commonly results in long-term ulcer remission.

Gastritis

This is inflammation of the gastric mucosa.
  Types:

- Acute gastritis is caused by drugs or chemicals
  - Alcohol, histamine, digitalis and certain metabolic disorder, e.g., uraemia, can all contribute to gastritis
  - Non-steroidal anti-inflammatory drugs (NSAIDs) such as aspirin, ibuprofen also cause gastritis
  - Clinical features include
    - Abdominal discomfort
    - Epigastric tenderness
    - Bleeding
  - Usually heals spontaneously over a period of days causative drugs should be discontinued and antacids given

- Chronic gastritis associated with *Helicobacter pylori* infection, atrophy of the gastric mucosa and tends to occur in the elderly
- Autoimmune attack of the parietal cells in the stomach and an inability to secrete intrinsic factor leads to pernicious anaemia

Peptic Ulcer

These ulcers occur as a result of the secretion of acid digestive juices. They can occur in the

- Oesophagus due to reflux
- Stomach as a GU
- Duodenum as a DU

Duodenal ulcer is the most common, now known that *H. pylori* is a factor and treated medically with the eradication of *H. pylori*
Other causes:

- Smoking
- Aspirin and NSAIDs
- Alcohol
- Stress which can lead to an over secretion of hydrochloric acid in the stomach

Clinical Features

- May be similar to other acute abdominal problems
- The pain is in the epigastrium and may be intermittent
  - DU eating relives the pain and so there is no loss of appetite
  - GU eating exacerbates the pain and there is weight loss
  - DU tends to be overweight and male
- Investigations include fibre-optic endoscopy; biopsy will show presence of *H. pylori*

Treatment is Mainly Medical

- H2 antagonist e.g., ranitidine, omeprazole
- If only H2 antagonist therapy is used there is a chance of relapse, but treating with *H. pylori* infection as well will reduce relapse by 80% and improve prognosis
- Sucralfate may be used to improve mucosal protection
- Occasionally surgery may still be necessary when complications such as haemorrhage or perforation occur
- Perforation
  - More common in a DU
  - Sudden and excruciating epigastric pain that rapidly spreads through the whole abdomen

- Rigid 'board like' abdomen that is due to generalized peritonitis
- Shock may be present, with a high or low BP, rapid pulse, cold and clammy to the touch; may present as haematemesis or melaena or both

Disorders of the Lower GIT

This involves the small intestine (duodenum, jejunum and ilium), the large intestine (ascending, transverse, descending and sigmoid colon) and the rectum. These disorders disrupt one or more of its functions:

- Structural and neural abnormalities are slowed, obstruct or accelerate movement at any level.
- Inflammation and ulceration conditions disrupt secretion, motility and absorption.

The Acute Abdomen

Symptoms are of acute onset admitted via A&E with severe abdominal pain being the most severe feature. May have a life-threatening condition or simple. Common causes include

- Nonspecific pain that resolves without intervention
- Acute appendicitis
- Acute intestinal obstruction due to strangulated hernia, adhesions, occlusion
- Peptic ulcer
- Gallstones acute cholecystitis
- Acute pancreatitis
- Urinary tract infections
- Renal colic due to stones in the ureter
- Retention of urine
- Constipation
- Leaking or even ruptures abdominal aortic aneurysm
- Gynaecological emergencies such as ectopic pregnancy

Bowel Obstruction

The small intestine from the duodenum to the ileum is where most of the nutrients are absorbed here.

Causes

- Adhesions or bands from previous surgery
- Strangulated hernia
- Tumours
- Inflammatory strictures such as Crohn's disease
- Impacted faeces

- Intussusception
- Strangulation of the bowel, leading to ischaemia of the bowel and infarction, can lead to perforation

Clinical Features

- Vomiting which may be in large amounts and depending on where the obstruction is may be faecal in nature
- Abdominal pain is usually colicky and more severe in strangulation
- If obstruction is complete, there is no flatus being passed rectally
- Dehydration can occur is vomiting or diarrhoea is present
- Abdominal distension due to collection of gas; the lower the obstruction, the more the distension
- Abnormal bowel sounds, which can be exaggerated, high pitched and sometimes tinkling but completely absent in some cases

Management

- Nil by mouth IV replacement commenced
- If vomiting NGT
- Analgesia
- If impaction use of enemas or drug therapy
- Operation may be necessary to relieve the obstruction

Inflammatory Bowel Disorders

Any condition of the GIT can lead to stimulation of the IR (Fig. 4.2). The most important mediators are

- Histamine
- Prostaglandins
- The cytokines

The release of these mediators is to

- Protect the body from invading microorganisms
- Limit the extent of blood loss and injury
- Promote rapid healing of involved tissues

The mediators act as a signalling system (chemotaxis) to attract nutrients, fluids, clotting factors and neutrophils and macrophages to the damaged site. The mediators cause a localized increase in

- Capillary permeability, swelling and pain
- Vasodilatation to increase blood supply, redness and heat
- The release of interleukin 1 (IL-1) from macrophages, which causes a small rise in body temperature

These conditions include

- Ulcerative colitis
- Crohn's disease
- Diverticular disease
- Peritonitis
- Appendicitis

Ulcerative Colitis

- Chronic inflammatory disease − inflammation and ulceration of rectum and sigmoid colon
- Oedema forms and narrows the lumen of the involved colon
- Mucosal destruction causes bleeding, cramping pain, urge to defecate, diarrhoea
- Dehydration, malnutrition, steroids/analgesia
- Periods of remission, with possible surgical resection if therapy unsuccessful

Crohn's Disease

- Difficult to distinguish from ulcerative colitis
- The rectum is seldom involved and the formation of cancer rare
- Few symptoms other than IBS, then inflammation, tenderness, weight loss
- May develop pernicious anaemia, deficiencies in folic acid and vitamin D absorption, hypo-albuminaemia
- Surgery to manage complications − fistula, abscess, relief of obstruction

Diverticular Disease

- Herniations or sac-like outpouchings of mucosa through the muscle layers of the colon wall
- Asymptomatic, diverticulitis with inflammation
- Appear in weak points in the colon wall and reduce the diameter and increases pressure − can lead to rupture of the diverticula
- Can lead to abscess formation and peritonitis
- Increase in dietary fibre frequently relieves symptoms
- Surgical resection may be required

Peritonitis Inflammation of the peritoneal cavity, covering of the

- Bowel and mesentery
- Omentum

- Lining of the abdominal cavity
- Perforation of any region leads to life-threatening peritonitis

  Causes:

- Appendicitis
- Crohn's disease
- Diverticulitis
- Cholecystitis
- Salpingitis

A patient can be seriously ill with generalized peritonitis as inflammatory fluid moves into the peritoneal cavity and causes hypovolaemia and may lead to toxaemia or septicaemia. This condition is most severe when contaminated with faeces, infected bile or pus and less severe in the absence of infection. The abdomen will be rigid and tender; bowel sounds will be absent. Treatment of peritonitis will depend on the cause.

Appendicitis Inflammation of the vermiform appendix, a projection from the apex of the caecum. Common surgical emergency – affects 7%–12%.
Causes:

- Obstruction of the lumen with stool, foreign bodies, bacterial infection
- Drainage of the appendix is reduced
- Increased pressure – appendix becomes hypoxic
- Bacterial/microbial invasion
- Inflammation and oedema
- Gangrene
- Classic sign is rebound tenderness

Conditions of the Accessory Organs of GIT
Liver Failure

Liver failure refers to a reduction in the functioning of the liver. The liver has great powers of regeneration and if injured can completely recover. When the process of regeneration is inadequate cells are being regenerated and damaged at the same time. Blood vessels and biliary ducts must be replaced as well as connective tissue; fibrous tissue is laid down to form the normal liver cells known as cirrhosis. Liver failure only occurs when 75% of liver cells have died.

As cirrhosis develops the blood supply becomes disrupted and collateral circulation develops from the hepatic portal vein; back pressure occurs in the portal system around the oesophageal/gastric junction, which may burst. Fluid can accumulate to cause ascites, discomfort and respiratory embarrassment.

Functions of the Liver

- Converts glycogen, fat and protein into glucose
- Stores protein
- Breakdown of worn out red blood cells and white blood cells and some bacteria
- Renders dangerous substances harmless to the body — either breaks them down or transforms them into less harmful compounds
- Produces bile salts used in small intestine for the emulsification and absorption of fats in the body
- Stores copper, iron and vitamin A, D (involvement of the kidneys), E and K
- Produces clotting factors — heparin, prothrombin, fibrinogen and albumin
- Forms urea — removal of ammonia

Classifications of Liver Failure

- Fulminant liver failure is severe in onset, rapid in progress, also known as acute liver failure. From onset to jaundice to development of encephalopathy is around 0—8 weeks
- Sub-fulminant liver failure occurs from jaundice to encephalopathy in around 8 weeks to 6 months
- Chronic liver failure occurs over a 6-month period

Causes of Liver Failure

- Poisoning due to overdose, e.g., paracetamol
- Drug-induced, e.g., isoniazid, sodium valproate, antidepressants, NSAIDs
- Viral hepatitis
- Miscellaneous, e.g., Wilson's disease, Weil's disease, Reye's syndrome

  Liver disease can also occur in

- Herpes simplex
- Varicella zoster
- Measles
- Rubella
- Coxsackie B virus infection
- Adenovirus infection

Clinical Features

- Varices — as pressure increases in the portal veins small veins in oesophagus and rectum vasodilate to equalize pressure. The increased pressure shunts blood, and the vessels get wider and if too large may rupture:
  - 70% of patients with liver cirrhosis will develop varices

- Cause of life-threatening haematemesis when they rupture
- Painless but extremely frightening for patient and relatives
- Encephalopathy occurs when amino acids burned for energy leave behind toxic nitrogenous waste (ammonia), generally converted to urea by the liver, while other organs cope the brain deteriorates (grades 1–5, Table 4.11)
- Jaundice urine testing is an early diagnostic method, as bilirubin will be present in urine
- Respiratory failure generally relates to coma grades 2–3 (Table 2.3), hyperventilation and respiratory arrest. Ascites makes lung expansion difficult
- Bleeding clotting factors are not being produced by the liver; bruising may be visible
- Renal failure 60% of patients with fulminant hepatic liver failure go into renal failure due to episodes of reduced BP and excretion of ammonia in urine damaging the renal tubules (converted into urea by the liver). Renal failure due to liver failure is often referred to as and hepatorenal syndrome
- Metabolic disturbances is whereby ammonia, which is acidotic to the body contributes to a metabolic acidosis; abnormal metabolism of glucose due to reduced vitamin intake of thiamine (B_1), riboflavin (B_2) and pyridoxine (B_6)
- Impaired drug metabolism in liver failure as drugs can act as double doses as they cannot be converted into harmless substances by the liver quickly; reduced enzymes that render some drugs harmless
- Ascites is often seen in chronic liver failure
- Portal hypertension is due to obstruction and liver cirrhosis

Blood Tests

- Serum bilirubin
  - Unconjugated
  - Conjugated
- Enzyme levels
  - Transaminases
    - Alanine
    - Aminotransferase (ALT)
  - Aspartate transaminase (AST)
  - Alkaline phosphatase (ALP)
  - γ-glutamyltransferase (GGT)
- Serum proteins
  - Clotting factors, coagulation screen
    - Prothrombin time
    - Vitamin K levels
  - Serum albumin
  - Serum immunoglobulins

- Transport proteins
- Full blood count

Complications

- Portal hypertension
- Ascites an accumulation of fluid in the peritoneal cavity and changes in capillary dynamics
- Hepatorenal syndrome whereby ammonia is excreted as the liver cannot convert ammonia to urea
- Jaundice occurs due to hyper-bilirubinaemia as the liver fails to make bile
- Hepatic encephalopathy leading to forgetfulness, drowsy, night and day reversal, semi-consciousness, coma, irreversible brain swelling

Hepatitis

The different types of hepatitis include

- Obstructive
- Drug induced
- Infectious: an acute viral hepatitis is a common and sometimes serious infection of the liver − there are five subgroups:

    A − enteric, faecal oral transmission incubation is about 28 days, usually sudden onset

    B − blood and sexual high-risk groups, incubation is 70 days, insidious onset

    C − 'delta agent' blood-borne transfusion

    D − parenteral transmission usually intravenous drug users and those who already have the hepatitis B virus

    E − enterically transmitted, non-A and non-B

Many other viruses affect the liver and cause hepatitis:

- Yellow fever virus
- Epstein-Barr virus (EBV)
- CMV

Investigations:

- Liver function tests (see Section 2)
- Pulmonary artery pressure measurement
- ICP monitoring
- Blood glucose level
- Liver biopsy
- Arterial blood gases
- Coagulation studies
- EEG

Patients with jaundice should always be assumed to represent a high risk for transmission of hepatitis.

Gallstones

- The gall bladder is a muscular sac that stores and concentrates bile, made in the liver
- It emulsifies fats prior to their digestion by lipase enzymes
- If bile does not arrive in the duodenum:
  - Fats are not digested or absorbed
  - Loose, foul-smelling, fatty stools are passed (steatorrhoea)
  - This leads to a lack of absorption of the fat-soluble vitamins (A, D, E and K)
  - Lack of vitamin K leads to inadequate synthesis of prothrombin and problems with blood clotting
- Most gallstones are cholesterol mixed with bile pigments and calcium salts
- Some are pure cholesterol
- Women are more affected four times as often than men

Clinical Features

- Most often the patient presents with pain in the epigastrium or the right hypochondria. It is often not severe or well defined
- May present with jaundice, if the gallstone passes into and blocks the common bile duct, thus obstructing the flow of bile into the duodenum
- Transient obstruction of the gall bladder by a stone may cause episodes of severe pain called biliary colic and can be accompanied with nausea and vomiting
- The obstruction may cause inflammation of the gall bladder called cholecystitis and in its acute form is a common cause of attendance to A&E

Investigations

- Ultrasound
- Gall bladder function can be determined by an oral cholecystogram
- Endoscopic retrograde cholangiopancreatography (ERCP)
- Small gallstones can be removed by slitting the sphincter at the lower end and using a balloon catheter to retrieve them
- Percutaneous cholangiography is used if ERCP is not available or unsuccessful

Treatment

- Cholecystectomy
- A low-fat diet is prescribed

Pancreatitis

Aetiology

- Alcohol, biliary disease, trauma, metabolic abnormalities, infection drugs etc.
- Initiating process
  - Spontaneous, obstruction, bile, reflux, duodenal reflux (oedema, vascular damage, rupture of pancreatic ducts)
- Activation of enzymes
- Auto-digestion
- Necrosis

Diagnosis Is difficult due to differential diagnosis:

- Pain
- Tenderness over the abdomen
- Reduced bowel sounds
- Abdominal distension
- Nausea/vomiting
- Pyrexia
- Hypotension
- Blue-brown discoloration of limbs (Grey Turner's sign) a late sign of pancreatitis

Complications

- Starvation/malnutrition
- Absorptive and post-absorptive states
- Absorptive state — process of eating/digestion
- Post-absorptive state — fasting no more than 12 hours:
- Glycogenolysis in the liver
- Glycogenolysis in skeletal muscles
- Lipolysis in adipose tissues and the liver
- Catabolism of cellular protein

4.8 IMMUNOLOGICAL

Human Immunodeficiency Virus/Acquired Immunodeficiency Syndrome

The Virus

- First reported in 1981
- Retrovirus — at least two types:
  - HIV-1 is less pathogenic, patients stay healthy and live longer than those with HIV-2
  - HIV-2: an HIV-1 mutation and differs genetically from HIV-1, a more virulent strain
- Only survives in living host cells, dying quickly once outside the body; it cannot survive on inanimate surfaces

Pathogenesis

- A versatile virus, it does not immediately initiate an immune response
  - Surrounds itself by a protein shell and is not recognized by the host's immune system
  - Attaches itself to the receptor of certain T-cells
  - Implants itself, replicates in antibody cells
  - Eventually reduces the effectiveness of the whole immune system
- Main receptor is CD4 (T-helper cells), expressed on most T lymphocytes
- Virus attaches via its surface proteins (gp120) on the surface of the T-cell
- CD4 plays a major role in establishing an immune response
- Destruction of CD4 cells occurs

Clinical Features

- Incubation 2—4 weeks following infection
- Initially there are no clinical signs; there might be some nonspecific illness 6—8 weeks after exposure:
  - Fever
  - Arthralgia
  - Myalgia, lethargy
  - Lymphadenopathy
  - Sore throat
  - Mucosal ulcers
  - Faint pink rash

HAART — Highly Active Antiretroviral Therapy

- Combinations of drugs that act against reverse transcriptase and protease enzymes
- Effective in controlling HIV replication
- May show marked improvement in 4—8 weeks
- Full improvement takes about 6 months
- Involves multiple drugs that have to be taken at the same time every day
- Psychological effects can be great for the patient, but compliance is generally good

Effects of HIV

- Neurological disease
- Eye disease
- Mucocutaneous manifestations
- Haematological complications
- Gastrointestinal effects
- Renal complications
- Respiratory complications
- Endocrine complications

Autoimmune Disease

- The response of the immune system against self, protected by self-tolerance
- Affects about 5%—7% of the population
- May be
  - Organ-specific
  - Systemic

Organ-Specific

- Immune response is directed to a target antigen unique to a single organ or gland.
- Manifestations limited to that organ.
- Organ may be subjected to direct cellular damage or may be stimulated or blocked by antibodies.
- Lymphocytes or antibodies bind to cell membrane antigen causing lysis and/or an IR.
- The cellular structure of the organ is replaced by connective tissue and the organ function declines.

Organ-specific diseases include

- Addison's disease — adrenal glands
- Haemolytic anaemia — red blood cells membrane protein
- Graves' disease — thyroid hormone; TSH over-stimulation of the thyroid gland
- Hashimoto's thyroiditis — thyroid proteins; uptake of iodine reduced production of thyroid hormones
- Type 1 diabetes — pancreatic β-cells
- Myasthenia gravis — ACh receptors
- Pernicious anaemia — gastric parietal cells

Systemic Autoimmune Diseases

- The response is directed towards a large number of target antigens and involves a number of organs and tissues
- A defect in immune regulation which results in hyperactive T and B cells
- Tissue damage is widespread both from cell-mediated immune responses and from direct cellular damage caused by auto-antibodies
- Systemic autoimmune diseases include
  - Ankylosing spondylitis — vertebrae
  - Multiple sclerosis — white matter in CNS
  - Rheumatoid arthritis — connective tissue immunoglobulin (Ig)G
  - Systemic lupus erythematosus (SLE) — DNA, nuclear protein, RBC and platelet membranes. The response is directed towards a large number of target antigens and involves a number of organs and tissues

Treatment

- Aimed at reducing the autoimmune response but leaving the rest of the immune system intact
- Current therapies palliative
- Reduce symptoms: reasonable quality of life
- Immunosuppressive drugs to slow down proliferation of lymphocytes
- Increased risk of infection and cancer
- Removal of thymus for myasthenia gravis
- Plasmapheresis may help some patients

Hypersensitivity

Cytotoxic Hypersensitivity

This type of hypersensitivity involves IgM or IgG antibodies directed against antigens on the surface of the body's own cells. Antibodies bring about the destruction of the cells in the same way as foreign bacteria are destroyed.

Mechanisms of Cytotoxic Hypersensitivity

Once the antibody has bound to the surface of a cell there are three ways the cell can be damaged:

- Phagocytosis — antibodies bind to the surface of the cell engage with Fc receptors on phagocytic cells, facilitated by complement.
- Direct lysis of the cell coated with antibody.
- Extracellular killing — due to the activation of phagocytosis, neutrophils and macrophages release mediators or cytokines that brings about lysis and death of the target cell.

Types of Cytotoxic Hypersensitivity

- Haemolytic disease of the newborn: the mother is Rh^2 and baby is Rh^1
- Reactions to drugs
- Haemolytic anaemia following penicillin (uncommon)
- Reactions to tissue antigens
  - Thyroid and endocrine tissues — antibodies directed against cells and molecules of a gland leading to damage or destruction
    - diabetes — antibodies to the insulin-producing islet cells
  - Basement membranes — antibodies against the kidney (nephritis) affecting filtration capacity of the kidney
  - Myasthenia gravis — antibodies deposited in the neuromuscular junction

Immune Complex Hypersensitivity

- When antigen combines with antibody in the body, immune complexes are formed
- These immune complexes can be eliminated through phagocytosis and macrophages
- The reaction can become exaggerated and lead to a tissue-damaging IR
- When localized in a particular tissue the response is called an Arthus reaction
- When spread throughout the body it is called serum sickness
- The formation of immune complexes is a natural and protective process
- Occurs only when the body is exposed to an excess of an antigen over a long period of time, e.g.,
  - Microbial organism
  - Foreign antigen
  - Autoimmunity to the body's own tissues

Mechanisms of Immune Complex Hypersensitivity

- When a large number of immune complexes are formed the phagocytes become overloaded leading to
  - Prolonged circulation of the complexes
  - Deposited at vulnerable sites, e.g., the glomerulus of the kidney
- Immune complexes trigger a variety of inflammatory processes
  - Degranulation of mast cells
  - Interaction with platelets to form a clot or thrombus
- Arthus reaction occurs in a variety of occupational lung diseases; the antigens are different but the mechanisms are the same:
  - Farmer's lung
  - Pigeon fancier's disease
  - Maple bark stripper's lung
  - Cheese washer's disease
  - Furrier's lung
- Allergic bronchopulmonary aspergillosis − a mixture of hypersensitivity and allergic reactions:
  - IgE-dependent allergic (type I)
  - An immune complex (type III)
- Serum sickness
  - Reaction like serum sickness can occur with some antibiotics
  - Immune complex glomerulonephritis following infection with certain strains of streptococci, malaria, chronic hepatitis B infections
  - Can also occur in systemic lupus erythematosus (SLE)
    - It may be because SLE is triggered by an infection of some sort

Delayed-Type Hypersensitivity

- This type of hypersensitivity is not mediated by antibodies
- Mediated by T-cells alone, and these initiate tissue damage
- The reactions are slow, may take up to 10 years to develop
- There are three types:
  - Contact hypersensitivity
  - Tuberculin reactions
  - Granulomatous reactions
- Contact dermatitis and eczema; the most common agents are
  - Nickel
  - Chromate (in cement)
  - Hair dyes (*p*-phenylene diamine)
  - Poison ivy and oak
- Tuberculin-type
  - Tuberculosis sufferers and immunized patients have T-cells that recognize tuberculin

- If tuberculin injected into the skin, T cells migrate to the site of injection
- Granulomatous hypersensitivity
  - Tuberculosis:
    - Immunological granulomas thought to be a physiological response to wall off the site of persistent infection
    - Can occur throughout the body wherever mycobacteria exist and not just in the lungs
  - Leprosy:
    - Granulomatous skin lesions observed in leprosy
    - Dependent on CD4 and CD8 cells which make different cytokines, e.g., IL-2, IL-4 and IL-10
    - The major cause of nerve destruction in this disease is the process of inflammation and cell infiltration

Hypersensitivities vary from

- Life-threatening and can be fatal (asthma, anaphylaxis)
- Degenerative, leading to severe debilitation, poor quality of life and may lead to death following a number of years coping with a particular disease/illness (autoimmune disease)
- An inconvenience and uncomfortable feelings of itching and upper respiratory swelling (eczema, hay fever)
- It can be due to occupational disease which can lead to chronic diseases/illness of the lungs (farmer's lung)
- It can mean that an injection or treatment is required that prevents the occurrence of the consequences (anti-D).

The broad focus of allergy and hypersensitivity denotes a variety of understanding and knowledge regarding its presentation, progress, mortality/morbidity and ultimately the interventions and treatments required.

The critical care nurse is at the forefront of caring for patients with these conditions and as they vary from being fatal to just an inconvenience a broad range of skills are needed.

4.9 BURNS

Severe burns lead to devastating physical and psychological effects. There is a massive loss of fluid from the circulatory system, due to tissue injury stimulating the IR. Therapy ranges from initial resuscitation to eventual surgery and rehabilitation. Burns patients are rarely seen in critical care areas as they are most effectively treated by specially trained staff in an isolated environment controlled in temperature and humidity.

Burns affect the

- Cardiovascular system through loss of circulating fluid volume by a combination of hypovolaemic and cellular shock

- Respiratory system leading to dysfunction due to
  - Airway injury
  - Lung injury
  - Cellular injury
- Inflammatory process – leading to the release of mediators
- Metabolism due to nitrogen loss
- Immune system response – the damaged tissue is easily colonized by bacteria
- Renal system – failure may occur due to renal hypoperfusion; if this occurs it is associated with a high mortality
- Gastrointestinal tract – stress ulcers can occur
- Psychological stability of the patient due to pain, severe illness, surgery, disfigurement, loss of independence and necessity for long-term care

The rule of nines to estimate body surface area burns in adults:

- Head – 9%
- Front and back – 18%
- Arms – 9% each
- Legs – 18% each
- Genital area – 1%

The Classification of Burns

Generally refers to the depth of the burn:

1. Superficial dermal wound (first-degree burn) only involves the epithelial layer, very painful, resolves within 2 weeks with no scarring.
2. Deep dermal wound (second-degree burn) involves epithelium and a varying degree of dermis; some scarring, healing is slow.
3. Full-thickness burns (third-degree burns) leads to scarring and contractures; wound closure by grafting.

The greater the body surface burned the greater the fluid loss. Fluid losses are caused by an increase in capillary permeability that persists for 24 hours after burn injury; because of this, fluid resuscitation is needed by intravenous infusion to restore the circulatory blood volume.

There are various recognized treatment options; here are just two:

1. The Muir and Barclay plan
   a. The first 24-hour period is divided into three 4-hour intervals followed by two 6-hour intervals.
   b. Albumin is the replacement choice in this regimen and is given at strength of 4.5%.
   c. The amount to be administered in each time interval is determined by formula 0.55 mL/kg/% total body surface area (TBSA) of burn.

2. The Parkland's plan
    a. This uses Hartmann's solution as the fluid of choice.
    b. The first 24-hour period is divided as follows:
        i. Half of the calculated amount is given in the first 8 hours and the remainder over the following 16 hours
        ii. The formula used to calculate the volume for the 24-hour period is 4 mL/kg/% TBSA of burns

The two fluids used have different properties: the Muir and Barclay plan uses albumin, which is a colloid and because of this stays in the body longer due to the increase in colloid oncotic pressure; the Parkland plan uses a crystalloid − a clear fluid with sodium chloride and other electrolytes. The colloid solution is administered more slowly, and a smaller amount is required.

The main physiological problems are

- Fluid output: which can be lost as fast as it is infused
- Pain: analgesia would be required depending on whether burns are first, second or third degree
- Risk of infection: antibiotics would be needed
- Input and output measure
- There is a massive water loss and flux of large amounts of fluids and electrolytes in the body tissues which manifests as oedema and circulatory hypovolaemia.

Rapid fluid replacement is paramount in burn patients.

Monitoring should include

- Temperature, pulse, respiration and BP
- Oxygen saturation
- Urine output
- CVP
- Blood tests − arterial blood gases
- Weight if possible.

Therapeutic intervention to sustain life is required urgently; the main three elements are

- Meticulous wound management
- Adequate fluid and nutrition
- Early surgical excision and grafting

Electrocution

Patients suffering from electrocution and associated burns occasionally require critical care intervention.

Considerations:

- For a current flow the body must complete a circuit
- Generally from sources to ground through the body
- The physiological effects depend on the
  - Size of the current
  - Duration of the current
  - Tissue traversed by the current
- Most cases of electrocution occur in the workplace (60%) or at home (30%).

Types of injury:

- The injury is generally burns to the skin and internal tissues and organs
- Depolarization of muscle cells leading to
  - Cardiac asystole if current is of significant strength
  - VF and other arrhythmias
  - MI has been reported
  - Tetanic contractions, which can lead to long bone fractures
- Vascular injuries – thrombosis or occluded blood vessels causing ischaemia and necrosis
- Neurological injuries – central or peripheral, spinal cord injuries, unconsciousness
- Renal failure – muscle necrosis
- Other injuries
  - May lead to falls or involve being thrown some distance from where the shock occurred
  - Clothing may catch fire
  - Rupture of the eardrum

Management:

- First aid and resuscitation
- Investigations – ECG, echocardiography, CT, EEG, X-ray of the spine and long bones, haemoglobin, serum electrolytes, creatine kinase and urine myoglobin
- Critical care management – burns, ischaemic and necrotic tissue and injured organs, fasciotomies and amputations

4.10 POISONING/OVERDOSE

Poisoning or overdose is frequently intentional, either accidental or deliberate or may result from criminal intent. Specific antidotes are available for only a very few poisons or drugs. Many patients will recover with supportive care.

Priority Poisons

- Paracetamol — Acetylcysteine is the antidote
- Benzodiazepines — Flumazenil is the antidote
- Narcotic drugs — Naloxone is the antidote
- Carbon monoxide
- Methanol
- Ethylene glycol
- Cyanide and paraquat are dangerous poisons

Paracetamol overdose can lead to liver failure.

Diagnosis

- The time to diagnosis is imperative; limiting the period from ingestion to supportive treatment is important
- Always considered in the unconscious patient
- Consult relatives, friends, general practitioners and pharmacists who may provide valuable information
- Administration of thiamine and glucose should be considered

Assessment and Resuscitation

- Airway and ventilation
- Haemodynamic status
- Conscious level and neurological signs
- Body temperature
- Body surface — head or body injury, venepuncture marks
- Investigations:
  - Urinalysis
  - Chest X-ray
  - Electrolytes and creatinine

- Osmolality − may indicate ethanol, methanol or ethylene glycol poisoning
- ABC analysis
- Drug levels, e.g., paracetamol and paraquat

Drug Manipulation

- Decrease absorption by the administration of
  - Emetics − ipecacuanha
  - Gastric lavage uncommonly used
  - Absorbent − activated charcoal (Carbomix, Medicoal)
  - Cathartics − magnesium citrate/hydroxide, magnesium sulphate (milk of magnesia), sorbitol (Sorbilax)
- Increased excretion
  - Forced diuresis − diuretics
  - Alkalosis − hyperventilation and/or sodium bicarbonate
  - Increasing the acid of urine may increase the elimination of phencyclidine and amphetamines
  - Extracorporeal techniques, e.g., haemodialysis
- Administration of specific overdose antidote:
  - Paracetamol − acetylcysteine, methionine (Parvolex)
  - Anticholinesterase − atropine
  - Narcotic − naloxone (Narcan)
  - Benzodiazepine − flumazenil (Anexate)
  - Heparin − protamine sulphate
  - Digoxin − anti-digoxin antibodies (Digibind), atropine, phenytoin (epanutin)
  - Warfarin − vitamin K_1

Continued Supportive Therapy

- Care of the unconscious patient.
- Vital functions are monitored and recorded.
- Organ function is supported where possible.
- The patient is rewarmed using humidified gases, space blankets and warmed infusion fluids.
- Antibiotics are started if aspiration has occurred.
- Fluid and electrolytes and nutritional support are maintained.

Common Side Effects Seen in Drug Overdose

On occasions when the drug taken or the dose is unknown and management of care is related to symptom management (Richards, 2009):

- Coma often seen in CNS depressant drugs.
- Convulsions due to CNS stimulation.
- Respiratory symptoms such as cough, cyanosis, hypoventilation, hyperventilation and pulmonary oedema.
- Cardiovascular symptoms such as tachycardia, bradycardia, dysrhythmias, hypotension, hypertension.
- Pupil changes small pinpoint is usually a sign of opioid overdose, dilated suggest other drugs.
- Body temperature hypothermia, hyperthermia.

Section 5

Psychological and ethical care

Section Outline

5.1 MENTAL EFFECTS OF CRITICAL CARE

The psychological needs of critical care patients are frequently overlooked as a great deal of time, and effort is allocated towards caring for the critically ill patient's physical needs. Although the physical aspect of critical care nursing is paramount, there is also a psychological dimension to critical care, which also needs to be discussed and understood.

Sensory Imbalance

Sensory imbalance occurs when the level of sensory stimuli received by the individual is either too great or too minimal to be recognized. Illness can replace familiar bodily responses with ones that are alien to the patient. There is then potential for the patient to interpret these responses incorrectly. In critical care, a patient's sensory balance becomes destabilized and, therefore vulnerable due to many and varied external stimuli.

Sensory imbalance involves a fluctuating state of consciousness that may be characterized by many factors (Table 5.1). An increase in sensory input, or when certain stimuli are above normal in amount, can lead to sensory overload and can contribute to sleep deprivation. Sensory deprivation is associated with the absence or decrease of normal stimuli, poor quality stimuli resulting in reduction in a patient's well-being.

Sensory Overload

Sensory overload occurs when a person receives multiple stimuli more than the brain can sort through and process. The input into the five senses cannot perceptually be disregarded or selectively ignored. Excessive sensory stimulation prevents the brain from appropriately responding to, or ignoring, certain stimuli. In critical care environments, this might include:

TABLE 5.1 Factors that influence fluctuating state of consciousness.

Environment	• Noise • Lighting • Unfamiliar sounds and noises • Constant disturbances • Impaired day and night rhythms • Isolation and confinement • Loss of familiar contact, for example, family
Communication	• Social isolation • Inappropriate touch • Conversation around or at end of bed • Reduced contact or stimuli
Medical and nursing interventions	• Medication • Constant/regular taking of observations • Turning and washing • Suctioning • Physiotherapy • Renewing dressings • Taking bloods
Physical condition	• Alcohol/drug addiction • Previous cerebral damage • Increasing age • Underlying chronic pathology • Altered conscious state • deranged acid–base balance • Hypoxia • Sleep deprivation

- Multiple conversations going on at the same time, staff talking
- Flashing overhead or bright lights
- Loud noises such as machines or alarms constantly going off or the bleeping of pumps
- Telephones ringing, the constant use of suctioning and the constant hum of the equipment

However, the majority of these noises are vital to caring for a patient on critical care.

Noise is considered to be an important factor in causing sensory overload. Consultants, doctors, anaesthetists, physiotherapists, electrocardiogram (ECG) technicians, visitors and nursing staff create a potential source of noise and disturbance to the patient. Noise can give patients extra anxiety, that is, alarms going off and patients thinking that they are in trouble, and constant noise can prevent patients from sleeping.

The recorded noise levels in a busy critical care setting averaged 70 dB during the day and 65 dB at night. The international noise council recommends an upper limit of 45 dB during the daytime and 20 dB overnight. Much of the noise in a critical care setting may be described as 'white noise', for example, a constant hum, which comes from equipment.

Due to the amount of stimuli leading to overload, the person may no longer perceive the surrounding stimuli in a way that makes sense, which can lead to serious complications (Table 5.2).

However, there are noises, which can be viewed as less vital, and these should be decreased with particular consideration for the patient's presence taken into account. Increased staff awareness could encourage a more sensitive and welcoming environment.

Ensure that noise is kept to a minimum in the critical care environment.

Sensory Deprivation

The normal conscious state requires a minimum level of sensory stimulation and/or variation in type of stimuli received. The normal type of sensations received by the reticular activating system would include auditory, visual, olfactory, tactile and kinaesthetic stimuli, that is, stimuli that relate to the position of joints in space and the degree of contraction of muscles.

When normal healthy individuals are deprived of all sensory input, that is, auditory, visual and touch, there is a detrimental effect on the individual's functionality (Wung et al., 2018). Some individuals become bored, restless, irritable and emotionally upset. Visual hallucinations, poor concentration and problem-solving difficulties also result from sensory deprivation.

Sleep Deprivation

The unfamiliar environment of critical care may be further compounded by a patient's altered conscious state, acid balance, hypoxia and sleep deprivation. The lack of sleep experienced by critical care patients has the potential to slow recovery and reduce patient's attention during postoperative teaching or respiratory weaning. These factors further highlight the importance of allowing patients to sleep for periods of at least 2 hour to complete all sleep cycles before nursing interventions are carried out. Other factors that can lead to sleep deprivation are sedation and analgesia, stress and technology.

Sedation and analgesia are administered to patients in critical care and are essential parts of modern treatment. This is because many interventions are

TABLE 5.2 Complications of sensory imbalance.

Sensory imbalance	Cause	Outcomes
Sensory overload	Increased noise level: • Phones ringing • Monitor alarms • Toilets flushing • Hand-washing • Conversation Unfamiliar sounds from infusion pumps, respirators and suction equipment Physical discomfort due to limitations of bed rest Loss of privacy due to removal of clothes and feared loss of belongings Stressful environment Uninvited touch Constant lighting	Restlessness Total body discomfort Agitation Loneliness Isolation Increased awareness of the noise level Loss of control over self and environment Poor perception of surrounding stimuli Sweating hands Numbness Fidgetiness Tachycardia
Sleep deprivation	Increased noise level and interruptions leading to: • taking longer to fall asleep • less time sleeping • more awakenings	Slow recovery Reduced patient attention Mood changes Depression Personality disorders Analgesia preparation Fear Restlessness Anxiety Fatigue Confusion Illusions Delirium Hallucinations Disorientation
Sensory deprivation	A reduction in the amount and variety of stimuli Perceptual deprivation – no variation in stimuli Isolation – physical or social Confinement – immobilization or restriction of movement Increased sensory input (sensory overload)	Problem-solving difficulties Boredom Restlessness Irritability Emotional upset Visual hallucinations Reduced concentration

uncomfortable, distressing and frequently painful, and lying in a fixed position for prolonged periods of time may lead to backache and muscular discomfort. Using sedation and various analgesic preparations can also lead to sleep deprivation, and efforts should be made to promote natural sleep. It is important, therefore, when using sedation to concentrate on the adequacy of sedation and analgesia and also to ensure that the patient is getting sufficient rapid eye movement (REM) sleep. Talbot et al. (2010) reported that sleep deprivation can lead to increased anxiety, negative moods and fatigue.

Within the critical care setting, patients undergo many events that may be perceived as being stressful. All critically ill patients are generally stressed to a greater or lesser degree during their time in critical care, recognizing that each person has their own limit to what they can tolerate. In most cases, the critical care setting involves incidences and environments, which the individual is not familiar with, contributing towards the stress and sleep deprivation. The effects of long-term sleep deprivation contribute to patients not understanding the procedures that have been explained to them contributing to threatening worry (Talbot et al., 2010). Thus, it is not only the unfamiliar environment and events that cause stress and sleep deprivation in patients in critical care settings, but the pain, medical conditions and alterations in social behaviour can become threatening leading to fear of what the patients might experience next.

Promoting Rest and Sleep

Sleep can be defined as an altered state of consciousness from which a person can be aroused by stimuli of sufficient magnitude. The function of sleep is far from clear. It is considered as restorative and energy conserving, as protein synthesis and cell division occur for the renewal of tissues, which takes place predominantly during the time devoted to rest and sleep. More importantly, sleep is needed to avoid the psychological problems resulting from inadequate sleep. Perpetual awakening and sleep interruption have been associated with increased anxiety, irritability and disorientation, which may have a negative influence on recovery. In addition, total sleep deprivation for 48 hour can result in changes such as:

- Aching muscles
- Confusion, disorientation
- Memory lapse or loss and development of false memory
- Depression
- Hallucinations during falling asleep and waking
- Headaches
- Malaise and lethargy
- Periorbital puffiness, minor visual misperceptions
- Reductions in motivation and willingness to perform tasks, which could include mobilisation and other aspects of care
- Increased blood pressure, stress hormones and risk of diabetes
- Reduction in immune response and increased susceptibility to illness
- Irritability

- Violent behaviour suspiciousness
- Slurred speech
- Later on, delusions and paranoia manifestations

All of which may hinder recovery. If the function of sleep is correctly assumed, then sleep deprivation could be considered as an added stressor, over and above those physical and emotional traumas already suffered.

Critical care nurses should use their knowledge of:

- The patient's normal sleeping patterns;
- Supportive family relationships to optimize environment for sleep and
- Analgesic and sedative administration, according to the patient's felt need and monitor events thereafter to promote sleep and rest.

Sound levels in a critical care setting impact negatively on the subjective quality of sleep. This is due to the fact that an individual does not enter the REM stage until 90 minute after the sleep begins, and therefore if awakening occurs before the 90 minute, they do not enter REM sleep. Furthermore, critical illness and major surgery can disturb sleep but exogenous factors, including noise and nursing interventions, can also disturb sleep.

During an average night's sleep, individuals pass through four or five sleep cycles, each cycle lasting about 90–100 minute. Within the sleep cycle, five successive stages have been defined by their distinctive characteristics. The first four stages of sleep are collectively named non-REM sleep and demonstrate a progressive increase in the depth of sleep. The final stage is called REM sleep, or paradoxical sleep, and is associated with dreaming, learning and memory.

Strategies that minimize sleep interruptions in critically ill patients are as follows:

- Turning off/down number of lights, especially at night
- Keeping noise levels to minimum, for example, switch off suction equipment
- Offering earplugs to protect patients from sensory overload
- Reassessing the need and value of continually interrupting patient's sleep to perform observations and care
- Centralizing of nursing duties so as to minimize touch and stimuli
- Charting amount of uninterrupted sleep time per shift as evidence of stages of sleep
- Communicating the patient's need to sleep to other health care professionals

Recommendations for minimizing patient's sleep interruptions are listed in Table 5.3.

TABLE 5.3 Minimizing sleep interruptions in patients.

- Turn off maximum number of lights especially at night
- Keep noise to a minimum (switch of suction equipment, reduce talking and whispering)
- Offer cotton wool balls for patient's ears
- Continually reassess the need to interrupt patient's sleep to perform observations
- Perform as many nursing observations as possible together
- Chart amount of uninterrupted sleep per shift and evidence of sleep stages
- Communicate the patient's need to sleep to other professionals
- Use knowledge of:
  - Patient's normal sleeping patterns
  - Supportive family relationships
  To optimize environment for sleep
- Administer analgesics and sedatives according to the patient's felt need and monitor events

Intensive Care Unit Syndrome

Interestingly, any single cause of sensory alteration, such as sensory overload, sleep and sensory deprivation, or any combination of these, may lead to the general condition referred to as intensive care unit (ICU) syndrome. It is believed that a significant proportion of critically ill patients between 15% and 80% will suffer from it. ICU syndrome is associated with poor patient outcomes, increased length of stay and impacts on morbidity and mortality. However, the processes, which lead to ICU syndrome, do incorporate additional factors:

- Multisystem illnesses — haemodynamic instability
- Patient/ventilator disharmony
- Alcohol/drug abuse
- Advancing age
- Medication — drug side effects, withdrawal
- Acidosis
- Hypoxaemia
- Pain
- Severe infection
- Frustration
- Immobilisation
- Cerebral illness, dementia, stroke

These are the effects of ICU syndrome that patients often remember or perceive their experiences in critical care as both torturous and inhumane. Amnesty International supports this view, and their literature clearly outlines some psychological torture techniques, including:

- Sensory and sleep deprivation
- Enforced stimuli — for example, noise or light

- Deprived people of food
- Psychotropic and paralysing drugs
- Immobility
- Isolation
- Reduced and forced communication
- Re-regulation of the biological clock by changing routines

Although patients receiving critical care experience similar interventions to those mentioned above, it is proposed that essential and specialized critical care nursing skills can prevent the development of ICU syndrome. Furthermore, the move towards prevention is imperative, as even though short-term effects of ICU syndrome — such as hallucinations, disorientation and tachycardia — are transient, they are nevertheless disturbing and prolonged with lasting psychological effects.

In comparison, long-term effects can delay recovery, lead to depression and, in some instances, develop personality changes. Therefore, essential nursing skills are crucial in reducing the incidence of ICU syndrome:

- Recognize the signs of sensory overload, sensory deprivation and sleep deprivation
- Continued reorientation, distraction, reduction on stimuli
- Minimize the contributing factors — maintenance of a normal sleep/wake cycle
- Therapeutic stimulation
- Consider psychiatric consultation
- Patient safety
- Medical management

Consideration of these psychological aspects should play a part in everyday nursing care of every critically ill patient.

Reducing Mental Effects of Critical Care

Changes in psychological well-being can have deleterious effects on the patient's physiological stability. Thus, all efforts need to be taken by the critical care nurse to reduce the mental effects.

Communicating With Patients

Communication strategies can either be verbal, non-verbal, conscious or unconscious. Nevertheless, they all play an important role in ensuring that the critically ill patient's psychological needs are met and addressed within the stressful critical care environment. Regardless of the communication strategy, adopted communication is an essential activity of living, which is as important as physical support and care. Patients often experience dissatisfaction with the level and mode of communication during their hospital stay; this is associated with the quality and amount of information received and with insufficient, confusing and contradictory information being disseminated by different health care professionals.

By giving information verbally, health care professionals can speed up recovery and reduce the number of complications and the need for continued pain relief. Furthermore, within the critical care setting, the development of verbal skills, the giving of information and additional use of listening skills are insufficient on their own to minimize patient dissatisfaction. In order to increase proficiency at monitoring and interpreting non-verbal cues from physically dependent patients who are unable to communicate verbally − due to speech loss brought on by the patients' condition or intubation or factors affecting speech, such as breathlessness, pain or stroke − health care professionals need to focus upon their communication strategies and work towards enhancing any shortfalls they may be experiencing.

Non-verbal communication is the term used to describe all forms of human communication not controlled by speech and can be used therapeutically by health care professionals. The non-verbal component of communication is five times more influential than the verbal aspect. In addition, stress can be actively reduced, using relaxation and soothing techniques, and caring can be conveyed through touch and sensitivity. Touch is an important means by which the giving and gathering of information can be achieved, but significant consideration should be given to the fact that people are individuals, so interpretation of tactile communication will differ from person to person. This mode of communication must therefore be assessed on an individual basis, and it must be decided whether this is the appropriate mode − hence, the nurses' demonstration of sensitivity is essential.

The communication process comprises five elements:

1. The sender or encoder of the message
2. The message itself
3. The receiver or decoder of the message
4. Feedback that the receiver conveys to the sender
5. The environment in which the message is transmitted

When planning to meet patient's communication needs, there are six classical essential areas:

1. Orientation to the time, day, date, place, people, environment and procedures
2. Specific patient teaching on any aspect of care
3. Adopting methods to overcome patient's sensory deficits
4. Comforting patients who are confused or hallucinating
5. Communication, which maintains the patient's personal identity
6. Helping the communications of voiceless patients

Always check the patient's hearing, speech and vision to determine what it was like prior to critical care admission.

It is important to remember that the critically ill patient medications may interfere with their ability to process and store information, and they may not remember the information given through verbal communication. In addition, the patient may be unable to assign meaning to or organize the information at the time of exposure to it. This may lead to confusion and lack of memory with regard to the occurring event.

Barriers to and interference with communication can occur at any point in the communication process. A summary of potential problems relating to the patient's reception of messages from the nurse the critical care setting is provided in Table 5.4.

Effective Communication

The critical care setting can dehumanize the individual patient experiencing hospital stay.

The Nurse and Other HCP

A great deal of importance is placed on the health care professional's role in treating the patient as a person and not as an appendage to a machine. This can be achieved using the necessary communication skills so that the critically ill patient's overall care and treatment are achieved. It is important to note that communication can make a major contribution to the patient's emotional stability while in a critical care setting.

A personalized approach to care supports the notion that patients should not lose touch with the outside world by suggesting that patients should be addressed by their preferred name, and conversation should mimic their normal conversation so that an environment, similar to their own, is closely resembled and experienced.

The importance of health care professionals maintaining effective communication with critical care patients is well recognized as a vital component of the delivery of quality health care. The communication that occurs between nurse and patient is probably the single most important way of relieving patient anxiety in critical care, and therefore, nurses should endeavour to talk to their patients as though they were awake even if they appear unconscious (Kisorio and Langley (2016a). A communication risk assessment tool is outlined in Table 5.5. It is vital that the nurse gives reassurance and explanation to the patient in order to limit anxiety, but

TABLE 5.4 Communication barriers within critical care.

Potential problem	
Distortion of message delivery	• Noise • Poor/bright lights • Vibration • Temperature
Distractions	• Other surrounding activities • Competing messages
Patient issues	
Psychological	• Perception altered by drug therapy and/or underlying pathology • Motivation and interest in message • Attitude/values/beliefs • Emotions/mood • Intelligence • Self-image

Physical	• Conscious level/sedation
	• Endotracheal tube ETT
	• Sensory deficits:
	  • Hearing
	  • Sight
	  • Movement
	  • Sensation
	  • Speech
	• Constraints to movement
	• Pain

Social	• Language • Culture/lifestyle • Isolation

communication is much more complex than telling the patient what has happened, what is happening and what will happen. The patient is an individual, and therefore, the nurse needs to ensure that they have acquired personalized information about them so that they may individualize their nursing care (see Case study in Box 5.1).

The Patient and Relatives

All procedures should be explained to patients and relatives so that there is effective communication and a reduction in stress and anxiety. Relatives play an important role in reducing patient's stress and anxiety levels by simply providing familiar touch and communication. Noome et al. (2016) stated that for relatives to be properly informed and understand their role in the patient's

TABLE 5.5 Critical care communication risk assessment tool.

Profound/severe difficulties (scores 2)	Intervention
Does the patient fulfil the criteria below: • Unconscious • Deeply/moderately sedated • Non-responsive/minimal response to deep pain • Fully ventilated • Profoundly withdrawn, passive, unwilling to communicate • Confused • Has a neurological disorder • Richmond sedation score −5 to −2?	Observe patient for any attempts to communicate/monitor their response Refer patient to speech therapist team if unsure about ability to communicate Can sedation be reduced? Can ventilation be reduced? Assess neurology Assess sedation score
Moderate difficulties (scores 1)	**Intervention**
Does the patient have: • Cuffed tracheostomy tube • COETT, but is alert • Facial weakness • Speech/language/voice problems • Minimal English • Visual or hearing impairment • Withdrawn, passive, unwilling to communicate?	Can cuff be deflated? Can patient have speaking valve trial? Liaise with interpreters Use of hearing aids/glasses Refer to speech therapists
Mild/no difficulties (scores 0)	**Intervention**
Does the patient have: • No tracheostomy or COETT • No speech/language or voice problems • No neurological impairments • Good spoken and written English • Alert and orientated • Richmond sedation score −0?	Encourage communication Use writing aids to support speech

recovery, they need to be properly informed. An environment needs to be created whereby relatives feel comfortable in expressing their concerns, ask questions and be reassured these will be answered. Listening to the family creates trust and provides comfort so they can then express these to the patient.

According to Kisorio and Langley (2016b), often relatives felt left in the darkness and did not understand when information was being explained to them. Relatives felt confused at what was going on and did not fully understand the seriousness of the situation. Arbour et al. (2013) stated that effective communication can be in the form of educating the family.

Developing a relationship with the family and patient requires work by the nurse assigned to care at the bedside. It is the nurse who spends most of the

---

BOX 5.1 Case study

Dave, a 55-y-old gentleman who was diagnosed with Guillain–Barré syndrome, was unable to communicate except by moving his eyes, up and down for yes, side to side for no. Dave had a continuing terror regarding his illness, he was stressed and found his surroundings uncomfortable and difficult to understand. His continuous stress was affecting his physical state, he was difficult to ventilate and was constantly agitated with a tachycardia and high blood pressure. His wife tells you that he enjoys gardening, has a dog and keeps owls.

This scenario gives insight into Dave's life and demonstrates that there is a man hidden beneath the highly technological equipment. It also provides a basis for conversation with his family and something to talk to Dave about other than the weather, time of day or regular reassuring or orientating communication. By talking about his garden, his dog, his owls and his family there is the chance that Dave will feel less alone and have the impression that the person caring for him knows him. It also assists in refocusing his mind on happier times and looking towards those times again.

---

time with the patient and families and is in constant communication regarding their well-being.

Music in Critical Care

Music therapy is an effective non-invasive intervention, which can be readily implemented within a critical care setting. The important role of music therapy within the critical setting is to primarily reduce anxiety levels and promote stress management strategies within the clinical area. In addition, music has often been used as a distraction from unpleasant feelings and is believed to offer internal empowerment and confidence. However, the notion of music therapy is often not widely accepted within the highly technological area of critical care. This holistic approach to patient care is unfortunate as often the introduction of music within such a stressful and unfamiliar environment can result in positive physiological and psychological benefits – for example, lowering of blood pressure, heart rate, respiratory rate, pain and anxiety levels.

An individual's response to music therapy is often linked to personal music selection and to whether they are able to relate to and familiarize themselves with the choice of music. Aimless blaring of music does not benefit patients but only the person who selected the music. This form of music therapy should not be promoted.

In the case of the unconscious patient, it is paramount that family members or friends are consulted and advised to bring in the patient's choice of music.

Furthermore, music therapy is a non-pharmacological aspect of care, which can be used as a supportive and complementary therapy to traditional and innovative treatments used.

Conscious patients should be given the opportunity to select their music preference and have periods of uninterrupted music listening throughout their day. This can promote a patient's autonomy within a highly technological environment where often autonomy is unnecessarily forfeited.

Music is a holistic, noninvasive therapy within the critical care setting that undoubtedly promotes an individualized approach to patient care and should be promoted, when appropriate, in the care of the critically ill patient.

Always ask the patient or family member what music the patient likes.

Follow-Up Clinics

Until recently, critical care environments paid little attention to the fate of their patients following discharge. A discharge of a patient from critical care marked a successful critical care stay and nursing, and medical focus was drawn towards the next critical care patient and their family. However, over the last decade, critical care has seen the creation of nurse- and physician-led follow-up clinics and what seems to be an interest in obtaining patient and family insight into critical care.

Follow-up clinics are useful and an integral part of care for patients and their families.

The primary purpose of follow-up clinics is to gain an insight into patient and family members' perspectives of critical care experiences, there also needs to be an understanding of quality of life and the effects of critical care treatments on the individual have also proven invaluable in questioning the ethical and moral aspect of critical care.

There are no hard or fast rules as to when the follow-up clinics should commence, but interestingly some institutions commence their follow-up service immediately after critical care discharge and often visit the longer stay patient (4 days) on the ward. This can prove beneficial in bridging the large void that critical care patients often experience when they become accustomed to 1:1 nursing in the critical care environment in comparison to ward care nursing.

Upon discharge from hospital, critical care patients are invited to attend nurse- or doctor-led outpatient clinics. The frequency of attendance varies locally, often patients are invited in periods of 2-, 4-, 6- and then 12-monthly intervals so that the critical care team can advise or assist with any physiological or psychological ailments or concerns.

Follow-up clinics provide an invaluable service for patients and families after critical care stay and assist critical care nurses and clinicians alike in improving the quality of care and service. It also proves to act as a platform to initiate changes in practice.

In addition to this support, follow-up is offered to bereaved relatives of patients in critical care. Support workers telephone relatives 4−5 days after the death and ask how they were coping; this gives survivors an opportunity to ask any further questions and to talk. Telephone follow-up is considered a useful way of contacting relatives to help with practical advice, show concern and identify those who may have needed referral to other agencies.

5.2 DEATH AND DYING IN CRITICAL CARE

Palliative Care

Palliative care is the active total care of those patients whose disease is not responsive to curative treatment, encompassing both the patients and their families/carers. Issues of death and dying are often not discussed with ease within a ward setting, but, within critical care, mortality is generally high. Therefore, health professionals who choose to work within a critical care setting need to develop skills and strategies for caring for the dying patient and their family.

Control of pain, or other symptoms, and psychological, social and spiritual problems is paramount. Palliative care emphasizes the care of people who have recently been diagnosed with advanced cancer, and Addington-Hall and Higginson (2001) also recognized those who have other life-threatening diseases such as:

- end-stage renal failure
- chronic heart failure
- chronic obstructive pulmonary disease
- multiple sclerosis

Palliative/end-of-life care can take place in hospital and is an integral part of all clinical practice. What it comprises has universal applicability and should be practised by all health care professionals.

Thus, critical care nurses have a fundamental role to play in supporting relatives when their loved one's condition moves from acute to palliative care.

Chochinov (2006) state that palliative care:

- affirms life and regards death as a normal process
- neither hastens nor postpones death
- provides relief from pain and other distressing symptoms
- integrates the psychological and spiritual aspects of patient care and
- offers a support system to help patients live as actively as possible until death.

The objective is to enhance personal satisfaction for both the individual and their families. Palliative care includes the control of pain and other symptoms, of psychological, social and spiritual problems and also recognizes the paramount importance of looking after those who are close to the patient. It is holistic and multifaceted. It emphasizes the care of those who have a life-threatening disease but are not imminently dying.

The key principles underpinning palliative care comprise:

- Whole-person approach
- Care, which encompasses both the patient and those who matter to them
- Emphasis on open and sensitive communication, including adequate information about diagnosis and treatment options
- Respect for patient and family autonomy and choice
- Focus on quality of life, which includes good symptom control and nursing care

What is so empowering about the care outlined above is that it can be adopted within a critical care setting as an integral part of clinical practice. The quality of palliative care in a critical care setting is of crucial importance; this is despite the rapid growth of hospices and home care schemes. Many critical care patients will be too ill to transfer to a hospice or home care scheme; therefore, it is the role of critical care nurses to enhance palliative care in their setting and promote the notion of palliative care.

The role of the critical care nurse is central to the care of the dying patient and their family. It requires the utmost sensitivity and attention to detail. Sadly, many dying critical care patients are unaware of their surroundings or plight as their condition is often critical, and it is then for the critical care nurse and doctors to offer:

- Skilled, supportive care to patients and families
- Sensitive nursing care
- Reporting of presenting symptoms and monitoring of symptom control
- Coordination of care between the multi-professional team

Critical care has adopted palliative care strategies in caring for patients with life-threatening illnesses. Many patients in hospital or in the community are suffering from a chronic/non-malignant disease. These patients might be coming to the end of their illness and, in effect, dying. The majority of these patients will die while still receiving active treatment. Yet, other interventions that will relieve some of the distressing symptoms − such as analgesia − may be withheld because of their side effects and the view that they may hasten death. Palliative care is a vital and integral part of all clinical practice, whatever the illness or its stage.

Death in critical care is a common occurrence; the adult person cared for in critical care areas requires curative, life-prolonging therapies. Sometimes patients are admitted with an acute illness unnecessarily with a chronic disease or to relieve distressing symptoms. The common assumption is that time needs to be determined when it is appropriate to shift from aggressive treatment to death-accepting care (Coombs et al., 2012). This is, however, misleading, as both may have to exist simultaneously.

Always allow time for the dying patient and family member to be together.

Improving Palliative Care in Critical Care

There is a need to develop clinical practices that continue to seek recovery and survival at the same time as the possibility of dying. Patients and families need to be helped to face dying even while pursuing every reasonable opportunity to live longer. An integrated model of practice is available in which all patients receive palliative care along with curative care where appropriate:

- Palliative care may gradually assume precedence when death is imminent.
- Palliative, curative, symptom and suffering relieving therapies may proceed in parallel until the patient either survives or succumbs.
- The next step is towards valuing a peaceful death, education and consultation with experts.

Obstacles to Implementation

Unrealistic expectations about prognosis for some patients lead to different views with regard to palliative care being undertaken in critical care. This is possibly due to patients in critical care:

- Having an impaired capacity to communicate their needs
- Being generally uninvolved in decisions
- Being given choices, but their preferences then subsequently being disregarded

In addition, there is a limited number of suitably qualified nurses, and there are competing demands on clinicians' time. Therefore, time should be spent with family members reviewing the patient's condition or prognosis or discussing treatment or limitation(s) of treatment.

Research agenda:

- The practice of forgoing life support
- Nurses' influence on the decision to withdraw or withhold limit life-support interventions
- Inconsistencies in the withdrawal or withholding of mechanical ventilation

Issues concerning symptom management:

- Pain control
- Assessment tools
- Perceptions/experiences of critical care nurses, patients and families
- Clinically important outcomes that can be changed

Identifying areas of conflict:

- Prolonging life or reducing complications
- Improving symptom management for those critical care patients who may be suffering

Fundamental Premise of Palliative Care in Critical Care

It is not appropriate to restrict critical care for those patients whose care is generally palliative, as critically ill patients and their families may all benefit from the systematic, comprehensive and integrated approach to comfort that palliative care offers. Critical care nurses must proceed with an integral approach in the face of prognostic uncertainty and incorporate palliative care in the plan for all their critically ill patients.

It would be unusual for critical care and palliative care practitioners to be involved in tending and caring for the same patients. All critically ill patients should receive both palliative care and intensive care. This strategy will hopefully improve the quality of death and care of the dying in critical care but also the quality of life and the care of those whose lives critical cares extraordinary technology can prolong. Considering both critical care and palliative care maximizes the humanity and the efficacy of the treatments provided to patients with critical illness.

Withdrawing and Withholding Treatment

The notion of withdrawing or withholding treatment within critical care is both complex and stressful for all concerned. The term withdrawing treatment involves the reduction and termination of organ support. This may take the form of reducing or terminating ventilatory support or not offering certain treatments that may prolong life.

The withdrawing or withholding of treatment within the critical care setting does include pain relief or methods of maintaining dignity, and this must be put to the patient and family. Withdrawing or withholding treatment is moving from maintenance of life to maintenance of dignity and prevention of torturous care and/or treatment. Pain relief, hydration and nursing care are a few of the treatments and care that will continue until death occurs. It is important to note that any decisions made may be modified and reversed depending on the patient's individual circumstances.

Ethnic, social and family influences play a major role in deciding the treatment pathway. Furthermore, it is important that the critical care team have discussed and are in agreement with the course of treatment before approaching the family members. Family members will inevitably be distressed by the information given to them and thus need committed and confident practitioners who are certain about their decision-making process and have the patient's best interest in mind. This process must take the form of considerable compassion towards the patient and family members so as not to cause further unnecessary distress.

Unfortunately, due to the very nature of the withdrawing and withholding situation, there are always going to be difficulties and problems surrounding the family dynamics. But factors such as truthful information giving, listening, promoting discussion and empathy are all important factors in minimizing the pain and anguish often experienced by patients and family members. The patient's wishes are paramount, and their best interests must always be at the forefront of any decision-making.

Upon receiving such information, family members can become aggressive and manifest episodes of irrationality. These are all normal signs of grief and must be taken into account when involved with such sensitive matters. It is important that the critical care team offer support and empathy during this difficult time so that their journey to acceptance is easier. Any discussions between the family and critical care team must be documented in the event that there are discrepancies about the giving of information.

Technological advances in the past 40 years have had an enormous impact on the way medicine is delivered today. This is particularly true within the critical care speciality, where intensivists possess the knowledge and tools to prolong life in many situations where patients may not have survived in the past. Before a decision is made to withhold or withdraw treatment, the treating doctor must carry out a thorough assessment of the patient's condition and determine the likely prognosis, taking into account current guidance on good clinical practice and seeking the views and assessments of the clinical team and family members.

Where there is significant disagreement within the clinical team and family, the treating doctor must try to resolve them and ensure clarity and consistency in the information provided to family members. In some instances, a second opinion may be beneficial where there is a significant disagreement within the clinical team about clinical aspects of patient care.

Decisions to withdraw or withhold treatment must be documented properly. This should include the relevant clinical findings, details of discussions with patient, family or other members of the clinical team and details of treatment given with any agreed review dates and outcomes of treatment or other significant factors surrounding the decision-making process, which may affect patient outcome.

Dying in Critical Care

The majority of critical care patients are admitted with the hope of reversing the immediate illness, avoiding a fatal outcome. Death is a common event in critical care − which treats a substantial number of patients who will ultimately die. Critical care generally has more deaths than anywhere else (Orban et al., 2017).

Patients are more likely to die on critical care as they may be admitted:

- For aggressive technological, invasive life-prolonging, curative interventions.
- Unnecessarily due to unknown patient's wishes for invasive treatment when the condition is at a certain stage.
- As death is uncertain for chronic illnesses, they are treated right up to the end of life.
- For relief of painful/distressing symptoms that can occur before death.
- To alleviate other symptoms and to improve quality of life, for example, cardiac surgery.

The Difficulties of Death in Critical Care

Many very sick patients, their families, physicians and nurses in critical care see the patients as individuals in need of treatment, not as dying. It is often difficult to predict with any certainty when a patient in critical care is going to die, and treatment may last right up to the moment just prior to death. In critical care, there might be a need to sometimes change from a primarily curative focus to a primarily palliative approach. This is often misleading, as what is omitted is time to make decisions with regard to the patient's wishes in the event of their coming to the end of life.

The Transition From Curative to End-of-Life Care

This transition often finds families in shock and grief when they are told that nothing further can be done. The family are often in denial and need:

- Time to accept what is happening
- To be allowed to spend uninterrupted time with the patient
- To be present at the patient's last moments
- To perform their own rituals

The Decision to End Life

There is sometimes confusion between:

- Voluntary euthanasia
- Assisted suicide
- Pain control/withdrawal of life support

There are concerns about:

- Addiction, which is unwarranted
- Limiting analgesia due to instability of condition
- It may hinder sensitivity to physical examination − when the Glasgow coma scale (GCS) is reduced
- Endurance of dyspnoea or the presence of an endotracheal tube (ETT)

Always involve the patient and their family in decision making.

The Difficulty in Predicting Death

Often a period of time cannot be relied upon in which dying is evidently near, which is long enough to allow those involved to embark upon planning for death.

- In critical care (CC), the line between life and death is blurred.
- The course of the disease is unpredictable.
- The time of death cannot be predicted with any certainty.
- Death in CC patients is harder to predict than it is in cancer.

The Situation is Unknown

- The patient has not had the opportunity to make the necessary choices and come to terms with their own demise.
- How long to continue with the aggressive interventions of life-support treatment.
- The justification of admission to CC in terms of provision of comfort, symptom control and/or quality of life.

The Differing Perceptions/Goals with Regards to Offering Palliative Care in Critical Care

- CC nurses suggest that, ideally, patients who are expected to die should not be admitted to critical care.
- If admitted, they should be transferred out as soon as the focus of care is palliative rather than curative.
- This presents with conflicting goals and who should have access to critical care interventions.
- Palliative care is often perceived as the domain of hospices rather than critical care, but if technological interventions such as noninvasive ventilation can be used to support and relieve the symptoms of discomfort, pain and/or suffering at the end of a person's life than should this not be used.
- Interventions are valued in CC − in PC, too much can be seen as a barrier.

The View of the Patient

- It is not known how welcome palliative care services would be for CC patients.
- The stigma and fear of cancer by patients with serious conditions are evident in patients with heart conditions who have often been known to state 'thanks goodness I do not have cancer', and as such to not see themselves as potentially dying or other similar statements:
- 'I may be ill but I do not need palliative care yet'
- 'There are people worse off than me, they mean people with cancer'

Brain Stem Death

The brain stem is collectively the midbrain, pons and medulla oblongata. It is between the cerebrum and the spinal cord, the medulla oblongata being a direct upward continuation of the spinal cord. It is a small but vitally important area of the brain, responsible for reflex control of essential functions, for example, cardiovascular and respiratory, sneezing, coughing, gagging all originate from the brain stem. In addition, all nervous impulses from the peripheral nervous system have to go through the brain stem to get to the higher centres for effect on the body. Ten of the 12 cranial nerves originate in the brain stem.

The midbrain

- Pupillary dilation
- Muscles and gland stimulation

The pons

- Cranial nerves pair off from here
- Controls breathing rhythm

The medulla oblongata

- The cardiac centre maintains force and rate of heart contraction
- The respiratory centre controls rate and depth of breathing
- Controls various other centres vomiting, coughing/sneezing, swallowing/hiccupping

Brain stem death occurs when structural brain damage is so extensive that there is no potential for recovery, the brain can no longer maintain its own internal homeostasis, and there is a complete loss of brain stem function.

- It is the permanent loss of the function of the brain stem; this results in a combined, irreversible loss of the capacity for consciousness and breathing.
- It is a diagnosis of death accepted by both the medical and legal profession.
- The most frequent causes of brain stem death are intracranial haemorrhage, cerebral hypoxaemia and trauma.

Always involve the patient and their family in decision making Every patient fulfilling the criteria for brain stem death is a potential organ donor.

Brain Stem Death Criteria

- The patient is brain stem dead and mechanically ventilated.
- Age is irrelevant to whether patients require brain stem death tests, but it is essential for the patient's clinical condition, blood results are within satisfactory parameters at the time the tests are taking place. This assessment is undertaken and checked by the relevant medical team.
- The medical and nursing staff have no known objections from the family, or coroner.

Brain Stem Death Tests

For brain stem death tests to take place, the patient will be deeply unconscious and require full ventilatory support. Prior to commencement of brain stem tests, the patient must meet certain preconditions. These preconditions are designed to ensure the patient's unconscious state is caused by irreversible structural brain damage, and their current status has not been influenced by other factors such as the use of muscle relaxants or an existing metabolic disorder. For brain stem death tests to take place, the patient has to have:

- Normal blood gases, urea and creatinine, potassium (K^1) and sodium (Na^1), temperature
- No sedation, analgesia or muscle relaxants for 24–48 hour (or longer)
- A specific condition that causes brain stem death
- A diagnosis of brain stem death that has been made and confirmed by two independent and suitably qualified doctors
- Two sets of tests are performed
- The tests have been designed to look at the most basic brain stem functions and assess their responses

The tests consist of the following:

- *Eyes*: Pupils do not react to light; eyelids do not move when the corneas are stimulated; there is no movement of the eyes when ice cold water is injected in the ear canals.
- *Cranial nerves*: There is no motor response within the cranial nerve distribution to stimulation of any somatic area.
- *Oral*: There is no gag or cough response to tracheal suction

- *Respiratory*: There is no respiratory effort when ventilation is discontinued, even when monitored arterial carbon dioxide (PaO_2) exceeds the threshold for respiratory stimulation.

If the patient is brain stem dead, there will be:

- No vestibulo-ocular reflex − 20 mL of ice-cold water is slowly injected into each ear: there will be no movement of the eyes in response.
- No corneal reflex − if the cornea is stroked with a piece of gauze, the patient will not blink.
- No brain stem reflexes:
  - No pupil response to light
  - No blinking or grimacing
  - No gagging or cough reflex
  - No motor response to painful stimuli
- No stimulation of breathing after a period of removal from the ventilator (pre-oxygenate with 100% to prevent hypoxia); if carbon dioxide has risen above 6.65 kPa, it can be assumed that no respiratory effort has taken place during the period of discontinuation of ventilation.

Two doctors, a consultant in charge of the patient's case and a second doctor of senior registrar status, carry out the tests either separately or together to make the diagnosis of brain stem death. Once brain stem death has been confirmed, the possibility of organ harvest for transplantation should be considered. If a patient is going to become an organ donor, it is necessary to continue ventilation until organ retrieval can take place.

All brain stem tests are carried out twice as a matter of law.

Potential Organ Donation

Many patients in the United Kingdom die or suffer prolonged dependency because of a lack of organs for transplantation. Therefore, if a young or middle-aged patient with a fatal condition has healthy kidneys, liver, heart and/ or corneas, it might be relevant to discuss organ donation with the medical team. Suitable organ donors include:

- Victims of severe head injury
- Severe subarachnoid or intracerebral haemorrhage
- In the case of corneal donation, any young patient with healthy eyes or a rapidly fatal illness

Patients who are unsuitable for organ donation are:

- Where brain stem death criteria fulfilment is uncertain
- Those aged older than 60 years
- Where there has been significant hypotension or a hypoxic episode during a fatal injury
- Where there is a history of previous disease affecting the potential donor (e.g. hypertension, diabetes, hepatitis B, alcohol abuse)
- Where the patient has received drugs or other treatments which might have affected the organs to be transplanted
- In the case of the kidneys, where there is persistent oliguria

Currently, people have to register their decision to be an organ donor by joining the NHS Organ Donor Register online and/or by carrying an organ donor card.

However, change to this system is underway with a new opt-out system for organ donation. This is being considered to be in place by 2020 in England. Wales have had this system since 2015, and Scotland is planning to do the same. Under these plans, adults will be presumed to be organ donors unless they have specifically recorded their decision not to be.

Involve the organ transplant coordinator and team as soon as possible.

Clinical Management of Potential Organ Donors

Following brain stem death diagnosis, significant pathophysiological changes will occur, which may lead to complications, and this may in turn lead to potential damage to the donor's organs. Once a family has made the decision to donate their family member's organs, it is the duty of the medical and nursing team to ensure the donor's organs have the best possible outcome.

Common complications of patients who have been diagnosed as brain stem dead include:

- Hypotension
- Hypothermia
- Hypernatraemia
- Hyperglycaemia
- Acidosis
- Diabetes insipidus
- Disseminated intravascular coagulation
- Pulmonary oedema

Routine monitoring of a brain stem dead patient should include:

- ECG, cardiac monitoring
- Arterial blood pressure
- Oxygen saturation
- Temperature
- Central venous pressure
- Fluid balance
- Arterial blood gases
- Pathology, for example, biochemistry, haematology

Care of the Donor and Family

The physiological manifestations of brain stem death are complex. Their effects include profound hypotension, cardiac arrhythmias, hypothermia, pulmonary oedema, diabetes insipidus and clotting abnormalities. Maintenance of a patient's status quo during this time can often prove to be difficult and multifaceted. Furthermore, organ donations are sometimes lost because of a rapid deterioration in the donor's clinical condition.

Potential donors need intensive nursing and complex medical care once brain stem death has been confirmed. Their combined care will ensure that the organs are maintained at a high-quality pre-donation and thus ensure that the family's wish for donation is fulfilled. It is important to note that the longer the time after the diagnosis of brain stem death, the more problems may arise in the patient's clinical condition and medical management.

Often family members of potential donors choose when and where they feel ready to say their goodbyes to their loved one. Some family members leave shortly after brain stem tests have been performed; others may stay until they go to theatre. This is managed on an individual basis, and the intensive care and organ transplant team help family members through this difficult time by offering intense support, empathy and compassion.

The Transplant Recipient

Organ transplantation is the treatment of choice for end-stage organ failure. Transplant recipients who may benefit from organ transplantation fall into the following categories:

- Heart — cardiomyopathy, ischaemic heart disease
- Lung — emphysema
- Heart and lung — cystic fibrosis
- Liver — primary biliary cirrhosis, chronic active hepatitis
- Kidney — polycystic kidney disease, glomerulonephritis
- Kidney and pancreas — diabetic nephropathy

Allocation of Organs and Retrieval

Prior to the retrieval of an organ, a transplant centre must have accepted the organ for a suitable waiting list patient. All organs are primarily offered to the local zonal centre. If they do not have any suitable recipients, the organ will then be offered to each of the country's other transplant centres. If none of the UK centres accepts the organ, it is then offered to a European centre. This is a reciprocal agreement, and it is important to note that the UK imports more organs than it exports.

In the event that the organ cannot be placed with a potential organ recipient, then the organ will not be retrieved.

Legal Issues

If the death would normally have been referred to the Coroner, then permission must be sought before organ donation can be performed. It is unusual for a Coroner to refuse all donations, but they have specific objections to certain organs and/or tissues being removed. On rare occasions, a Home Office pathologist may attend organ retrieval.

It is unnecessary for family members to sign a formal document but often the organ transplant coordinator will document their lack of objection within the patient's medical notes.

All potential organ donors will be required to have a virology screen to exclude HIV and hepatitis B and C. Furthermore, the organ transplant coordinator is required to ask family members about the patient's social behaviour so that they have a detailed history of the patient's past. Once again, this information will be documented within the patient's medical notes.

What to Do after the Patient Has Died

- The family should be able to spend as much time with their loved one as they want; this should not exclude children
- The ICU doctor may be called to certify the death
- Date and time of death are recorded in the patient's notes
- Inform surrounding patients/visitors of the patient's death

Last Offices

This is the care given to a deceased patient, which is focused on fulfilling religious and cultural beliefs as well as health and safety and legal requirements. It should be remembered that this is the final demonstration of respectful, sensitive care given to the patient.

- It is important that the critical care nurse knows in advance the cultural values and religious beliefs of the patient and family, as there are considerable variations between people from different faiths, ethnic backgrounds and national origins in their approach to death and dying.
- Individual preferences should be determined and patients should be encouraged to talk about how they wish to be treated upon dying. In the case of the unconscious patient in ICU, the critical care nurse should consult the family members.
- Catheters and other appliances should be removed (except in a Coroner's case where local guidance should be sought) and any dentures replaced.
- Relatives should be asked whether jewellery should be left on or taken off the patient.
- Wash the patient unless requested not to do so for religious/cultural reasons. It may not be acceptable for the nurse to undertake this task — or sometimes a relative or spouse may want to help.
- The body is dressed in a shroud or other garment (refer to local policy).
- Local policy should be followed with the identification of the body and their property identified and stored.
- The patient is then wrapped in a sheet and the sheet secured with tape.
- A notification of death card is taped outside the sheet (refer to local policy).
- Request the portering staff to remove the body.
- Screen off appropriate areas from view of other patients and visitors to ICU when the body is being removed.
- Update nursing records, transfer property and patient records to appropriate administrative staff.
- Give bereaved family members an information booklet regarding contacting hospital about viewing the body, collection of death certificate etc.

Refer the family members to the patient affairs team for ongoing support after the patient has left ICU.

Emotional Care

Emotional care relies on openness and sharing the truth about the illness. Often the conscious critical care patient will feel loss and grief for the lack of:

- Independence
- Self-esteem
- Status, job and income
- Role and relationships
- A future

Thus, it is important to provide emotional support for families and patients while experiencing critical care. Despite it sometimes being difficult for critical care nurses to find time to provide emotional support, it is your responsibility to meet the demands of patients and their families. However, sometimes it is enough that the nurse is in attendance at the bedside as much as possible (Noome et al., 2016).

Spiritual Care

Spiritual care gives the patient and family an opportunity to examine the impact of the illness on their belief systems. They need to be given the opportunity to ask questions:

- Why me/us?
- Why now?
- What have I done to deserve this? This is a question that the dying may ask themselves and others.

As a critical care nurse, staying with this sort of spiritual pain and not being afraid of the questions asked by the patient or their family is a helpful and sensitive response. Offering the support of a relevant religious figure may not be appropriate for all but listening and being present will be appreciated.

Cultural Diversity

Making nursing practice relevant to people of many cultures is a constant challenge to the critical care nurse (Table 5.6). Cultures differ with regard to:

- The meaning of an illness
- Attitude to pain, symptoms and medication
- Ways of coping with illness
- Attitude to place of care, physical and emotional care
- The roles of the family
- Rituals around death, the funeral and bereavement

Social Needs

The critical care nurse needs to ensure that patients and families have adequate information regarding the benefits to which they may be entitled. These include:

- Housing benefits
- Income support
- Council tax
- Drawing up a will

Often referral to the Patient Advice and Liaison Service (PALS) group or palliative care team is beneficial.

TABLE 5.6 Last rites and religious influences.

Religion	Last rites
Baha'i	• Treat body with great respect after death as believe in afterlife. • Routine last rites are appropriate. • Cremation is not permitted. • Burial should take place within an hour's journey from place of death.
Buddhism	• Believe in rebirth after death; therefore, state of mind at moment of death is important in determining the state of rebirth. • Some form of chanting may be used to influence the state of mind at death so that it may be peaceful. • May not wish to have sedatives or pain-killing drugs administered at this time. • peace and quiet for meditation and visits from other Buddhists are appreciated. • If Buddhists are not in attendance, then a Buddhist minister should be informed of the death as soon as possible. Routine last rites are appropriate. • Cremation is preferred.
Christian science	There are no rituals to be performed.
Christianity • Anglican • Roman catholic • Protestant • United reform • Methodist	Routine last rites are appropriate for all Christians.
Hinduism	• Want to die at home. This has religious significance and death in hospital can cause great distress. • May wish to call in a Hindu priest to read from the Hindu holy books and to perform holy rites. These may include tying a thread around the wrist or neck, sprinkling the person with water from the Ganges, or placing a sacred tulsi leaf in their mouth. • Their belief in cremation and body being returned to nature may involve a dying person asking to be placed on the floor during their last moments.
Islam	• May wish to sit or lie with their face towards Mecca. Moving the bed to make this possible is appreciated. • Family may recite prayers around the bed. If no family are available, any practising Muslim can assist. • May wish the imam (religious leader) to visit. • After death, the body should not be touched by non-Muslims. Health workers should wear disposable gloves to touch body. • The body should be prepared according to the wishes of the family.

TABLE 5.6 Last rites and religious influences.—cont'd

Religion	Last rites
	• If family are not available, the following procedure should be followed: • Turn the head towards the right shoulder before rigor mortis begins. This is so that the body can be buried with their face towards Mecca. Do not wash the body or cut hair or nails. • Wrap the body in a plain white sheet. • Muslims are always buried, never cremated. • The body will be ritually washed by the family, and Muslim undertakers before burial. • Funerals take place as soon as practicable, as delay can cause distress. If a delay is unavoidable, explain the reasons carefully to the relatives. • If the death has to be reported to the Coroner, they should be informed that the patient is a Muslim and be asked if the procedures can take place as soon as possible. • If the family wish to view the body, staff should ask the mortician to ensure that the room is free of any religious symbols. • Post-mortems are forbidden unless ordered by the Coroner, in which case the reasons for it must be clearly explained to the family. • Family may request that organs removed should be returned to the body after examination.
Jehovah's witness	• No special rituals for the dying but they will usually appreciate a visit from one of the elders of their faith. • Routine last rites are not appropriate.
Judaism	• In some cases, the son or nearest relative, if present, may wish to close the eyes and mouth. • The body should be handled as little as possible by non-Jews. • Depending on the sex of the patient, a fellow male or female washes and prepares the body for burial. Usually three members of the community are present. Traditional Jews will arrange for this to be done by the Jewish burial society. • If, however, members of the family are not present, most non-orthodox Jews would accept the usual washing and last rites performed by hospital staff. • The body should be covered with a clean white sheet. • The family may wish for the body to be placed with the feet pointing towards the doorway and to light a candle. • Some orthodox Jewish groups may wish to appoint someone to stay with the body 'watcher' from the time of death to the burial, which usually takes place within 24 hour. • If family wish to view the body, staff should ask the mortician to ensure that the room is free of any religious symbols. • If the death has to be reported to the Coroner, they should be informed that the patient is Jewish and be asked if the procedures can take place as soon as possible.

Continued

TABLE 5.6 Last rites and religious influences.—cont'd

Religion	Last rites
	• Orthodox Jews are always buried but non-orthodox Jews allow cremation. • The funeral has to take place as soon as possible.
Mormons	• There are no rituals for the dying, but spiritual contact is important. • The Church has 'home teachers' who offer support and care by visiting church members in hospital. • Routine last rites are appropriate. • The sacred garment, if worn, must be replaced on the body following the last rites. • Church burial is preferred, although cremation is not forbidden.
Rastafarianism	• Visiting the sick is important, and visits are often made in groups. Family members may wish to pray at the bedside. • Apart from this, there are no rites or rituals, before or after death. • Routine last rites are appropriate. • Burial is preferred.
Sikhism	• May receive comfort from reciting hymns from the Guru Granth Sahib, the Sikh holy book. Family or any practising Sikh may help with this. • Generally, Sikhs are happy for non-Sikhs to attend to the body. However, many families will wish to wash and lay out the body themselves. • If members of the family are not available, in addition to the normal last rites hair or beard should be left intact and not trimmed. • If the family wish to view the body, staff should ask the mortician to ensure that the room is free of all religious symbols. • Apart from stillbirths and neonates, who may be buried, Sikhs are always cremated. This should take place as soon as possible. • There are no objections to post-mortem examinations.

Bereavement in Critical Care

Over the last decade, care of critical care patient's relatives has increasingly been seen to be of growing importance in the holistic approach to nursing care. Critical care nurses working within this setting need to have an understanding of bereavement and how to recognize abnormal grief and to refer to specialist members for guidance and assistance with aiding bereaved family members.

Historically, critical care professionals focused primarily on:

- Close patient assessment
- Obtaining observations

- Close monitoring for complications
- Management of technology

In the past, less emphasis was placed on the nurse's perception of what was deemed important to relieve anxieties experienced by bereaved family members in critical care. However, today critical care nurses play an important role in caring for the bereaved in critical care.

The concept of bereavement is a subject area that many choose not to explore or understand. The death of a family member can evoke many feelings of denial, guilt, anger and hopelessness. Furthermore, the admission of a 'loved one' to critical care can seriously disrupt the dynamics of a family and close friends, and families' needs on a cognitive, emotional and personal level are very high.

Grief is not an illness; it is a pattern of reactions that take place while the person adjusts to the death of their loved one. The critical care nurse is not expected to be a bereavement counsellor but to be there for the family member before the patient has died. A well-managed death will help with the emotional health of a family. Listening and understanding imply concern and care while acknowledgement of their pain and sorrow may also help family members move forward:

- The family need the nurses' presence at the bedside as much as possible being with the patient
- Attending the family's basic needs showing empathy and compassion
- Ensuring the patient is comfortable and pain free

Recognizing abnormal grief:

- Are grief reactions prolonged, excessive and seemingly incapable of resolution?
- Are grief reactions absent?
- Has grief been displaced or masked, for example, by illness, drugs, alcohol or overwork?
- Was the relationship with the deceased person particularly ambivalent or dependent?
- Were the circumstances of the death unexpected or violent?

Sudden Death

Sudden death refers to any patient who has died unexpectedly from accident or illness. This area of bereavement is vast, and sudden death itself covers many modes of death. Sudden death includes suicide, murder, accident, illness, 'cot death' or sudden infant death. Sudden death(s) robs relatives of any preparatory grief. The relatives left behind may require more support and counselling than those who have known for some time that their relative is dying. Accidental deaths are more likely to be unexpected by the family.

The Needs of Survivors Bereaved by Sudden and Unexpected Death

Death and loss are an unavoidable part of life. As critical care nurse practitioners, responding to death is frequently encountered, yet the deceased is not the only 'patient': those left behind should also be the focus of care. When survivors are notified of a death, their grief begins. People may show no manifestations of grief at the time of death but experience normal grief prior to death occurring (McInroy and Edwards, 2002).

With sudden death in mind, it is imperative that critical care nurses are aware of the family's distress, acknowledge this and have an understanding of the needs of those who are suddenly bereaved. After sudden death, families' experiences may have a powerful effect on their process of grieving and professionals' responses to them play a valuable part in the crisis.

- Viewing the body — equipment should, if possible, not be in view, and there should be privacy and a member of staff staying with them in the room being supportive and compassionate.
- Signing of papers is necessary but not an initial priority.
- Meeting the family immediately upon arrival in the critical care area; a member of hospital personnel should accompany the family, offer support, give information and provide a separate room for them to wait.
- Knowing patients' condition — survivors need accurate information about death and to talk about their experiences.
  - Breaking bad news of the death of a family's relative is one of the most difficult and sensitive things a critical care nurse has to learn to do.
  - Poor communication skills can leave families confused and angry at the way news was broken.
  - Families need to be reassured that all appropriate actions were taken to save their loved one.
- Recommending sedation is the least helpful because it inhibits the bereaved person's expressions of grief.
- Consistency with usage of words — critical care staff often use a variety of words/language to describe a relative's notification of death.
  - Explanations should be clear of medical jargon, gentle and sincere.
  - The word 'dead' should be used, instead of terms such as 'passed away'.
  - The word 'dead' or 'died' can help the bereaved person not to deny the death and leads to less confusion.

Encourage family members to view the deceased as this aids the process of closure and promotes progress in the grieving process.

Caring for Relatives

Involving Relatives in Care

Commitment to individualized patient care requires considerable emotional involvement and commitment from critical care nurses. Critical care nurses need to involve and support patient families in their care. One way of ensuring this takes place is to engage relatives in the essential care needs of the patient. This may help alleviate any feelings of detachment, isolation and helplessness they may feel.

Involving family members in the nursing care of critical care patients can sometimes be seen as a major challenge for critical care nurses, in that they are not familiar with letting family members assist with nursing care (Table 5.7). However, what critical care nurses must ask themselves is: is it unreasonable to let a loved one assist with essential care when they have been together or known each other for a significant period?

Nurses' fears are often associated with not wanting to be watched or assessed when at work by family members. However, care in critical care is often extended to family members − involving them in their loved one's care can often alleviate both their and their loved one's anxieties (Table 5.8). In addition, this can prevent the development of ICU syndrome and thus improve recovery.

Visiting in Critical Care

The need for family members to visit their loved ones when they have been admitted into the critical care unit has long been identified as a requirement for maintaining family unity and closeness. Few topics have generated as much controversy as visitation policies in critical care units.

TABLE 5.7 Summary of the needs of family members of critically ill patients.

Molter's (1979) study	Mitchell et al (2019) and Kiwanuka et al (2019) studies study
• To feel that there is hope	• Information - the need to know - explanations, assurance, open and transparent communication
• To feel that hospital personnel care about the patient	• To know the treatment being given and to be part of the discussion
• To have a waiting room near the patient	• Comfort, amenities, close proximity to patient and spiritual support
• To be called if the condition changes	• The opportunity to be involved in care of the patient
• To be told of the patient's prognosis	• Trust in and support from the nurse

TABLE 5.8 Johns model for structured reflection (10th edition).

Write a description of the experience

Cue questions

Aesthetics	What was I trying to achieve? Why did I respond as I did? What were the consequences of that for: • The patient? • Others? • Myself? How was this person feeling? (Or these persons?) How did I know this?
Personal	How did I feel in this situation? What internal factors were influencing me?
Ethics	How did I feel in this situation? What factors made me act in incongruent ways?
Empirics	What knowledge did or should have informed me?
Reflexivity	How does this connect with previous experiences? Could I handle this better in similar situations? What would be the consequences of alternative actions for: • The patient? • Others? • Myself? How do I now feel about this experience? Can I support myself and others better as a consequence? Has this changed my ways of knowing?

The visitation policy of critical care units has been liberalized in recent years. This change has been progressive in seeing critical units move from a restricted to an open visiting policy. The belief is that open visiting generates positive effects on patients, family and nurses. Kisorio and Langley (2016) discussed the importance of allowing open visitation for family members at any time. However, it cannot be ignored that within critical care worldwide, there are still two forms of visiting strategy within critical care. There is the liberalized visiting policy, which is open visiting, and then there is the restricted policy, which imposes a more structured and rigid visiting policy.

Familiarize yourself with the critical care unit's visiting hours and plan your patient's care around these set times.

Critical care literature has highlighted the importance of visitation in critical care units and its beneficial effects on patients and their families alike. However, nurses' attitudes and beliefs about visitation have not always correlated with those of patients and their families nor do actual visitation practices correlate with the critical care unit's written local policy.

Factors that influence visitation practices within critical care are as follows:

- The patient's need for rest
- Nurses' workload
- Doctors' ward rounds
- The beneficial effects of visitation on patients
- The patient's condition
- Rapport between nurse, patient and family member

In comparing restricted versus open visitation, restricted hours were perceived to:

- Decrease noise
- Promote patient's rest

and open visitation practices were perceived to:

- Beneficially affect the patient
- Beneficially affect the patient's family
- Decrease the anxieties of patient and family

In evaluating the ideal visitation policy that should be implemented within a critical care environment, the main factors that should be taken into accounts are as follows:

- Restrict the number of visitors allowed at any one time.
- Restriction on hours that patient has visitors, for example, to allow for rest and sleep.
- Allow visits by children.
- There should be no restriction on visitation by immediate family members, but they should be aware of the patient's condition and take this into account when visiting.

Interestingly, the literature suggests that critical care nurses do not, in fact, restrict visitation, regardless of whether restrictive policies are in place. Most nurses base their visitation decisions on the needs of the patient and the need for nurse and medical interventions.

The Cost of Caring to the Critical Care Nurse

Working closely with critically ill and dying patients can cause emotional distress for the critical care nurse and can be painful, difficult and challenging.

Continued Education and Support

Kisorio and Langley (2016) stated that there is often not enough emotional support available for critical care nurses, and this can have an emotional effect.

Thus, critical care management needs to ensure regular updates and training on breaking bad news and have a shared professional goal with reflections, discussions and feedback about the caring aspect of critical care work. In addition, a support group for staff. Being exposed daily to stressful, emotional and death requires further education, which is important. However, these topics are difficult to teach but issues need to be explored in a safe environment. Training should include knowledge about emotional intelligence, death, grief and bereavement, communication skills either at breaking bad news or dealing with discomfort felt by staff when they were dealing with relatives showing extreme emotions.

Support From Colleagues

Critical care nurses can often feel distressed when caring for a challenging or dying patient when colleagues do not support them. Kisorio and Langley (2016) mention that some staff members can be 'desensitised' or 'switched off' or they should 'just get on with it'. Kisorio and Langley (2016) reported that some critical care nurses do not communicate well with other staff members. However, other nurses in critical care are also dealing with pressure and workload and as such cannot find the time to support others. However, when difficult and challenging patients are being cared for, it is important that staff members are aware and ensure they feel supported.

Critical Care Nurses' Support Systems

Nurses working within the critical care environment need adequate support systems in both their professional and personal lives. It is imperative that all staff members working in critical care realize their needs following the death of a patient.

Critical care nurses must always remember to look after yourself.

The critical care nurse needs to recognize internal signs of stress and develop strategies for coping:

- Spacing for holidays and time off is important to recharge lost energy
- Continuous training and education for mental stimulation
- Take time to debrief with colleagues

- Concisely written recording can be therapeutic and assist in the letting go of particularly stressful situation
- Keeping a reflective diary

Being honest and sharing vulnerabilities will help a team relate and work well together.

5.3 PROFESSIONAL PRACTICE ISSUES

Consent

Consent is to voluntarily agree to receive a particular treatment based on an adequate knowledge of the purpose, nature and likely risks of the treatment, including likelihood of its success and alternatives to it. Permission given under any unfair or undue pressure without sufficient knowledge or information is not consent.

Consent Criteria

In order for consent to be obtained lawfully, the patient must

- be competent
- be conscious
- be mentally capable
- have the relevant information to give consent
- have understood information given
- have given consent voluntarily

If a patient is unconscious, then a family member cannot consent on their behalf.

Battery and Medical Law

In the absence of consent all, or almost all, medical treatment and all surgical treatment of an adult are unlawful; however, beneficial such treatment might be apart from the criteria outlined above; three other important areas control the law on consent; these are:

- Case law, whereby previous cases taken to court set precedence on future cases, for example, Sidaway *v* Bethlem (1985).
- Statute law, whereby the government passes a law which governs the area concerned, for example, Family Law Reform Act 1969, section 8.
- Rules, where professional codes of conduct, guidelines and protocols should be followed in practice; this is referred to as 'quasi law'.

Types of Consent

There are different types of consent used within the health care setting, which allow treatment to be undertaken without there being an issue of 'unlawful touching'. These are as follows:

- Express consent. This is usually written, although there is no legal requirement for this to be so — only governmental and employment guidelines advise that this should be written.
- Implied consent. This usually takes the form of action undertaken by the patient, for example, holds out an arm to have blood taken.
- Consent forms. This is particularly so for people detained under the Mental Health Act 2005.

All critical care practitioners must familiarize themselves with the different types of consent, as this is fundamental to your patient's care.

Different categories to take into account when obtaining consent:

- Is the patient conscious and are they able to consent for themselves?
- Adults can refuse treatment at any time before and during the procedure.
- Is the patient temporarily or permanently incapacitated?
- When an adult has an impaired capacity, the decision to refuse treatment is based on the patient's rights versus the protection of their best interest.
- Is there an advance directive?

Advance Directives

An advanced decision to refuse treatment is governed by statutory rules. This legal framework gives clear safeguards that confirm the notion that people may make a decision in advance to refuse treatment even if they should go on to lose their mental capacity in the future. Furthermore, the Act clearly states that an advanced decision will have no application in an emergency situation to sustain life unless strict formalities have been followed.

These formalities require that the decision must

- be in writing
- be signed and dated
- be witnessed
- contain an express statement that the decision stands 'even if life is at risk'

If you are unsure about what category your patient falls into or what their current position might be, then consult your clinical governance department.

Informed Consent in the United Kingdom

There is no such doctrine of informed consent in the United Kingdom; however, the medical standard of what information should be given is set out in the landmark case of Bolam (1957). It is also important to note that English law states that it is a doctor's 'therapeutic privilege' to withhold information from a patient during the process of obtaining consent if the doctor deems it to be detrimental to the mental or physical health of the patient.

Non-Disclosure of Risk

The law states that patients must be informed of risks associated with their treatment; the leading case is Sidaway *v* Bethlem (1985) whereby the doctors were at fault for not disclosing the material risks associated with a particular procedure. This case has been recently challenged in Chester *v* Afshar (2002) where the courts upheld that not only must the clinician disclose risks but they must offer alternative treatments.

Good practice states that:

- Obtaining consent should not be seen as obtaining a signature but should be viewed as a process.
- Doctors should have an understanding of patient's perceptions.
- Clinicians should document, document, document.
- Consent should be written and translated, if necessary.
- Clinicians should review their consent-obtaining practices.
- Clinicians should give time to their patients/families to ask questions and discuss the procedure.
- There should be enhanced communication links between the multidisciplinary team to aid effective consent.

Mental Capacity Act 2005

This Act governs the way in which decisions are made on behalf of people lacking mental capacity. It also includes provisions for advanced decisions to refuse treatment. It also sets out a framework in which health care professionals can assess the best interest of a patient who lacks capacity, together with provisions relating to medical research. In addition, the act now makes it a criminal offence to ill-treat or neglect a person who lacks mental capacity, and such a person may be liable to a term of 5 year imprisonment.

This Act is underpinned by a set of five key principles set out in Section 1. These are that:

1. There is a presumption of capacity, and that every adult has the right to make his or her own decisions, and they must be assumed to have capacity.
2. The rights of individuals are to be supported to make their own decisions; therefore, all appropriate assistance must be given before anyone may conclude that they cannot make their own decision.
3. Individuals retain the right to make decisions even if eccentric or unwise.
4. The 'best interest' notion prevails for incapacitated individuals.
5. Only the least restrictive intervention should be performed on an incapacitated individual to minimize their infringement of basic rights and freedoms.

The Act also sets out clear parameters for research. These are that:

- Research involving incapacitated persons may be lawfully carried out if an appropriate body (normally research ethics committee) agrees that the research is safe, relates to the person's condition and cannot be undertaken as effectively on people who have mental capacity. If the research is to enhance new scientific knowledge, it must be of minimal risk to that individual and carried out with minimal interference or intrusion on their rights.
- Carers or nominated third parties must be consulted and agree that the individual concerned would want to join an approved research project.

www.dca.gov.uk/capacity.http://www.dca.gov.uk/capacity

Applications to the High Court

Applications to the High Court are made by hospitals when there is serious:

- Uncertainty about a patient's capacity to consent to treatment, or their best interest is being jeopardized
- Unresolved disagreement between a patient's family and health professionals

The Human Rights Act 1998

This Act highlights the issues concerning patient's human rights and the issues faced when they refuse treatment. This is outlined in the Acts below.

- Article 3 – opposes any degrading treatment, which is against the patient's will

- Article 8 – upholds the respect for private life and therefore opposes non-consensual treatment
- Article 9 – reinforces freedom of religion and objects to a patient's belief being ignored in order to give non-consensual treatment

Professional Issues

NMC (2018) Standards of proficiency for registered nurses

The new NMC (2018) proficiencies specify the knowledge and skills required by registered nurses when caring for people. They identify the role of the nurse in the 21st century is:

- Person-centred
- Accountable for their own actions
- Able to work autonomously
- An equal partner with other professionals
- Emotionally intelligent and resilient
- Able to manage their own personal health and well-being
- To know when to access support when needed
- To take a role in contributing to health, health protection and health prevention
- To provide leadership
- Able to work in the community and care for patients in their own homes
- Able to work in a changing, challenging environment
- Confident and think critically, apply knowledge and skills
- Able to incorporate evidence-based practice (EBP)

Accountability

Accountability within a critical care setting can be exercised by following Platform; one of the new NMC (2018) standards combined with The Code (NMC, 2015). In addition, accountability can be served in a number of ways within the critical care environment.

- The interests of the critically ill patient are paramount.
- Professional accountability must be exercised in such a manner as to ensure that the interests of the critically ill patients are respected and are not overridden by those of professionals or members of the multidisciplinary team.
- The notion of accountability requires the practitioner to seek, achieve and maintain a high standard of care delivery, at all times.
- Advocacy on behalf of the critically ill patient is an essential feature of exercising professional accountability on behalf of their patient's care; this is especially so if the patient is unconscious.

- The role of other persons who are involved in the delivery of health care to critically ill patients must be recognized, respected and honoured provided that the interest of patients is paramount.
- Public trust and confidence in the professional workforce must be upheld, and professionals must be seen to exercise their accountability in accordance with their code of professional conduct.

Responsibility

Responsibility, within a critical care setting, takes three major forms:

- Responsibility for self is often captured in a professional practice code (www.nmc-uk.org). Wilful failure to adhere to these responsibilities may result in legal action to exclude the individual from the right to practise.
- Responsibility for others is a far more complex issue, which varies according to position, degree of authority delegated and the nature of accountability to be exercised. It includes:
  - Concern for the safety of all in a shared working environment
  - The need to be explicit with all colleagues about authority and accountability issues as they affect both oneself and others
  - Working only within your scope of knowledge and ability
  - Professional responsibility entails the legitimate freedom to choose one course of action or intervention over another, combined with the responsibility for making correct choices in each circumstance.
- Professional responsibility, in particular, is an important issue as all professionals can be required to provide a service in areas in which they are not adequately prepared. This can occur because of work pressure and service pressure whereby funding restraints may require staff to work within another area. Being open about one's limitations must not be seen as a weakness but rather a key indicator of a mature and caring practitioner.

Autonomy

The notion of autonomy relates to the independence of action, meaning that one can perform one's total professional function on the basis of one's knowledge and judgement. It consists of making decisions and acting upon them. Furthermore, to be autonomous, one must be accountable. Autonomy is defined as:

- Self-rule
- A patient is free to make up their mind and act on their decisions
- A patient has the right to be given all the information required to make an informed, autonomous decision about care or treatment received or being offered
- Ethical principles of self-determination and self-governance with concomitant responsibility for one's actions

The ethical principle is important as no one has the legal right to impose their views upon another. Furthermore, everyone has the right to determine their actions and fate. By adopting a legal stance, one must realize that all surgical and medical interventions and delivery of nursing care are permitted because a patient has consented them to be carried out. The principle of autonomy underlines concerns about informed consent for surgical, medical and nursing interventions. All patients have the right to be respected as autonomous beings capable of making informed decisions for themselves and take responsibility for their own actions. Therefore, patients have the right to be kept informed of their condition and options available to them while undergoing treatment. Informed consent therefore consists of:

- The patient's right to know
- The patient's right to refuse treatment

In addition, patients have the fundamental right to give or withhold consent before an examination or treatment. The following must be borne in mind when giving information:

- Is something being withheld so that the patient makes the decision required by the doctor/nurse?
- If all the information were given, would the patient refuse treatment?

If information is withheld in order to ascertain consent to treatment, then truth-telling and honesty have been compromised; this places patient autonomy under threat.

Arguably, most consent is implied, such as a patient holding out an arm for blood to be taken; however, one cannot rely on this form of consent. In today's legal climate, it is important that all health care professionals who are able to obtain patient consent do so in an informed manner or they may face the legal repercussions if they fail to do so.

Ethics and Morality

Whether we are addressing nursing, medical or health care ethics, the critical care environment is likely to rate quite highly in terms of an ethical minefield. The arrival of 'life-support' machinery, advances in technology and the initial development of organ transplantation practices have prompted healthcare professionals to support their practices by developing strategies which allow, for example, brain stem death to be diagnosed correctly and prevent the misdiagnosis of brain stem death.

One of the reasons that nursing ethics in a critical care setting might be thought to be different from nursing ethics in a wider sense is the tendency to consider ethics in terms of dilemmas. Critical care dilemmas are often emphasized by the fact that the person concerned is frequently incapable of expressing a view because of their unconscious state.

Nurses and Morality

Self-development is an important area of morality for those in the caring profession, and it is the most important in that its neglect can seem a virtue. It is quite common for professional carers to live a life of devotion to their patients, and as a result, their own lives become empty and impoverished.

The duty of self-development can also be justified in terms of its benefits to other people. Since so much of the success of a nurse depends on a patient's perception of the helper, it is vital that the nurse be seen primarily as a human being who happens to be a nurse, and not vice versa. Furthermore, most nursing judgements are imbued with a moral element, and so it is important that the nurse is a morally developed person who happens to follow a given professional pathway.

Privacy and Dignity of the Critical Care Patient

Critical care patients are often totally dependent on the nurse looking after them for all their needs. Many of these needs are extremely personal, and it, therefore, falls to the bedside nurse to ensure that privacy and dignity are maintained as far as possible.

As health care professionals, we should all be skilled in maintaining the dignity of patients who are unable to do so for themselves, but it is important to remember that we are obliged to protect their privacy as well.

Maintaining privacy goes beyond simply ensuring that the patient is not visible to other visitors, patients and staff when a procedure is carried out. It is also about the information that we give out to those who enquire and the conversations that we hold about a patient in areas where what we say might be overheard.

As health care professionals, we are governed by our Professional, Legal, Employers and Personal Code of Conduct to maintain our patient's confidentiality at all times. The policing of confidentiality can often be difficult when caring for critically ill patients; they are often unconscious and thus unable to explain whom they would wish information to be disclosed to in what detail. Despite this dilemma, we are obliged to protect the patient's confidentiality as a first principle.

When dealing with privacy issues in critical care, it is important that you follow the guidelines:

- Except in exceptional circumstances, never give specific information about a patient's condition over the telephone. Generally, the decision about what constitutes exceptional circumstances will need to be made by senior members of the critical care team.
- Never give information about a diagnosis or potential diagnosis unless you know that the person enquiring has already been told.

- Always remember that your conversations in the critical care environment are likely to be overheard by others. Never discuss issues that would compromise a patient's privacy or dignity where they may be overheard.

Confidentiality

The health care practitioner is under a legal obligation not to disclose confidential information without the patient's consent. Disclosure of information may occur in the following ways:

- With patient consent
- Without patient consent, when the disclosure is required by law
- By accident
- Without patient consent, when disclosure is considered necessary in the public interest

Confidentiality is now incorporated in The Code NMC (2015) standards of proficiency, whereby confidentiality is not so much stated, as embedded throughout (nmc.org.uk).

Never discuss your patient's condition or identify them to non-medical/nursing colleagues.

Advocacy

Advocacy is defined as the act of pleading a cause on behalf of another. It is a process of acting for or on behalf of someone. The word advocacy is mentioned in The Code (NMC, 2015), which are the professional standards for nurses (nmc.org.uk).

Advocacy is an important principle in nursing adult patients because it makes it clear that generally adults are rational. Adults are capable of making choices and making decisions; however, some illnesses and specific situations, for example, admission to an ICU, may mean that the patient may temporarily lose their autonomy and a person will need to speak on their behalf. That person might be the nurse.

Always ensure that you are representing your patient's best interest when decisions are being made on their behalf.

Compassion

The term compassion is commonly used in the NHS today (Darzi, 2008). Often compassion is associated with being a human being. Compassion is often used interchangeably with caring, empathy, sympathy and compassionate care creating some confusion (Schantz, 2007). What can also be added to the words is the compelling need to act when someone is suffering. Dewer (2011) and Cole-King and Gilbert (2011) combined suggest four dimensions to compassion:

- Identifying that someone is suffering
- Understand that person
- Aim to alleviate that suffering
- Take action to prevent it

These four areas are shared with most views and definitions of compassion.

Compassionate Care

This is the act of a critical care nurse showing compassion in an act that benefits the patient. It is expressed through empathy, developing a therapeutic relationship, providing practical help, for example, the nurse often acts selflessly. The act of compassionate care involves:

- The character of the nurse
- Competence in knowledge and skills
- Ward leadership

Compassion Fatigue

This is sometimes seen as a type of burnout. Often in busy clinical areas such as critical care nurses provide high levels of compassion, which is associated with patient satisfaction. In addition, this contributes to high levels of fatigued nurses. On busy clinical areas, nurses' compassionate ideals and values can become compromised.

A way of preventing compassion fatigue and burnout is about finding appropriate interventions:

- Debriefing of challenging and difficult situations.
- Change of work situation when they become too challenging and difficult recognizing the signs and symptoms.
- Caring for yourself – self-compassion, kindness toward yourself, you cannot be selflessly concerned providing compassionate care towards others until the nurses look after themselves.

Professional Practice

Reflection

Dewey (1933) noted that the human brain often engages in cognitive processes that consist of mental streams of 'uncontrolled coursing of ideas'. Dewey defined these thought patterns as reflective thinking and maintained that their function was to 'transform a situation in which there is experienced obscurity, doubt, conflict, disturbance of some sort, into a situation that is clear, coherent, settled and harmonious'.

Dewey believed that reflective thinking arose out of situations of doubt, hesitation, perplexity and/or mental difficulty, and that it prompted the person to search, hunt or enquire to find material that will resolve doubt and settle or dispose of the perplexity.

Schon (1983) developed two key concepts reflection-in-action from reflection-on-action. However, since these were developed, hybrid models have been created in an attempt to tie the two together. Edwards (2017) reconceptualized reflection to further aid understanding of reflection using a four-dimensional approach:

1. Reflection before action — requires practitioners to reflect in advance of a learning event
2. Reflection in action — the moment-to-moment decision-making that it is taking place during care.
3. Reflection on action — occurs after the experience has taken place.
4. Reflection beyond action — relates to how the practitioner had developed/improved as a consequence of the previous three.

Reflective Thinking

This is essential for self-evaluation and improving one's clinical competency. It is argued that to reflect effectively and to practise reflectively are now requisite skills for all pre- and post-registration nurses. Reflection has become so integrated into mainstream nursing that it is easy to forget its radical origins. Reflection is a source of knowledge. Reflection offers a challenge to technical rationality, the straightforward application of context-free prepositional knowledge to practice.

Reflective accounts involve the practitioner paying attention to significant aspects of experience in order to make sense of them within the context of their work. By reflecting on and taking action to resolve the contradictions that occur in practice, practitioners come to know themselves and, as a consequence, learn to become increasingly effective in achieving desired work.

Reflection is a way in which professionals create new understandings of knowledge in practice. It pulls together disparate thoughts, attitudes and opinions and gives them focus (Rolfe, 2000). This results in new learning, a new angle, further reading to improve and develop knowledge. Therefore, there is a potential to write down and use reflection as a means of developing unique nursing knowledge.

Approaches to Guide Your Reflective Thinking and Writing

Gibbs reflective cycle (1988; Fig. 1.1)

- Description
- Feelings
- Evaluation
- Analysis
- Conclusion
- Action plan

Boud et al. (1985).
What − returning to the situation:

- Is the purpose of returning to the situation?
- Exactly occurred in your own words?
- Did other people do?
- Do you see as key aspects of the situation?

So what:

- Were you feeling at the time?
- Are your feelings now?
- Were the effects of what you did or did not do?
- 'Good' emerged from this situation?
- Were your experiences in comparison with those of your colleagues?
- Are the main reasons for feeling differently from your colleagues?

Now what:

- Are the implications for your colleagues and clients?
- Needs to happen to alter the situation?
- Are you going to do about the situation?
- Happens if you decide not to alter anything?
- Might you do differently if faced with a similar situation again?
- Are the best ways of getting further information about the situation should it arise again?

Johns model for structured reflection (1995; Table 5.8)

- Aesthetics (the art of what we do)
- Personal (self-awareness)

- Ethics (moral knowledge)
- Empirics (scientific knowledge)
- Reflexivity (how does it connect with previous experience)

To facilitate reflection upon an incident:

- Identify what you did well and what were your weaknesses
- Are you pleased with what went well — why?
- How can you improve your weaknesses?
- Identify your learning needs
- Compile an action plan
- Dialogue with others
- Identify future professional development needs
- What you did well and why
- Learning needs
- How can you resolve the learning needs?
- Professional reflective behaviour
- Reflection brings ideas of changes of action
- Changes of action
- Identifying learning needs
- Satisfying learning needs
- Changes in practice

Reflective Practice

The reflective processes enable the person to learn from experiences. The questions and possible action that results from the new perspectives that are taken:

- What was I trying to achieve?
- Why did I intervene as I did?
- What were the consequences of my actions for:
  - Myself?
  - The patient/family?
  - The people I work for?
- How did I feel about this experience when it was happening?
- How did the patient feel about it?
- How do I know how the patient felt about it?
- Influencing factors:
  - What internal factors influenced my decision-making?
  - What external factors influenced my decision-making?
  - What sources of knowledge did/should have influenced my decision-making?
- Could I have dealt with the situation better?
- What other choices did I have?

- What would be the consequences of these choices?
- How do I feel now about this experience?
- How have I made sense of this experience in the light of past experiences and future practice?
- How has this experience changed my ways of knowing:
  Empirics
  Aesthetics
  Ethics
  Personal
  Reflexivity
- Does this situation connect with previous experience?
- How could I handle this situation better?
- What would be the consequences of alternative actions for the patient/others/myself?
- Can I support myself and others better as a consequence?
- How 'available' am I to work with patients/families and staff to help them meet their needs?

There is a need in nursing for the development of competent practitioners who are flexible, adaptable and reflective. It has also been highlighted that competence is an important consideration for determining the scope of practice. A competent practitioner is deemed to have many attributes, including critical thinking and the ability to solve problems; a sub-skill of these is reflection. Continued professional development is essential in nursing, and reflective practice is suggested as one method of achieving this. Given the increased focus on reflection, it is intended to review the implications of these directives.

The Dangers of Reflection

Reflection in its many guises does not accurately verbalize or articulate the complex activity of psychologically and emotionally processing the issues that trouble us as nurses in everyday clinical practice from time to time. How do we deal with and process, psychologically and emotionally, the very real issues of critical care nursing, much of which is often left unspoken.

These events often result in a kind of ferocious emotional and psychological assault on nurses in their everyday work. Can reflection offer a solution? There is no doubt that carefully coached thinking can clearly help and offer therapeutic respite.

However, the more experienced and successful the practitioner, the less incentive there might be to acknowledge the need to analyse or theorize about their practice (Edwards, 2014), as there are many more pressing demands on critical care nurses time. This implies that less experienced critical care nurses could be mentored or taught by experienced professionals who cannot or do not reflect. Other problems have been levelled at reflection and reflective practice (Edwards, 2014):

- Reflective practice remains poorly defined
- The individualistic orientation of reflective accounts
- The realities of reflective practice as a confessional
- Reflection requires professional support
- Reflective practice: the challenges of reflection 'as not seeing yourself good enough'
- The impact of reflection on assessment during postgraduate critical care study

Critical Thinking

To deal effectively with rapid change, the health care professional needs to become skilled in higher-level thinking and reasoning. Critical thinking is relevant to all forms of nursing practice and can be used when situations or problems arise for which there is no definitive answer or to make it easier to find solutions. There is not always the theoretical evidence to support practice, therefore, critical care practitioners need to incorporate critical thinking processes into their practice in order to provide new answers to practical questions, which may not be answered with traditional research methods (Edwards, 2007). Every day critical care practitioners sift through an abundance of data and information to assimilate and adapt knowledge for problem clarification in an attempt to find solutions. Health care professionals need to be equipped and ready to find solutions, make decisions, and solve unique and complex problems within their clinical environment.

Critical thinking is essential and plays an important part of developing students, newly qualified and qualified health care professionals to critical care to interpret the often-complex issues in relation to practice. The explanations of critical thinking processes outlined in the literature are often complex. The concepts that interrelate with critical thinking are critical, analysis, thinking, synthesis and creative. Explanations of these interrelating concepts can be viewed in Table 5.9.

Professional bodies are promoting the concept of health care professionals being analytical practitioners, who are able to demonstrate critical thinking in the clinical setting (Roberts and Ousey, 2004). Similarly, critical thinking is widely recognized as an important part of nursing and equally essential to students and critical care practitioners alike.

The development of these cognitive processes encourages the individual to become open-minded, consider alternative perspectives, and respect the right of others to hold different opinions (Clarke and Holt, 2001). It is about equipping health care professionals with the tools needed for independent and life-long learning.

TABLE 5.9 Definition of the concepts in critical thinking.

Concept	Definition
Critical	• Often associated with fault finding, criticism, exercising negative judgement. • Uncovering hidden assumptions, individual values and beliefs, opinions. • Positive role to enhance the position of an argument. • Situations, practices and innovations can be interpreted, judged and preferred choices determined to bring about change.
Thinking	• A mental process whereby all the sorting and organizing of information takes place. • The formation of patterns is logically assembled, in the mind or on paper. • It is not a method that can be learned, but a process, an orientation of the mind. • It is the ability to consider all possible descriptions of a problem or situation and includes other people's perspectives. • The thinking process considers individual assumptions and past experiences and then expands perspectives by continual questioning.
Analysis	• Breaking down of material into parts. • Discovering the relationships between the parts. • Searching for and identifying evidence, and interpreting that evidence following a detailed examination.
Synthesis	• Once all sources have been identified, summarized and critiqued, the abstract summaries begin to create a synthesized product. • Identify common ideas within selected areas. • Sort all the ideas into reasonable divisions – conceptual thinking of ideas/solutions until they become organized. • What might be the result of implementing the different ideas/solutions? • What changes could be made? • How would people adapt/cope?
Creative	• Creativity is drawn from all of the above and is the ability to generate from them new ideas by combining, changing, or making additions to existing ideas. • Implementation of the decision/solution, which may involve changing, refining or developing something new.

The current and future critical care practitioner needs to be inquisitive, curious and enthusiastic, willing to seek the truth, be courageous about asking questions to obtain the best action for patients. It is not easy to challenge and question decisions, but it can be made possible if the question is thought through with all the arguments and rationale before the challenge takes place.

TABLE 5.10 Main areas to consider as part of critical thinking in critical care.

Phase 1		
1.	Interpretation and organization of the information	• Descriptions of the situation or problem • Logically assemble the information in the mind or on paper • Use a concept or mind map starting with a broad concept with linking words that are interrelated and connected • If possible, attempt to apply a systematic, organized and diligent approach to the situation (disorganized and abstract is also satisfactory at this time)
2.	Hidden assumptions	• What are these? • Values, attitudes and beliefs held by all those involved – are they opposite to your own beliefs or interests? • Consider positive and negative judgements that might be included • Try to be open-minded
3.	Nursing knowledge involved (both objective and subjective)	• Look for the evidence (theoretical and research) • The ethical principles involved • Knowledge from past experiences (personal or professional) • Practical knowledge/skills • What are your gut feelings about this? – Use your intuition
4.	Break down the situation/information into parts	• Is there a relationship between the parts? • How does one affect the other? • Analysis – examination of the ideas/arguments and possible courses of action
5.	Consider all of the options	• Include other people's views/perspectives • Continual questioning of the issues involved • Consideration of all of the possibilities • Flexibility – view the situation in many different ways with a variety of ideas • Be inquisitive, curious, courageous about asking questions to obtain all of the information

6.	Are there any conflicting issues?	• What are they?
		  • Nurse–patient
		  • Professional–ethical
		  • Nurse–nurse/doctor–nurse/other HCP–nurse
		• Air the concerns with each other
		• Team-working, communication, negotiation skills to resolve conflicts

Continued

TABLE 5.10 Main areas to consider as part of critical thinking in critical care.—cont'd

7.	Consider all of the options again, synthesizing of ideas	• Try to make sense of the muddle that is formulating in your mind or on paper • Put them in some type of order with the preferred solution and consider the consequences of one decision over another • Delete the ones that no longer apply or for which there are no resources • What is the best way forward and why?
8.	A decision has to be made	• A decision/solution/conclusion has to be reached • Self-confidence and trusting own reasoning when making decisions/solving problems
Phase 2		
9.	Defending the decision	• A reason why that decision was made • How the decision was reached • Justification has to be given
10.	Accountability and responsibility for the decision made	• Taking/accepting responsibility for the decision that has been made • Being accountable legally, ethically and professionally
11.	Evaluation of the process	• Critical reflection/reflective practice • Self-regulation/changing practices in the light of new insight and knowledge • Correcting oneself if found to be wrong • Learning from the situation/process/action plan for future learning needs • Personal learning and continuous professional development
12.	Creativity and innovation	• Implementation of the decision/solution • Implementing change, doing things in a different way, being creative and innovative (may go back to the start) • Changing, refining or developing new policies/procedures • Moving practice forward, doing things differently as a result of knowledge gained

Edwards, S.L., 2007. Critical thinking: a two phase framework. Nurse Education in Practice 7, 303–314.

Table 1.5 details some of the phases involved in critical thinking. By adopting this approach to care delivery, health care professionals can be seen as being in a better position to put forward the arguments and therefore influence change and subsequent practices.

Dealing with questions of quality of life and death, the lived experiences of patients suffering, in pain, breathless, and healing, health care professionals are continually weighing up the alternatives. They are looking at reasons for choosing one alternative over another in an open, flexible and attentive manner and considering what actions to follow. Professional, independent knowledge helps us to understand our patients better and is an integral part of critical thinking. The concept of nursing knowledge has been explored to demonstrate an example of how health care professionals' knowledge can best be applied to practice.

EBP/Health Care

For some time, there has been preoccupation with EBP in the health care setting. This term is now being replaced by the phrase evidence-based health care (EBH) by some authors. However, there does not appear to be any overarching principles that have been set to guide health care professions in the quest for achieving EBP. The underpinning key concepts include:

- Clinical effectiveness, practice development, (clinical) audit.
- Problem-solving, decision-making, clinical judgement and expertise.
- Research-based practice.

EBH brings responsibilities and issues for critical care nurses, health care organizations and patients alike, which are currently measured in respect of clinical effectiveness and quality. So as well as needing to take account of all of the key concepts, any guiding principles must also reflect the need for patient involvement and the drive for clinical effectiveness and quality.

EBH is a highly complex concept based upon the value judgements for nursing; this will focus on the patient experience encompassing the development of a wide range of knowledge. Best evidence comes from a variety of sources. The main source is generally considered to be research. In the absence of a gold standard for generating and judging nursing research evidence, other mechanisms are necessary to ensure that best evidence is developed and used in practice.

Nursing Knowledge

Nursing knowledge covers those aspects of knowledge that are relevant to nursing (Edwards, 2002). The different types of knowledge in nursing are many and varied; the generation of knowledge therefore becomes complex. Carper (1978) identified four ways of knowing: practical, scientific, personal (including experiential and intuition) and ethical.

Aesthetic Knowledge

- The importance of the art of nursing — it is expressive and viewed through action.
- Aesthetic knowledge is about expert practice and the motivation to care — the desire to care for someone and to enable them to cope with their illness or disability or to recover fully and perhaps enjoy an increased level of wellness and quality of life.
- It is about the understanding of human experience, insight into the dimensions of the human condition and the lived experiences of illness, suffering, dying, healing, pain and disability.

Sadly, generally only the patient witnesses it. Nursing practices that are encountered in everyday practice are deemed 'simple' yet are complex. Giving bed baths and getting patients to the bathroom are often cited as 'basic' tasks and are often delegated or taken for granted; their complexity and importance to nursing expertise are frequently overlooked. As a consequence, these 'simple' tasks are qualities that separate nursing from other disciplines, but often are not accorded the value they deserve.

Empirical Knowledge

- This includes empirical research, scientific enquiry, reductionism and positivism.
- This is often viewed as the only 'true' or 'valid' knowledge as it has been subjected to rigorous empirical testing utilizing mainly quantitative approaches to research.
- It includes theoretical knowledge from books, journals and conferences and draws on traditional ideas of science, including biology, sociology, psychology and pharmacology.

The use of empirical knowledge means that skill and knowledge of a particular situation must be supported by well-validated scientific knowledge. This implies EBP and highlights that empirical knowledge needs to inform practice. Empirical knowledge is often broadened to include inductive methodologies.

Personal Knowledge

- Is about becoming self-aware.
- It does not emanate from books, journals, lectures or academic conferences. It is also about 'we know more than we can say' or 'understanding without rationale'.
- It can be as valid as scientific knowledge and nurses can be confident in using it as a justification for actions.

However, personal knowledge is not utilized to support practice, as its credibility is of little or no consequence in relation to that of empirical knowledge. It includes both experiential knowledge and intuition.

Experiential Experiential includes gaining inner personal meaning from life experiences. Health care professionals have personal experiences such as having a baby, bereavement or a close family member or friend spending a period of time ill in hospital. These experiences develop experiential learning, which can form part of an individual's knowledge base so that they may draw upon clinical situations in the future. It is also knowledge that is gained from the experience of professional practice. Health care professionals have many clinical experiences during their years in practice, and it is these that can inform future practices when similar situations are met.

Intuition: 'Just Knowing'

- Intuition or tacit knowledge is widely accepted within health care.
- Intuition has been cited as an integral part of clinical practices.
- It helps to develop creativity and often it is not directly communicable in language.
- This type of knowledge is just a hunch, gut feeling.

Everyone can remember an intuitive tacit moment when caring for a patient. The health care professional has intuitively felt that something was wrong with a particular patient that they were caring for but could not express it in words. The patient's heart rate, blood pressure, respiratory rate, temperature, oxygen saturation and urine output were all normal. These intuitive feelings might be communicated to the doctor, who might suggest that the patient 'is all right'. You return from your coffee break to find that the patient has had a cardiac arrest.

Ethical Knowledge

- Is often thought to include questions about when to withdraw treatment, when to and when not to resuscitate a patient, allowing relatives to be present during resuscitation.
- It is also about making everyday clinical decisions, such as should you take the patient requesting to go to the toilet first or change and clean the patient who has been incontinent in the bed.
- It is about moral knowledge, decision-making and prioritizing. It includes what is good, right and responsible and involves confronting conflicting values.
- In ethical knowledge, there may be no satisfactory answer to the dilemma.

Emotional Intelligence

Emotional intelligence is generally described as the ability to manage your own emotions and the emotions of others (Raghubir, 2018). There are generally four attributes placed into two categories, which are accepted across disciplines, including nursing:

Personal

- Self-awareness – understanding and recognizing your own emotions, motivations, identifying achievements and emotions, strengths and weaknesses
- Self-management – control or redirect emotions, non-judgemental

Social

- Social awareness – observe and understand emotions, the needs and concerns of others, see other people's views
- Social/relationship management – management emotions of self and others to create good relationships, communication, inspire and influence others.

Emotional intelligence can influence critical nursing practice, as it focuses on meeting the needs of individuals, families, colleagues and addresses the nurses' own emotions in order to help understand how they may influence and improve their own professionalism and care. Emotional intelligence identifies the nurses' sensitivity to mood and emotions as an integral part of care to help critical care nurses enhance their competence as a nurse to benefit patients.

Resilience

The concept of resilience has had a lot of interest in psychology and concentrates on personal traits such as:

- Personality and adaptation in high-risk situations
- An individual's reaction to events, building up of coping strategies
- The capacity to respond and endure despite stressors and misfortune
- Stress resistance that can help guard against mental illness
- Human agency and survival
- The power of individuals to make use of resources that help nurture well-being
- The capacity of individuals to use social networks, families and communities to provide resources during difficult situations
- Creative problem-solving and the capacity to be flexible and accurate
- Being able to see different perspectives
- Continuing with daily life despite obstacles
- The capacity to be open-minded

The promotion of these skills in nursing can be beneficial in equipping critical care nurses with coping strategies to help with the difficult and challenging experiences they encounter on a day-to-day basis.

However, there is a danger in giving too high a significance on critical care nurses' obtaining a high level of resilience. For example, when critical care nurses are unable to find effective ways of coping, it would be easy for those in managerial positions to blame the individual for not being resilient enough, rather than their lack of providing appropriate support, education and training.

Decision-Making in Critical Care

Decision-making within a critical care setting is both complex and challenging to the health care team; therefore, a team approach is often adopted so that the views of all staff members may be sought — in doing so promoting the best possible outcome for the patient, staff and department.

Within the realms of decision-making, there are a number of areas where the expertise of the critical care team is sought. These include issues concerning common matters faced by the critical care team, uncommon matters rarely encountered by the critical care team and matters of extreme emergency where decision-making process is cut short and made by individuals rather than the team. However, this is not to say that the situation is not reflected upon later when a team discussion takes place.

In relation to seeking patient's views in the decision-making process, critical illness imposes severe limitations on the validity of patient autonomy, which requires a patient to be mentally competent and fully informed. In such cases, the views of the patient are sought via close family members, friends and critical care staff members so that their views are taken into account when making decisions about treatments and care issues.

Health Promotion

Health-promoting activities have long been an integral part of nursing care. The nurse's primary focus is to assist individuals to achieve a positive state of health, well-being and improved quality of life.

The notion of health promotion may be applied at all levels of patient care from a ward-based setting to a critical care setting. Therefore, within a critical care setting, health promotion activities will be aimed at restoring health or helping the individual to achieve an improved state of well-being and functioning. The promotion aspect is aimed at helping individuals to positively change their behaviour and to alter lifestyle in order to improve their health. Individuals with chronic health problems may never achieve the feeling of improved health, but they have the right to obtain the knowledge, skills and resources needed to maximize their quality of life.

The concept of patient teaching is important in educating the patient so that they are best positioned to make an informed decision about their health and well-being. It must be accepted that patients have the right to make their own decisions and assume responsibility for their health − effective patient education strategies should follow this aspect of care as a natural sequence.

Section 6

Pharmacology

Section Outline

6.1 MEDICATION MANAGEMENT

It is important for critical care nurses to understand and grasp the complexity of pharmacology. Medication management is one of the interventions that can contribute to patients' positive outcomes and recovery. Critical care nurses are at the forefront of medication management interventions and need to understand the purpose of prescribing drugs, what the body does to the drug and the action of the drug. The administration of drugs is not without problems, drugs can be poisonous and dangerous, and mistakes can be made.

Adverse Effects — Drug Toxicity

Adverse Effects

- There is no drug that is 100% safe.
- All drugs have side effects.
- These are usually predictable and dose related.

Drug Toxicity

- Drugs are more toxic in the very elderly and very young.
- Underlying pathologies also affect drug toxicity, for example, liver or renal disease whereby the drug may be allowed to build up in the system.
- Other drugs the patient may be taking have to be taken into account — polypharmacy.

Adverse Drug Reactions

These are becoming increasingly common (Richards, 2009). Some of these reactions can be minor (side effects), whereby others can be life-threatening (adverse reactions). Common drugs involved in adverse drug reactions are as follows (Richards, 2009):

- Nonsteroidal antiinflammatory drugs (NSAIDs)
- Psychotropic drugs
- Antimicrobials
- Diuretics
- Analgesics
- Antihypertensive
- Tranquillizers
- Antidepressants
- Hypoglycaemic agents
- Cardiovascular drugs
- Warfarin
- Digoxin

Some common side effects and adverse drug reactions are as follows:

- Constipation – common with narcotics, analgesics, antacids, tricyclic antidepressants
- Diarrhoea – antibiotics, antacids containing magnesium
- Nausea – common side effects of narcotic analgesics and anticancer drugs.
- Flatulence – a problem with metformin
- Rash – antibiotics, benzodiazepines, aspirin
- Dizziness – sensation of imbalance or faintness, confusion, blurred or double vision, narcotic analgesics, decongestants, antihistamines, vasodilators
- Hypertension – sympathomimetics, corticosteroids, monoamine oxidase inhibitors (MAOIs)
- Hypotension – postural hypotension, calcium channel blockers, anti-parkinson drugs, diuretics
- Thrush – antibiotics, corticosteroids
- Dry mouth – antimuscarinics, antihistamines, phenothiazine and antidepressants
- Drowsiness – often due to overdose
- Respiratory depression – narcotic analgesics, barbiturates, phenothiazine and general anaesthetics
- Allergic liver disease
- Haematological reactions – agranulocytosis NSAIDs, sulphonamides

- Anaphylaxis — a severe life-threatening condition that leads to difficulty in breathing and circulatory failure. A bodywide stimulation of the inflammatory immune response, commonly caused by penicillin leads to:
  - Urticaria
  - Angioedema
  - Laryngeal oedema
  - Bronchospasm
  - Hypotension
  - Rhinitis
  - Conjunctivitis
  - Gastroenteritis

All drug reactions need to be reported.

Classification of Adverse Reactions

- Type A — dose-related excessive or normal, but predictable, pharmaco-dynamics effects greater than expected
- Type B (idiosyncratic) — unpredictable and not usually part of the normal action of the drug, includes anaphylaxis (rapid action needed, stop drug, administer adrenaline), more common in patients with allergies
- Type C (continuous) — found in drugs that are used long-term
- Type D (delayed reaction) — includes teratogenesis (effects foetal development) and carcinogenesis (can lead to cancer)
- Type E (ending of use) — drug should be reduced gradually, for example, steroids

Margin of Safety

Some drugs such as Digoxin, Aminoglycoside antibiotics, Gentamycin and Tobramycin have a narrow margin of safety, and as such, blood levels of these drugs need to be monitored. Thus, the dose range of some drugs need to be within the drugs effective level:

- The minimum effective drug concentration to have an effect
- The maximum safe concentration

Poisoning/Overdose

This can be intentional, accidental or iatrogenic or criminal intent. There are only specific antidotes available for very few poisons or drugs. Consult either the National Poisons Information Service or TOXBASE (BNF, 2018).

Common Overdoses are as Follows (Richards, 2009):

- Alcohol
- Aspirin
- Opioids
- Paracetamol
- Antidepressants
- Antipsychotics
- Benzodiazepines
- Beta-blockers
- Calcium-channel blockers
- Lithium
- Others poisons
    - Noxious gases — carbon monoxide, sulphur dioxide, chlorine, phosgene, ammonia
    - Nerve agents
    - Pesticides
    - Snake bites and animal stings

General Principles

- Diagnosis — time is imperative limiting the period for ingestion
- Unconscious patient
- Relative involvement

Assessment

- Airway
- Vital signs — respiration may be impaired, hypotension is common, cardiac conduction defects
- Conscious level — convulsions
- Temperature — hypothermia may develop
- Body surfaces — needle sites
- Investigations — blood for drug levels

Drug Manipulation

- Decrease absorption of drug — emetics, gastric lavage, absorbent (activated charcoal), cathartics (magnesium citrate, magnesium sulphate)
- Increase excretion — forced diuresis (diuretics), alkalosis (hyperventilation, sodium bicarbonate), and haemodialysis, an antiemetic to induce vomiting is not encouraged as it may reduce the efficiency of charcoal treatment

- Administration of specific overdose antidote — paracetamol (Parvolex), narcotic (naloxone/NARCAN), heparin (protamine sulphate), warfarin (vitamin K)

Medication Errors

1 in 10 patients experiences medication-related errors. Most drug errors go unreported. A drug error can occur at any point along the medication trajectory and may involve the patient coming into contact with a variety of health care practitioners (HCPs), both inside and outside the hospital environment. This might include doctors, pharmacists and allied health professionals not just nurses administering the drug.

Factors That Contribute to Drug Errors
Faulty System Error

- Heavy workloads, poor teamwork and communication
- Lack of staff
- Poor management/leadership
- A blame culture when mistakes are made
- Complex error reporting systems
- Limited access to technology, electronic databases
- Poor storage of drugs, crowded preparation area and medication trolley

Condition of the Environment Where Clinicians Work

- The distractions, noise and poor lighting
- The environment where clinicians work
- Lack of awareness of circumstances of when and where an error can occur

Human or Personal Factors

- Poor calculation competency, lack of confidence
- Inadequate knowledge of medication, lack of experience
- Fatigue/illness, poor communication
- Prescriber's poor handwriting, prescriptions unclear, use of abbreviations
- Violation of double-checking practices (if a recommended hospital protocol)
- These factors are unintentional and unpredictable
- Nurses' preparation and administration of drugs

A number of issues related to the causes of drug errors give the sense that it is not just one factor but also a combination of failures that lead to a change in drug practice behaviour compounded by intense resource and workforce pressures. Edwards and Axe (2018) discuss the importance of combining the knowledge already accumulated of how drug errors occur is needed to better understand medication management mistakes and take action.

Strategies to Mitigate Drug Errors

Critical care nurses can take action by implementing strategies to prevent the occurrence of drug errors:

- Interruption minimizing strategies — nurses modifying their practice to enhance patient safety to reduce drug errors.
  - Visual reminders — the use of visual reminders has been used as a means to guide medication management (Edwards and Axe, 2015).
  - Protected time — when undertaking drug preparation, administration and management interruptions can be reduced by ensuring nurses wear a tabard or provide a reminder to other staff this is taking place.
  - Team communication — ensure that all team members are aware that drug preparation, administration and management are being performed to reduce distractions.
- Information technology — to reduce medication errors factors have included the introduction of information technologies.
- Drug error reporting — all drug errors need to be reported, so these can be collated, and common causes identified and learned from.
- Clear definitions of a drug error, which can lead to misconceptions and nonreporting of the error, as it was not clear which errors need reporting and those that do not.
- Implementing an evidence-based approach.
- The use of evidence to support medication management — utilizing research studies that provide evidence of the risks of drug errors to patients in hospital or by applying pathophysiological principles and would be able to omit a potassium supplement on the grounds that the patient's potassium level is too high (by checking daily blood results); or Digoxin, as the apex and radial pulses were below 60 bpm or the patient has a bradycardia.
- Improving knowledge and understanding — critical care nurses need to have an in-depth knowledge and understanding of pharmacology, which can contribute to reducing the occurrence of drug errors during medication management.
- Questioning practice/challenging — to prevent risk and ensure safety.
- Medication reviews — frequent medication reviews of patients' medications undertaken at regular intervals.
- Identifying complacency and attitudes towards safety — reduce the blind trust in clinical support systems, overconfidence in knowledge and familiarity of patients, which can lead to poor safety attitudes.

6.2 PHARMACOKINETICS AND PHARMACODYNAMICS

This is about the essential principles of drugs following their administration (Richards, 2009). Patients within critical care rely on specialist nurses to ensure that medicines are administered appropriately. It is vital for critical care nurses to have a sound understanding of the two classes of pharmacology: (1) pharmacokinetics, the way the body affects the drug with time (absorption, distribution, metabolism and excretion of drugs), and (2) pharmacodynamics, the effects of the drug on the body.

Pharmacokinetic Process

Absorption

With the exception of intravenous (IV) drugs, drugs must be absorbed across a cell membrane before entering the systemic circulation. Oral drugs are absorbed in the upper small bowel because of its large surface area.

- Drugs absorbed from the gastrointestinal tract (GIT) enter the portal circulation, and some are extensively metabolized as they pass through the liver.
- Drugs that are lipid soluble are readily absorbed orally and are rapidly distributed throughout the body water compartments.
- Many drugs are bound to albumin, and equilibrium occurs between the bound and free drug in the plasma. The drug that is bound to albumin does not exert a pharmacological action.
- The bioavailability is the fraction of the administered dose that reaches the systemic circulation; IV drugs have 100% bioavailability.

Drugs administered orally have to overcome the physical barrier of the gut wall. The absorption process is affected by many factors:

- Formulation
- Stability to acid and enzymes
- Motility of gut
- Food in the stomach
- Degree of first-pass metabolism (see later)
- Lipid solubility

Distribution

Distribution around the body occurs when the drug reaches the circulation to travel to its site of action. It must then filter through the capillaries and penetrate tissues to act. Factors that affect drug distribution are as follows:

- Plasma protein binding sites albumin − competition can occur if two-protein binding drugs are prescribed, for example, aspirin and NSAIDs, the bound drug will not reach the tissues, but the unbound free drug will, enhancing the combined drug effect leading to potential side effects.

- Specific drug receptor sites in tissues.
- Regional blood flow.
- Reduced in diabetes.
- Enhanced flow, for example, liver.
- Lipid solubility.
- Membrane of GIT.
- Highly water-soluble drugs, for example, gentamicin.
- Disease.
- Liver disease — low plasma protein levels.
- Renal disease — high blood levels.
- The blood–brain barrier — prevents the entry of harmful drugs into the brain; some drugs can pass through and lead to drowsiness.
- The first-pass effect — drugs absorbed from GIT pass into the bloodstream:
  - Some drugs are inactivated the first time they pass through the liver, and this affects drug doses given by different routes:
    - Propranolol, if given IV, is given in a dose of 1 mg, but if administered orally the dose is 40 mg.
    - Can also affect possible routes of administration such as glyceryl trinitrate (GTN), as this cannot be given orally except by bypassing the liver, for example, sublingually.

Metabolism

Metabolism of drugs takes place before the body excretes them and is the first stage of drug clearance. The metabolism of drugs occurs in the liver and involves a group of enzymes:

- The microsomal mixed function oxidases (cytochrome P450 system of enzymes). These transform drugs into products that are more water soluble and easier to excrete. The majority of drug metabolism occurs in the liver. It involves two general types of reaction:
  - Phase 1 reaction — the biotransformation of the drug — oxidations are the most common reactions, and these are catalysed by the mixed function oxidases that increase water solubility.
  - Phase 2 reactions — drugs from phase I cannot be excreted efficiently by the kidneys and are made more hydrophilic by conjugation with compounds in the liver.

Metabolism also occurs in the gut lining, kidney and lungs. The majority of drugs that are metabolized are as follows:

- Inactivated (propranolol) — slowed in liver failure.
- Activated (enalapril).
- Remain unchanged (atenolol).
- The products of metabolism (metabolites) are longer acting than the original drug (diazepam).

Concomitant drug administration may influence metabolism:

- Phenytoin can induce liver enzymes − increasing the metabolism of other drugs.
- Cimetidine can inhibit liver enzymes − reducing metabolism
- These can have serious consequences if the patient is already on other drug therapies.

Other factors can affect drug metabolism:

- Age (including elderly and paediatrics)
- Alcohol consumption
- Disease (impaired liver function, dose reduction may be necessary for drugs metabolized in the liver), for example, chlormethiazole
- Smoking

Excretion

Main route of excretion is the kidney in the urine either unchanged or as metabolites. Excretion can occur in the faeces, whereby it first circulates from the small intestine to the liver then passes into the bile and into the GIT. If renal or liver impairment is present, reduced dose may be required (digoxin or gentamicin). It can be reabsorbed and reenter the liver. Metabolism has been reversed (by enzymes present in the gut or by gut microflora), converts the drug so that it can be reabsorbed. This can lead to a cycle known as the enterohepatic recirculation and accounts for the prolonged effect of some drugs. Excretion varies with age and can lead to discoloration of the urine or faeces.

Frequent blood samples may be required for some drugs; in order for some drugs to be effective, a certain blood level has to be obtained. Drugs are generally poisonous and, at higher blood level concentrations, can lead to serious consequences, even death. For all drugs, there is also a minimum effective concentration, below which there will not be a therapeutic effect.

Make sure that you are aware of the patient's drug blood levels before administering drugs in patients with liver and/or renal impairment.

Factors affecting excretion are as follows:

- Renal failure
- Blood flow to the kidneys
- Glomerular filtration rate (GFR)

- Urine flow rate and pH, which indirectly alters:
  - Passive reabsorption and
  - Active tubular secretion.

The processes involved are drug absorption, distribution, metabolism and excretion change across the lifespan. This is because the body systems of young children are still developing and maturing; the manner in which their bodies handle drugs can be quite different to that of an adult. The effects of drugs may be either stronger or weaker than those observed in adults given the same treatment. At the other end of the lifespan, the elderly experience age-related changes in body structure and function that alter the behaviour of drugs after administration.

Pharmacodynamics

This is the study of the effects of drugs on the body or the biological processes. It is concerned with the pharmacological effect of drugs at their site(s) of action and considers mechanisms of action for both therapeutic and adverse effects of the drug.

- Pharmacological responses are initiated by the molecular interactions of drugs with cells, tissues or other body constituents.
- Drug molecules must exert some chemical influence on one or more cellular constituents to produce a pharmacological response.
- To affect functioning of cellular molecules, the drug must approach the molecules closely.
- Another requirement is that the drug must have some sort of nonuniform distribution within the body or the chance of interaction if the drug molecules distributed at random would be negligible. This means that a drug must bind in some way to constituents of the cell to produce an effect.

Drugs That Act on Receptor Sites

Most drugs produce their effects by acting on specific protein molecules usually located in the cell membrane. These proteins are called receptors and normally respond to endogenous chemicals in the body. A chemical that binds to a receptor is known as a ligand.

- For most drugs, the site of action is at a specific biological molecule − the receptor. A receptor is the primary site of action of a drug.
- Various types of receptor exist, and each responds to a different chemical or hormone, for example, histamine, acetylcholine (ACh), adrenaline and dopamine.
- When these receptors are bound to a certain chemical, this directs a change to occur in the cell, which then alters an activity of the cell.

Drugs That Act on Neurotransmitters

- Many endogenous hormones, neurotransmitters and other mediators exert their effects as a result of high-affinity binding or specific macromolecular protein or glycoprotein receptors in plasma membranes or cell cytoplasm.
- Some psychotropic drugs act on the brain and central nervous system (CNS) and reduce the reuptake/destruction of neurotransmitters, for example, dopamine, serotonin, noradrenaline to allow them to remain around for longer.

Many drugs cause their effects by combining with receptors or neurotransmitters and are either:

- Agonists interact with a receptor mimicking the effect of a natural mediator:
  - Adrenaline is a beta-receptor agonist, which stimulates the cardiac beta-receptors — increases heart rate.
  - Psychotropic drugs can increase the production of particular neurotransmitters or can interfere with the reuptake of neurotransmitter substances forcing them to remain in the synapse and interact with receptors longer.
- Partial agonists — maximal response falls short of the full response.
  - Pindolol and oxprenolol — block access of the natural agonist
- Antagonists block a receptor to prevent such an effect.
  - Atenolol is a beta-receptor antagonist — slows heart rate by blocking the cardiac beta-receptors and reducing physiological stimulation.
  - Interfere with the release of neurotransmitters into the synapse, blocks neurotransmitter receptors from being activated and can make less neurotransmitters available.

The Commonest Ways in Which Drugs Produce Their Effects

Not all drugs work via receptors for endogenous mediators or via neurotransmitters and many drugs exert their effect by combining with other regulatory proteins and interfering with their function:

- Ion channels — physical blocking of channel by the drug molecule — sodium channel blocking by local anaesthetics or by binding to accessory sites to facilitate opening of channels.
- Enzymes — many drugs are targeted in this way:
  - Acting as competitive inhibitors, either reversible inhibitors (neostigmine on acetylcholinesterase) or irreversible inhibitors (aspirin on cyclooxygenase), known as substrate analogues.

- Many act as a false substrate — fluorouracil replaces uracil and blocks DNA synthesis.
- Some drugs are prodrugs and need enzymic degradation to convert them to the active form, for example, diamorphine to morphine.
- Transport proteins — drugs may interfere with the uptake of ions or small molecules across the cell membrane:
  - Cocaine interferes with the reuptake of noradrenaline.
  - Digoxin interferes with the sodium/potassium pump.
- Other cellular macromolecules — these do not involve regulatory proteins:
  - Chemical action, for example, antacids (magnesium hydroxide).
  - Drugs which act by physical action — osmotic diuretics (mannitol).
  - Drugs which act by a physicochemical action — inhaled anaesthetics, which act by altering the protein of cell membranes.

Potency of Drugs

This is the amount of drug necessary to produce a given effect (Richards, 2009). The more potent a drug is, the smaller the amount required to produce an effect. The interaction between a drug and the binding site of the receptor depends on the 'fit' of the two molecules. The closer the fit and the greater the number of bonds, the stronger will be the attractive forces between them:

- If a drug is potent, it produces effects at low concentration.
- If a drug has a high potency, it is a consequence of high affinity for a specific receptor.
- Affinity is the tendency to bind to receptors.
- Efficacy is the ability, once bound, to initiate changes that lead to effects.
- If a drug is specific, small changes in drug structure lead to profound changes in potency or cause a change from agonist to antagonist:
  - Selectivity is the phenomenon that allows drugs to be useful; a drug must act selectively on particular cells and tissues.
  - Specificity is reciprocal — individual classes of drug bind only to certain targets, and individual targets only recognize certain classes of drug.
  - No drug acts with complete specificity — will only produce an effect.
- Potency is independent of efficacy, and efficacy is usually more important than potency when selecting a drug for clinical use.
- The lower the potency of a drug and the higher the dose needed, the more likely that sites of action other than the primary one will assume significance:
  - This is often associated with the appearance of unwanted side effects, of which no drug is free — varies from trivial to fatal.
  - Pharmaceutical companies try hard to manufacture drugs that are more selective and thus less dangerous to other tissues.

Mode of Action

- If the basic mode of action of a drug is via a receptor, then it is likely that:
  - It will be potent;
  - It will have biological specificity and may produce opposite effects on apparently similar tissue type;
  - It will have chemical specificity, and changes in the chemical structure of a drug molecule may have a large or small effect on its pharmacological activity.
- Specific antagonists abolish the effects of the drug on the tissue.
- If plasma concentration of the drug is too high (outside the therapeutic range), toxicity will occur.
- If plasma concentration is too low, treatment will fail.
- The aim of treatment is to keep the plasma concentration within the therapeutic range.
- The plasma levels of certain drugs are measured in practice for these reasons.

Drug Interactions

Drugs are chemicals and may interact with one another. When this happens, a drug's action may be:

- Suppressed
- Rendered completely inactive
- Increased

The therapeutic action of one drug may interfere with the therapeutic action of another — either cancelling out or amplifying effects.

Combinations of drugs must be carefully considered to avoid drug interactions. As the number of medications prescribed for a patient increases (polypharmacy), so does the potential for drug interactions. With so many drugs given at the same time and so many drugs available, it is impossible to predict the interactions that can occur. Any adverse reaction needs to be reported to the appropriate authorities. The *British National Formulary* (BNF, 2018) contains lists of known interactions, and these should always be consulted before drug mixtures are administered. Some produce minor problems, and others can be fatal. The types of drug interactions that occur are:

- Outside the body — generally due to storage conditions, too much light, oxygen or moisture, interactions with containers whereby the chemicals contained within the drug are prone to degradation.
- In the GIT — some food chemicals may react with drugs.
- After absorption — where the most known interactions take place, usually when more than one drug is administered concurrently.

Pharmacogenetics

After taking into account all the issues related to pharmacokinetics and pharmacodynamics, and the age, level of nutrition, occupation and state of health of the patient, there are still individual differences in drug metabolism. This is described in terms of a person's genetic make-up and how this affects the body's response to drugs. How some patients metabolize or inactivate drugs and facilitate their excretion is to a large extent determined by inheritable traits — our genes. In addition, different ethnic groups show different pharmacokinetic profiles for a number of drugs.

There are many issues to consider when administering individual patient therapy. A good understanding of the fundamental principles of drug therapy should help critical care nurses to optimize patient care. An increase in critical care nurses' contribution to multidisciplinary care in relation to drug administration/therapy is currently being explored (Edwards and Axe, 2015).

6.3 CLASSIFICATION OF DRUGS USED IN CRITICAL CARE

The classification of drugs (Table 6.1) is massive and is thus too huge to do it justice. The classes of drugs outlined in this section are brief. However, there are many texts (Galbraith et al., 2007; Neal, 2005; Richards, 2009; BNF, 2018) that go into much more detail regarding the drugs used in critical care. For further information, it is recommended that you use these and/or other sources for more in-depth information.

Adrenergic Drugs

These drugs are within the domain of sympathetic nervous system function. In the peripheral nervous system, only the sympathetic postganglionic fibres are adrenergic (a nerve that releases noradrenaline). Adrenaline affects adrenergic receptors. Stimulants that induce effector responses of a 'flight' or 'fight' character are sometimes referred to as sympathomimetics (drugs which mimic the sympathetic nervous system), while blocking, agents prevent these responses and are termed sympatholytics (drugs which block or inhibit sympathetic stimulation).

Sympathomimetics (Adrenergic Receptor Stimulation/Agonist)

- Direct-acting — they act directly on beta$_1$ adrenoreceptors — adrenaline, noradrenaline, isoprenaline, dopamine and dobutamine (Table 1.9):
  - Increase rate and force of contraction of the heart, increase cardiac output and exact positive chronotropic and inotropic effects.

TABLE 6.1 Classes of drugs.

Class of drug	Action of drug class
Antiemetic	Nausea, vomiting
Anticoagulant	Prevents or reduces clotting of the blood in blood vessels, e.g., heparin or warfarin
Antiplatelet	Decreases platelet aggregation – aspirin and dipyridamole
Antihypertensive	Used to reduce blood pressure – examples are beta-adrenergic antagonists (beta-blockers) such as atenolol, ACE inhibitors such as captopril, calcium channel blockers, e.g., nifedipine and diuretics such as bendroflumethiazide
Analgesic	Relieves pain
Hypnotic	Induces sleep – dependency-producing, e.g., triazolam
Anxiolytic	Relieves anxiety – used to alleviate acute and severe anxiety states, e.g., diazepam
Anaesthetic	Insensible stimuli – loss of sensation. Local anaesthesia – sensory nerve impulses are blocked, and the patient remains alert. General anaesthesia – loss of consciousness, and patient is unaware of and unresponsive to painful stimulation, can be maintained by inhalation of anaesthetic gases.
Antibiotic	Antibacterial – length of treatment depends on the nature of the infection and the response to treatment, e.g., penicillin, ampicillin, erythromycin, metronidazole and vancomycin
Antacid	Neutralizes the acidity of the gastric juice, given in dyspepsia, gastritis, peptic ulcer and oesophageal reflux
Antiarrhythmic	Given to prevent or reduce cardiac irregularities of rhythm, e.g., digoxin, amiodarone
Antihistamine	Blocks the release of histamine – released in an allergic reaction, used for insect bites and stings to reduce irritation and inflammation.
Antispasmodic	Relaxes smooth muscle as found in the gut – useful in abdominal colic and distension as in irritable bowel disorder
Antidepressant	Relieves depression – these may be tricyclics such as amitriptyline and imipramine or monoamine oxidase inhibitors
Antipyretic	Reduces temperature – such as aspirin, paracetamol
Antiepileptic	Epilepsy control – to prevent the occurrence of seizures, only one drug and combinations to be avoided, e.g., phenytoin, sodium valproate, carbamazepine

Continued

TABLE 6.1 Classes of drugs.—cont'd

Class of drug	Action of drug class
Bronchodilator	Dilates airways – relaxes the bronchial smooth muscle and causes dilatation of the air passages, e.g., salbutamol, ipratropium bromide
Cytotoxic	Used in the treatment of cancer, e.g., methotrexate and vincristine
Corticosteroids	Synthetic steroid hormones synthesized by the adrenal cortex – antiinflammatory and suppress the immune system
Diuretic	Increases urine output – best given in the morning, e.g., furosemide, bendroflumethiazide, reduces the circulating volume in heart failure and hypertension
Fibrinolytic	Digests fibrin in blood clots – used to dissolve the blood clot and restore circulation to the heart following myocardial infarction, e.g., streptokinase
Immunosuppressive	Suppresses the immune system and used in autoimmune disorders or following transplantation to reduce rejection of the donor organ, e.g., azathioprine
Inotrope	Affects the contraction of the heart muscle, e.g., digoxin
Laxative	Promotes a softer or bulkier stool or encourages a bowel action and given for constipation, e.g., lactulose
Miotic	Constricts the pupil of the eye – used in glaucoma to open up drainage channels, e.g., pilocarpine
Muscle relaxant	In conjunction with general anaesthetics to produce complete muscle relaxation, prevent muscles from contracting, stop respiration for ventilation, e.g., atracurium and vecuronium
Neuroleptic	Acts on nervous system; antipsychotic
Vasodilator	Dilates blood vessels reducing BP
Hypoglycaemic agent	Glucagon to treat hypoglycaemic states
Hyperglycaemic agent	Insulin for intravenous and subcutaneous use in type I diabetes. Oral drugs for use in type II diabetes.

ACE, angiotensin-converting enzyme; *BP,* blood pressure.

- Increase the level of lipid concentration in blood and convert into energy.
- Depress digestion and gastrointestinal motility.
- Release renin into the renal blood, resulting in the formation of angiotensin II, potent vasoconstrictor and increase GFR.
- Indirectly acting − by causing a release of noradrenaline from the stores at nerve endings (amphetamines)
  - Preventing reuptake of noradrenaline (tricyclic antidepressants − amitriptyline)
  - Preventing destruction of noradrenaline − MAOIs
  - Preventing the release of noradrenaline − guanethidine
  - Causing nerve ending to synthesize a false transmitter − methyldopa
- Prolonged use of local anaesthesia − causes vasoconstriction of the skin; this delays reabsorption from the injection site and prolongs the anaesthetic action.
- Acute anaphylactic reactions − gross swelling of the skin and mucous membranes; intramuscular adrenaline is effective as an emergency measure.
- Heart block − beta$_1$ agonists − isoprenaline

Adrenoreceptors (Adrenergic Receptor Blocking/Antagonists)

The Uses of Adrenoreceptor Antagonists

- These drugs act selectively on alpha and beta receptors; they do not usually act on both
- Hypertension − phentolamine, phenoxybenzamine, prazosin and terazosin

Alpha-Receptor Antagonists

Alpha-receptor antagonists result in:

- Vasodilatation and a drop in blood pressure;
- Relaxation of bladder and prostate gland inhibiting hypertrophy;
  They are used for:
  - Control of hypertension
  - Tumours of the adrenal gland
  - Urinary retention
  The following are the side effects:
  - Nasal congestion
  - Postural hypotension
  - Inhibition of ejaculation
  - Lack of energy

Beta-Receptor Antagonists

Block the beta receptors in the heart, peripheral vasculature, bronchi, pancreas and liver:

- At rest, they have little effect on heart rate, cardiac output or arterial pressure; they reduce the effect of excitement or exercise on these.
- Reduce coronary blood flow, but less oxygen consumption; oxygenation is improved, useful in angina.
- Reduce the force of cardiac contraction and slow the heart rate lengthening coronary artery perfusion time during diastole; can precipitate heart failure in patients with weak contractility.
- Antihypertension effect − produce a gradual fall in blood pressure over a period of several days.
- Increased airways resistance − dangerous in asthmatics and can produce severe asthma attacks.
- Have an antidysrhythmic effect.

They should not be used in:

- Severe bradycardia, heart block, cardiogenic shock, left ventricular failure (LVF)
- Severe asthma
- Severe depression
- Raynaud's disease

Cardioselective Beta-Blockers

There is some selectivity possible now with cardioselective beta-blockers; however, these are not absolutely cardiac specific and still block the beta$_2$ receptor to some degree. They have less effect on airway resistance but are not free from this effect. There is still a risk of inducing bronchospasm.

- These drugs include:
  - Atenolol
  - Betaxolol
  - Bisoprolol
  - Metoprolol
  - Acebutolol
- Some beta-blockers have intrinsic sympathomimetic activity − they are partial agonists, which stimulate as well as block the receptor, for example, oxprenolol, pindolol and acebutolol cause less bradycardia and less coldness of the extremities.
- Some beta-blockers are lipid soluble, and some are water soluble (excretion by the kidneys reduced in renal impairment).

Some drugs are photosensitive so ensure that you take adequate precautions when they are being infused.

Use of beta-blockers are as follows:

- Hypertension — may be combined with other drugs
- Cardiac dysrhythmias — ventricular arrhythmias
- Cardioselective beta-blockers should be used in diabetics as others may precipitate hypoglycaemic attacks
- Angina — reduce cardiac work and so oxygen consumption
- Myocardial infarction (MI)
- Thyrotoxicosis — propranolol
- Anxiety states
- Glaucoma
- Migraine

Parasympathomimetic Drugs

They act similar to that of the parasympathetic nervous system and act on cholinergic receptors (Table 6.2):

- Carbachol — used in urinary retention and causes contraction of the bladder muscle.
- Anticholinesterases potentiate the transmission of ACh at the neuromuscular junction:
  - Physostigmine prevents the breakdown of ACh by inhibiting the enzyme cholinesterase, causes constriction of the pupil, used in glaucoma, use replaced in myasthenia gravis by neostigmine.
  - Neostigmine — synthetic substance, direct effect on the neuromuscular junction of voluntary muscle, and less effect on the eye.
- Muscarinic antagonists: a weak central stimulant but at high doses cause a tachycardia — atropine.

Cholinergic Drugs

ACh is a neurotransmitter that acts in the central and peripheral nervous system. ACh binds to cholinergic receptor sites:

- Muscarinic receptors — action on the parasympathetic nervous system
- Nicotinic receptors — found at the neuromuscular junction, reacts to adrenaline and noradrenaline.

TABLE 6.2 Cholinergic receptors.

Neurotransmitter	Receptor type	Major locations	Effects of binding
Acetylcholine	Nicotinic	Centrally in autonomic ganglia and the neuromuscular junction of skeletal muscles	Feeling of relaxation and well-being; an increase in skeletal muscle tone; release of adrenaline and noradrenaline.
	Muscarinic subtypes	Centrally and peripherally: M_1 — brain and higher cerebral functions; M_2 — stomach; M_3 — visceral smooth muscle and exocrine glands	Pupil constriction; relations of GIT sphinchters, increased GIT motility and secretions; promotion of micturition and defaecation; promotes glycogenesis, gluconeogenesis, increases insulin secretion; promotes tears; bronchoconstriction and mucus production.

Muscarinic Agonists

Effects similar to that of activation of the parasympathetic nervous system:

- Cardiovascular — slows down heart rate
- Reduces cardiac output
- Systemic vasodilatation
- With an overall reduction in blood pressure

Muscarinic Antagonists

This includes atropine and other drug therapies:

- Increases heart rate and can be used to treat a bradycardia
- Reduces the production of secretions — eyes, mouth, sweating
- Dilates pupils
- Relaxes smooth muscle in the:
  - Lungs — ipratropium used in asthma and chronic obstructive pulmonary disease
  - Biliary tract and urinary smooth muscle
- Reduces peristalsis

Nicotinic Receptor Agonists

This group of drugs is known to cause muscle relaxants used during theatre and mechanical ventilation. Most common drug is suxamethonium. They can lead to some serious side effects:

- Bradycardia
- Painful movements
- Hyperkalaemia
- Prolonged paralysis
- Malignant hyperthermia

General Anaesthetics

These drugs lead to the absence of sensation associated with a reversible loss of consciousness. Anaesthesia depresses all excitable tissues, including central neurones, cardiac muscle, smooth and striated muscle. However, it is possible to administer anaesthetic agents at concentrations that produce unconsciousness without unduly depressing the cardiovascular and respiratory centres of the myocardium:

- Thiopental and propofol — unconsciousness occurs within seconds and is maintained by the administration of an inhalation anaesthetic such as halothane.
- Halothane — unconsciousness maintained by this inhalation anaesthetic, replaced by less toxic agents such as desflurane and isoflurane.
- Nitrous oxide at concentrations of up to 70% oxygen is a widely used anaesthetic agent — causes sedation and analgesia but not sufficient alone to maintain anaesthesia.

Muscle Relaxants

Anaesthetists in theatre and critical care use muscle relaxants to relax skeletal muscles during surgical operations and to prevent movement and breathing during mechanical ventilation. These drugs are given intravenously and distributed in the extracellular fluid.

Neuromuscular blocking agents compete with acetylcholine for muscle receptors but do not initiate ion channel opening; these include:

- Pancuronium — long duration of action, has an atropine-like action on the heart and can lead to a tachycardia.
- Vecuronium depends on hepatic inactivation and recovery takes 20–30 minutes; popular for short procedures.
- Atracurium — duration of action 15–30 minutes, only stable when kept cold and at low pH, at body pH and temperature it decomposes spontaneously in plasma and does not depend on renal or hepatic function for its elimination, good for patients with renal or hepatic disease.

Depolarizing blockers act on acetylcholine receptors, but trigger the opening of ion channels, and are not reversed by anticholinesterases; the only drug of this type used is:

- Suxamethonium — rapid onset and very short duration of action (3–7 minutes)

Always check that your patient is adequately sedated before administering a muscle relaxant.

Analgesic Drugs

Many medical or surgical conditions, for example, wound(s), can stimulate pain receptors and lead to severe/moderate/mild pain. The role of the critical care nurse in this situation (if applicable) is to assess the level of pain using a pain assessment tool and administer prescribed medication. However, when there is severe pain together with other changes observed, narcotic analgesia may be prescribed. These drugs mimic endogenous opioids by causing prolonged activation of the opiate receptors. The body produces endogenous opioids, which suppress centrally controlled pain mechanisms:

- Endorphins
- Enkephalins
- Dynorphins

Centrally, acting analgesics all act upon receptors within the CNS; there are at least three different receptors for these compounds (Table 6.3). This produces analgesia, respiratory depression, euphoria and sedation. Assessment tools and patient-controlled analgesia may be added as soon as the initial emergency is over.

Morphine

Morphine is an analgesic that can be used for severe pain, such as the pain following the injury caused by a coronary thrombosis and MI. Morphine not only relieves pain but also relieves the anxieties related to it and gives a sense of euphoria. This is because morphine is an agonist of all three types of opioid receptors named mu (μ), kappa (κ) and delta (δ). The analgesic effects start within 20 minutes when given by subcutaneous injection and within 10 minutes of IV infusion. Morphine has a short half-life of about 4 hours, so frequent dosing is required. Therefore, morphine has been superseded by a more potent agent, diamorphine, which requires smaller doses.

TABLE 6.3 Endogenous opioid receptors.

Endogenous opioid	Receptor type	Major locations	Effects of binding
Not known	Delta	Limbic system – emotions	Behavioural changes; hallucinations
Dynorphin	Kappa	Hypothalamus	Hypothermia Miosis sedation Analgesia
Endorphin	Mu	Dorsal horn of spinal cord Thalamus	Analgesia Respiratory depression Euphoria

Effects of morphine are as follows:

- Analgesia
- Euphoria
- Respiratory depression
- Depression of cough reflex
- Pupillary constriction
- Nausea and vomiting

Codeine

Related to morphine but less potent, codeine is partly converted into morphine in the liver. Approximately 10% of the population is lacking the enzyme responsible for this conversion (Galbraith et al., 2007); this explains why some patients gain little pain relief from high doses of codeine. Thus, codeine is not commonly used on its own, but it is prescribed as an antidiarrheal and enhances the analgesic activity of paracetamol and aspirin and is often combined with them.

Diamorphine (Heroin)

Diamorphine is metabolized to morphine but is twice as potent. Depresses the exaggerated respiratory effort, reduces the patient's distress and helps to redistribute some of the increased cerebral blood volume to the peripheries. Diamorphine is generally given intravenously for a rapid effect; orally, it is less effective as it is almost completely converted into morphine. Diamorphine is generally the analgesic of choice for severe chest pain in MI or by subcutaneous syringe driver if oral morphine sulphate (MST) can no longer be tolerated.

Pethidine

The analgesic effect of pethidine is not as strong as morphine, but it is widely used for moderate to severe pain as it causes less respiratory depression. Useful in labour as it does not suppress uterine contractions, but foetal respiratory rate can be affected. Pethidine is not recommended for long-term use because of its metabolite norpethidine, which can lead to serious convulsions.

Other Narcotic Analgesics

- Methadone − used as a morphine or heroin substitute as it produces fewer withdrawal symptoms.
- Fentanyl citrate − commonly used as a neuroleptanalgesic due to its short duration of therapeutic action, allows patients to recover quickly from the drug's effects and popular in the use of maintenance of ventilation.

Naloxone

Pure antagonist at the opioid receptors can be used to reverse narcotic analgesia in the case of overdose. The result can be quite dramatic, but the drug has a half-life of only 1 hour, and therefore, in cases of overdose, the patient needs to remain under observation for a considerable time.

Nonsteroidal Antiinflammatory Drugs

This group of drugs has in various degrees analgesic, antiinflammatory and antipyretic actions. NSAIDs have the ability to inhibit cyclooxygenase, and the resulting inhibition of prostaglandin synthesis is responsible for their therapeutic effects. Unfortunately, because of this action, NSAIDs should only be used in the short-term:

- These drugs are acid and need to be taken with food as they can result in gastric intestinal irritation.
- Lead to bleeding of gums, increased bleeding during menstruation − the inhibition of prostaglandin as part of the inflammatory immune response also blocks the clotting cascade.
- Should not be given to patients with:
  - Renal impairment as prostaglandins enhance GFR
  - Coagulation defects
  - Severe heart failure
  - Gastric or peptic ulcers
  - Asthma

Available in various strengths and so can be used for:

- Mild analgesic − ibuprofen and aspirin
- Moderate analgesic − diclofenac and naproxen
- Strong analgesic − indomethacin

Other analgesic drugs available are as follows:

- Paracetamol — no antiinflammatory action, usually tried first.
- Codeine and dihydrocodeine — stronger than paracetamol but more side effects.
- Paracetamol 1 codeine phosphate (co-codamol, co-dydramol and co-proxamol)
- Morphine sulphate for acute pain over short periods; MST (modified release formulation of morphine) not suitable for acute pain (12 hourly)

Anxiolytics and Hypnotics

These groups of drugs are used for sleep disorders (hypnotics) and acute anxiety states (anxiolytics) dominated by the benzodiazepines which:

- induce sleep when given in high doses and
- provide sedation and reduce anxiety when given in low, divided doses during the day.

Benzodiazepines:

- Short acting — temazepam or zopiclone preferred to avoid daytime sedation.
- Long acting — nitrazepam.
- Adverse effects — drowsiness, impaired alertness, agitation and ataxia.
- Dependence — a withdrawal syndrome may occur including anxiety, insomnia, depression and nausea.
- IV infusion — diazepam and lorazepam.
- Midazolam is used as an IV sedation during endoscopic, dental and ventilation procedures.
- All have an amnesic action, and patients have no recollection of an unpleasant experience.

Antidepressants

Antidepressants are used in patients with depression and anxiety; they are mood stabilisers and do not cause dependence.

- Tricyclic antidepressants — block the reuptake of serotonin and noradrenaline — amitriptyline
- MAOIs — not used as much as other groups due to the dangerous dietary and drug interactions, used when other drugs have been unsuccessful in controlling depression

- Selective serotonin reuptake inhibitors — these are the most frequently used antidepressant

Inotropes

The positive inotropic effect of these drugs is to increase the contractility of the cardiac muscle and so improve cardiac function and increase cardiac output (Table 6.4).

Inotropic drugs work by increasing intracellular calcium concentration by a variety of methods; the force generated by cardiac muscle is proportional to the amount of intracellular calcium present during contraction.

These are powerful drugs, which can lead to some serious side effects:

- Increase myocardial oxygen consumption
- Vasoconstriction can lead to reduction in blood supply to other organs

TABLE 6.4 Guidelines to cardiovascular effects of inotropic drugs.

Drug	DA	Alpha	Beta-1	Beta-2	HR	MAP	CI	SVR
Dopamine								
Low dose	+++	+	+	0	+/=	+/=	+/=	+/=
Moderate dose	+++	++	++	+	+	+	+	+
High dose	+++	+++	++	+	++	++	+	++
Dobutamine	0	+	+++	++	+	+/=/-	++	=/-
Dopexamine	++	0	+	+++	++	=/-	+	=/-
Noradrenaline								
Low dose	0	++	+	+	-/=	+	+/=/-	++
High dose		+++	+	+	-	++	=/-	+++
Adrenaline								
Low dose	0	+	+	+	+/=	+	-/=/+	++
High dose			+	+	+	++	-/=	+++
Isoprenaline	0	0	+	+++	++	-	+	-
Milrinone	0	0	0	0	+	-	++	-
IABP	0	0	0	0	=	+/=/-	+	-

+, increased; =, unchanged; −, decreased; *CI*, cardiac index; *DA*, dopamine receptor activation; *HR*, heart rate; *MAP*, mean arterial pressure; *SVR*, systemic vascular resistance.

- Dopamine − naturally occurring neurotransmitter, beta$_1$ receptors in cardiac muscle:
  - Increases cardiac contractility of heart with little effect on heart rate
  - Low dose acts on dopamine receptors in the kidneys and increases renal perfusion
  - Increased dose causes vasoconstriction and exacerbates heart failure
  - Increases systolic pressure
  - Titrated to blood pressure
  - Dosage is calculated in mg/kg/min
  - The drugs should be changed if no satisfactory results
- Dopexamine − artificial, primarily effective on beta-receptors, improves renal blood flow, increases mean arterial blood pressure and cardiac output without causing vasoconstriction
- Dobutamine − artificially formulated beta$_1$ agonist; inotropic effect without increase in heart rate and makes the heart work faster, has a more inotropic effect than chronotropic effect, sometimes used in cardiogenic shock and following cardiac arrest.
- Isoprenaline − increases heart rate and contractility and used for short-term treatment of heart block and bradycardia.
- Adrenaline − acts on both alpha and beta receptors and increases both heart rate and contractility, overall increases systolic blood pressure, heart rate, force of contraction.
- Noradrenaline − contraction of all smooth muscles and receptors, causes reduced vascular compliance, increases central venous pressure and systemic vascular resistance and blood pressure; used for acute hypotension and/or sepsis.
- The only inotrope used in cardiac failure is digoxin, which is also an antiarrhythmic drug:
  - Increases the force of cardiac contraction in the failing heart
  - Particularly effective in heart failure caused by atrial fibrillation
  - Can lead to drug toxicity

Ensure that you take extra care when changing infusions carrying inotropic drugs as there may be a considerable drop in your patient's blood pressure − consider using a two-pump approach.

Antihypertensive Drugs

Angiotensin-Converting Enzyme Inhibitors

- These drugs act by inhibiting the renin—angiotensin aldosterone system by preventing the conversion of angiotensin I to angiotensin II by the angiotensin-converting enzyme (ACE), therefore preventing the formation of angiotensin II. This process is overactive in heart failure, stimulated in hypovolaemic and low blood pressure states:
  - Captopril
  - Enalapril
  - Cilazapril
  - Lisinopril
  - Perindopril
  - Quinapril
  - Ramipril
- They reduce aldosterone and so increase sodium loss and thus water loss.
- They also vasodilate, which reduces the strain on the failing heart by reducing the preload and the afterload.
- Proven beneficial in heart failure:
  - Dyspnoea reduced
  - Exercise tolerance increased
  - Hospital care reduced
  - Life expectancy is increased in moderate to severe heart failure
- Other potential value:
  - Reduce left ventricular dilatation post-MI
  - Reduce the incidence of arrhythmias post-MI
  - May improve coronary blood flow at the same time as decreasing oxygen demand

Adverse effects are as follows:

- Hypotension
- Renal damage — regular monitoring is essential
- Cough — dry productive, worse at night
- Skin rash
- Aplastic anaemia — but this is rare

Vasodilator Drugs

These drugs act directly on the smooth muscle of the blood vessels or block the calcium channels in the muscle membrane.

Calcium Channel Blockers

These have actions on the heart by increasing the refractory period in the cardiac cell, lengthening the period of time calcium remains in the cardiac cell during depolarization. They relieve angina mainly by causing peripheral arteriolar dilatation and afterload reduction. The drugs include:

- Nifedipine in patients who have a related bronchospasm or left ventricular failure
- Diltiazem — only a slight negative inotropic effect; less potent than nifedipine
- Verapamil — used in SVT in addition to angina

   They can lead to flushing, dizziness, headaches and oedema of the ankles.

Nitrates

The main effect is to cause peripheral vasodilation, especially in the veins, by a direct action on the vascular smooth muscle. A patient suspected of an MI or suffering from angina may be commenced on a nitrate infusion.

Glyceryl Trinitrate It is generally short-acting and lasts for about 30 minutes:

- The aim is to diminish the infarction ischaemic zones and thus limit the size of infarct.
- GTN is a rapid-acting drug that causes coronary vasodilatation and ventilation promoting more oxygen-rich blood to move towards the heart.
- GTN by dilating both veins and arteries reduces the filling pressure of the heart as well as the resistance against which the heart has to pump; consequently, myocardial work and oxygen demand are reduced.
- GTN suffers a very large first-pass effect when given orally and is thus given by other routes:
  - Sublingually
  - Transdermally
  - Intravenously
- It has a very short duration of action, but the onset of action is rapid — within 2 minutes.
- There are nitrates that take longer to have an effect, for example, onset of action is later than 30 minutes:
  - Isosorbide mononitrate
  - Isosorbide dinitrate

Mechanism of Action

- Act by relaxing smooth muscle by converting nitrates into nitric oxide, which is a powerful vasodilator

- Have their main effects on cardiovascular system
- Veins are dilated more than arteries, and this reduces preload.
- There is a reflex tachycardia but even so oxygen demand is reduced.
- Systemic arteries are dilated — reduces afterload.
- The collateral coronary arteries are dilated resulting in a better blood flow to the heart.
- In atherosclerosis of the coronary vessels, nitrates do not cause dilatation of these vessels; they do reduce myocardial oxygen demand by reducing cardiac output and arterial pressure, but more than this they divert the blood to the ischaemic area by dilating the collateral circulation

Adverse Effects

- The vasodilator effect of GTN can produce a headache and flushing — these can be severe
- Palpitations and hypotension due to a reduction in peripheral resistance and may cause syncope — blood pressure should be continually monitored via an arterial line. If blood pressure falls, the infusion rate can be altered according to the condition of the patient.

Nitroprusside This is used for severe hypertension crisis; it acts directly by causing vasodilatation of smooth muscle, quick acting, reduces systemic vascular resistance of both veins and arteries.

Diuretics

It causes increased secretion of urine in the kidneys. They all produce their effect by decreasing the reabsorption of water and electrolytes by the renal tubules and thus allowing more to be excreted. The kidney filters about 100 L of fluid per day, but only 1500 mL is lost as urine.

It is useful in the following conditions:

- Heart failure
- Hypertension
- Nephrotic syndrome
- Cirrhosis of the liver
- Acute pulmonary oedema
- Oedema formation from heart disease and cirrhosis
- Hypercalcaemia and occasionally in hyperkalaemia

Types of Diuretic

- Water (atrial natriuretic factor/peptide) — fails to work in heart failure.
- Osmotic diuretics — mannitol increases osmotic pressure in filtrate and causes more water to be excreted, used in:
  - forced diuresis in drug overdose,
  - cerebral oedema and
  - maintaining diuresis during surgery.
- Xanthines — theophylline, caffeine, a weak diuretic action.
- Thiazide diuretics — relatively weak diuretics, inhibit sodium/chloride reabsorption in the early segment of the distal tubule, chlorothiazide, hydrochlorothiazide, bendroflumethiazide. It may lead to hypokalaemia, increased uric acid and cholesterol levels.
- Loop diuretics — most powerful of all diuretics — capable of causing 15% —25% of the sodium filtrate to be excreted. It acts similar to thiazide, but sodium/chloride reabsorption takes place in the ascending loop of Henle, a very rapid onset of action but of fairly short duration, powerful and can cause electrolyte imbalance, dehydration and hypovolaemia, for example, furosemide, bumetanide, ethacrynic acid.
- Potassium-sparing diuretics — weak when used alone, but cause potassium retention, often given with a thiazide or loop diuretic to prevent hypokalaemia.
  - Triamterene, amiloride — work on the distal tubule and the collecting ducts.
  - Frumil is a combination of furosemide and amiloride.
  - Spironolactone — an aldosterone antagonist.

Always check a patient's urine output after giving diuretics and monitor their electrolytes.

Antiarrhythmic Drugs

The rhythm of the heart is generally determined by the pacemaker cells in the sinoatrial node, but it can be disturbed in many ways leading to discomfort to heart failure or even death (Richards and Edwards, 2014):

- Serious arrhythmias, for example, ventricular tachycardia, are associated with heart disease.
- Supraventricular arrhythmias arise in the atrial myocardium or atrioventricular node.

- Ventricular arrhythmias may be caused by ectopic focus, which starts firing at a higher rate than the normal pacemaker.
- Reentry mechanisms can occur, where action potentials are delayed for some pathological reason, reinvade nearby muscle fibres leading to a loop of depolarization.

Many antiarrhythmic drugs are local anaesthetics or calcium antagonists, but they are generally classified into those which are effective in:

- Supraventricular arrhythmias
  - Adenosine − hyperpolarizes the cell membrane in the atrioventricular node and, by inhibiting the calcium channels, slows conduction in the atrioventricular node.
  - Digoxin − stimulates vagal activity, which slows conduction and prolongs the refractory period in the atrioventricular node and bundle of His. It is used in atrial fibrillation when the atrial beat is so high, and the ventricular rate is unable to follow so appears irregularly.
  - Verapamil acts by blocking calcium channels and has powerful effects on the atrioventricular node; has a negative inotropic action; largely replaced by IV adenosine because it is safer.
- Ventricular arrhythmias
  - Lidocaine − given IV to treat ventricular arrhythmias, usually after an MI
- Both supraventricular and ventricular arrhythmias:
  - Disopyramide − lengthens the refractory period of the action potential of cardiac cells; used to prevent recurrent ventricular arrhythmias; a negative inotrope and can cause hypotension and aggravate cardiac failure.
  - Quinidine − use is limited due to the danger of cardiac and frequent noncardiac side effects.
  - Flecainide − strongly depresses conduction in the myocardium; has a negative inotropic action.
  - Amiodarone − blocks several channels; is often effective when other drugs have failed.

Ensure that patients receiving cardioactive drugs are being cardiovascularly monitored, for example, regular 12 lead electrocardiogram and/or cardiac monitoring.

Bronchodilators

Beta-Agonists

These drugs act on the $beta_2$ adrenergic receptors in bronchial smooth muscle. Currently available beta-agonists include salbutamol, formoterol (eformoterol), terbutaline, salmeterol and fenoterol. They are used both in asthma and chronic obstructive pulmonary disease.

Stimulation of these receptors results in:

- Bronchodilatation
- Increased skeletal muscle excitability
- Vasodilatation of blood vessels in the brain, heart, kidneys and skeletal muscle
- Stabilization of the membrane of mast cells, preventing the release of inflammatory mediators

$Beta_2$-adrenergic receptor agonists:

- are used to dilate the bronchioles and help breathing;
- are associated with cardiac acceleration, leading to a tachycardia, and may compromise heart function;
- are generally given by inhalation as this route causes less marked $beta_1$ cardiac stimulation;
- can be given systemically (oral or parenteral route), but this causes greater cardiac stimulation, and systemic $beta_2$-agonists should therefore be used with caution.

Adverse effects include:

- A fine tremor
- Palpitations
- Peripheral vasodilatation resulting in hypotension and headache
- Increase in blood glucose level
- Warm limbs
- Decrease in serum potassium levels.

Antimuscarinic Agents

Muscarinic (M_3) receptor agonists are synthetic atropine-like agents, for example, ipratropium bromide (Atrovent) and tiotropium, and block muscarinic receptors associated with the parasympathetic stimulation of the bronchial air passages. Onset is slower than with $beta_2$-agonists (maximum effect in 30–60 minutes), but the duration of the effect is prolonged (3–6 hours; Galbraith et al., 2007).

Adverse effects include:

- Dry mouth
- Constipation

- Reduced gastric juice secretion
- Urinary retention
- Blurred vision

Methylxanthines

These include theophylline and aminophylline and induce bronchodilatation through a mechanism that bypasses interaction with an extracellular receptor, either adrenergic or cholinergic (Galbraith et al., 2007). Methylxanthines are phosphodiesterase inhibitors that prevent the degradation of cyclic adenosine monophosphate, which results in an increase in bronchial smooth muscle cell activity, leading to bronchodilatation.

Adverse effects:

- Mainly related to nervous system overstimulation – insomnia, anxiety, nervousness, epigastric distress, nausea, vomiting and tachycardia
- More serious and in higher doses – convulsions and dysrhythmias

Glucocorticoids

Glucocorticoids effectively increase the airway calibre in asthma; steroids act by reducing bronchial mucosal inflammatory reactions (e.g. oedema, mucus hypersecretion) and by modifying the allergic reactions of asthma and anaphylaxis. These include:

- Hydrocortisone – can be given orally, more commonly used intravenously (shock, status asthmaticus) or topically (eczema)
- Prednisolone – orally for inflammatory and allergic diseases

  The adverse effects are as follows:

- Metabolic effects such as redistribution of fat to the face and trunk, tendency to bruise easily, disturbed carbohydrate metabolism may lead to hyperglycaemia and occasionally diabetes, wasting and weakness, osteoporosis
- Fluid retention
- Adrenal suppression
- Infections due to immunosuppressive effects of glucocorticoids
- Peptic ulceration

Antihistamines

The term antihistamine is usually reserved for the H_1 blockers or antagonists (Table 6.5). It is used in the treatment of:

- Allergies
- Nausea

TABLE 6.5 Histamine receptors.

Receptor	Receptor abb.	Major locations	Effects of binding
Histamine	H₁	Smooth muscle and exocrine glands and respiratory tract	Used in the treatment of allergies and prevent release of histamine from mast cells, acid production
	H₂	Parietal cells of the stomach	Prevent the release of acid from the stomach H₂ antagonist

- Symptoms of the common cold
- Influenza
- Topical treatment for skin allergies, or insect bites

A common side effect of these drugs is drowsiness; patients should be advised not to drive or operate hazardous machinery:

- Astemizole, cetirizine, loratadine and terfenadine are less likely to cross the blood−brain barrier and lead to drowsiness.
- Promethazine and trimeprazine are so good at promoting drowsiness that patients commonly use them as sedatives.
- Doxylamine − used in combination with analgesia.

Antibacterial Drugs

Antibiotics work in three different ways:

1. Inhibit nucleic acid synthesis:
   a. Sulphonamides
   b. Trimethoprim
   c. Rifampicin.
2. Inhibit cell wall synthesis:
   a. Penicillin − benzylpenicillin, flucloxacillin, broad-spectrum (amoxicillin, ampicillin)
   b. Cephalosporins − cefadroxil (urinary tract infections), cefuroxime (prophylactic in surgery), ceftazidime and ceftriaxone
   c. Vancomycin − septicaemia or endocarditis; can cause renal failure and hearing loss.
3. Inhibit protein synthesis:
   a. Aminoglycosides − gentamicin, amikacin, netilmicin, streptomycin
   b. Tetracyclines

 c. Macrolides — erythromycin and clarithromycin
 d. Chloramphenicol

Antifungal and Antiviral Drugs

Fungal infections may be superficial or systemic, the latter occurring in immunocompromised patients such as AIDS patients.

- Amphotericin is highly toxic
- Nystatin is too toxic for parenteral use; mainly used in the treatment of thrush and applied to mucous membranes as a cream or ointment or suspension in the mouth or pessaries in the vagina
- Flucytosine
- Imidazoles
- Triazoles — fluconazole

Viruses are small and replicate by entering living cells as they lack independent metabolism and can therefore only reproduce themselves within living host cells. Vaccines are generally the major method for controlling viral infections (poliomyelitis, rabies, measles, mumps, rubella). Some effective antiviral drugs have been developed and act in two different ways:

1. Stop the virus entering or leaving the host cell
 a. Amantadine
 b. Zanamivir
2. Inhibit nucleic acid synthesis
 a. Aciclovir — selectively antiviral
 b. Antiretroviral drugs — used to suppress the replication of human immunodeficiency virus in patients with AIDS.

Drugs Used on the Gastrointestinal Tract

Antiemetic

- Metoclopramide — a dopamine antagonist that stimulates gastric emptying, used to treat nausea and vomiting.
- Prochlorperazine is a phenothiazine that is widely used as an antiemetic; less sedative than chlorpromazine.

Antacids

These are all weak bases and rapidly combine with hydrochloric acid and neutralize it.

- Antacids − raise the gastric luminal pH, provide effective but short relief of many dyspepsias and symptomatic relief in peptic ulcer, gastritis and oesophageal reflux and heartburn. These are usually basic compounds of:
  - Aluminium hydroxide
  - Magnesium carbonate
- Omeprazole − can produce virtual reduction in acid production by blocking the H^1/K^1-ATPase, which pumps H^1 ions out of the parietal cells

Histamine H_2 Receptor Antagonists

- Histamine H_2-receptor antagonists (Table 6.5) − cimetidine and ranitidine block the action of histamine on the parietal cells and reduce acid secretion.
- Cimetidine has been found to slow down metabolism of many other drugs, resulting in enhancement of their effects.
- There are others such as nizatidine and famotidine.

Sucralfate

A combination of sugar sucrose and aluminium compound, which only acts in the presence of acid. Once ingested, it forms a thick paste-like substance, which adheres to the gastric mucosa protecting it from acid. Effective in healing duodenal ulcers, with minimal side effects, but can lead to constipation.

Antispasmodics

Cholinergic antagonists − pirenzepine with a relatively selective action on the gut − directly relax smooth muscle and reduce gastrointestinal motility and are used to reduce spasm in irritable bowel syndrome (antispasmodics).

Antidiarrhoeal Drugs

- Infectious diarrhoea is a common cause of illness or a complication of some interventions, for example, antibiotics, enteral feeding
- Antimotility drugs are used to provide symptomatic relief
- Loperamide or Imodium are generally used; codeine also reduces bowel motility

Laxatives

Laxatives are used to increase motility of the gut and encourage defaecation:

- Bulk laxatives − increase the volume of intestinal contents stimulating peristalsis.

- Stimulant laxatives – increase motility by acting on mucosa or nerve plexuses, which can cause damage in prolonged use.
- Lubricants – promote defaecation by softening and/or lubricating faeces and assisting evacuation.

Antiepileptics

Epilepsy is a chronic disease in which seizures result from the abnormal discharge of cerebral neurones. The seizures are classified empirically, and the correct classification is important as it determines the choice of drug treatment. The aim of treatment is to control the seizures with one drug:

- Phenytoin or carbamazepine – will control tonic-clonic and partial seizures.
- Valproate is an alternative agent.
- The benzodiazepines, for example, phenobarbital and clonazepam, also can be used but have a sedative effect.

Antiplatelet Drugs

In the instance where there is some formation of clotting disorder, it is possible to use drugs that interfere with blood coagulation processes and thus reduce or prevent further thrombus formation.

Aspirin

- Used to reduce platelet aggregation, thus reducing the chances of increasing or causing clots in critical care patients with MI or at risk of MI and stroke.
- Works by inhibiting the production of thromboxane produced by the platelets from prostaglandin precursors, which is a powerful inducer of both aggregation of platelets and vasoconstriction.
- Can be used as an adjunct to fibrinolytic therapy and is effective in reducing the incidence of death in acute MI.

Fibrinolytic Agents

Critical care nurses may be involved in initiating, giving, assisting in the administration of or receiving patients from accident and emergency following fibrinolytic therapy. This treatment is given intravenously via infusion to break down clots that have led to the occlusion of coronary arteries and the MI.

Current fibrinolytic agents in patients can receive include streptokinase, alteplase (tPA), anisoylated plasminogen-streptokinase activator complex (APSAC), and urokinase. Streptokinase is often the fibrinolytic therapy of choice. The use of APSAC and urokinase is restricted due to cost. Although their mechanism of action differs, they all function by producing active plasmin, which dissolves fibrin clots and promotes vasodilatation.

Streptokinase

Streptokinase is an exotoxin from beta-haemolytic streptococci and a potent plasminogen activator, and when given in large doses as a short infusion, it accelerates the conversion of plasminogen to plasmin. This breaks down fibrin within the clot forming soluble fibrin degradation products, leading to the dispersal of the thrombus.

The treatment must preferably be performed as soon as possible after the onset of infarction and can reestablish blood flow in approximately 3 minutes. It is administered via IV infusion over a period of 1 hour. Streptokinase has a half-life of approximately 20 minutes.

Patients may have antibodies to streptokinase from a streptococcal infection or if they have received streptokinase previously. There is a general agreement that streptokinase should not be administered again within 2 years. In 1%−2% of patients, signs of an allergic reaction may develop, such as urticaria, wheezing or even hypotension and anaphylaxis.

Streptokinase is contraindicated in patients with severe hypertension and in those with a history of blood disorders or stroke. The main risk factor with treatment is the risk of bleeding as fibrinolysis is increased.

Alteplase (tPA)

Alteplase is an endogenous enzyme found in vascular endothelium. Alteplase activates plasminogen and is used to dissolve clots, salvage myocardium and hinder new thrombosis formation to help reduce mortality. The sooner it is given after the start of symptoms, the more likely it is to reduce the size and severity of the MI. The plasma half-life is 5−8 minutes and unlike streptokinase, repeated dose is possible. Alteplase is the agent of choice for patients who have previously received streptokinase.

When the coronary flow is successfully restored by fibrinolytic therapy, ST-segment elevation returns to baseline, and creatinine kinase falls as it is washed out by reperfusion. Fibrinolytic therapy is generally followed by a course of IV heparin to prevent immediate vessel reocclusion. However, in some cases, reperfusion after thrombolysis may fail to occur. Fibrinolytic failure has been associated with more complex plaques and with more extensive haemorrhage into the plaque. Other options after failed thrombolysis include:

- Rescue angioplasty
- Insertion of an intraaortic balloon pump (only if there is severe left ventricular failure)
- Repeat thrombolysis (Davies and Ormerod, 1998)

Fibrinolytic therapy is often followed by the administration of beta-adrenergic blockers. Early beta-blockade reduces mortality and decreases the incidence of ventricular fibrillation and infarct size. However, these drugs are contraindicated in severe heart failure, hypotension, bradycardia, second- or third-degree heart block or asthma.

There is an ongoing debate regarding which of the fibrinolytic therapies is more beneficial. Research evidence suggests that it does not necessarily matter which fibrinolytic agent is given compared to how soon it is administered. Fibrinolytic therapy can cause haemorrhage, particularly in females, older patients, those with low body weight and hypertension, and with fibrinogen depletion. Blood transfusion, heparin reversal and other corrective measures such as cryoprecipitate, fresh frozen plasma (FFP) and platelet transfusion may be needed.

Anticoagulants

Heparin

Heparin works faster than warfarin because it binds to plasma antithrombin III, which is a natural anticoagulant in the blood; in so doing, it inactivates thrombin, plasmin and other serine proteases of coagulation, including factors IXa, Xa, XIa and XIIa. Heparin also inhibits additional coagulation by inactivating thrombin thus preventing the conversion of fibrinogen to fibrin. The amount of heparin required to produce anticoagulant effect depends on each individual and their activated partial thromboplastin time (aPTT). A coagulation test is carried out to measure heparin activity. The normal APPT is 40 seconds. The concentration of heparin will prolong APTT from 2 to 2.5 times over the control value; this should be maintained and measured six hourly.

Some 10% of people on heparin suffer from haemorrhage, cytopenia and hypertensive reactions. This means that patients on heparin therapy require regular measure of BP and heart rate. Urine and stools are closely monitored for any signs of blood. If overcoagulation of heparin occurs, the effect may be rapidly reversed by administration of protamine sulphate. The protein protamine sulphate neutralizes a heparin overdose. It combines with the heparin molecule to form a complex that suppresses the pharmacological activity of the anticoagulant. A combination is formed to dissociate the heparin and antithrombin III. This will reduce the anticoagulant action of heparin because protamine is a protein and inactivates them.

Dalteparin

Dalteparin is a low-molecular-weight heparin (LMWH), which can be used for prophylaxis. It has been identified that the advantage of LMWH is that it does not need close monitoring of blood coagulation tests. It has a longer life and so requires once-a-day dosage.

Warfarin

Once the clotting stabilizes, warfarin may be started because of the time it takes to be effective. Warfarin inhibits the synthesis of clotting factors produced by the liver from vitamin K and thus active clotting factors decrease by binding to the albumin. This explains why it is given in low doses. Warfarin acts in the liver to prevent synthesis of vitamin K-dependent clotting factors (i.e. factors II, VII, IX and X). Warfarin acts as an antagonist to hepatic use of vitamin K, but it takes about 8−12 hours to deplete clotting factors. This is because its anticoagulant effect results from a balance between partially inhibited synthesis and unaltered degradation of vitamin K clotting factors. The resulting inhibition of coagulation is dependent on their degradation rate in circulation.

Degradation of vitamin K clotting factors of VII, IX, X and II to half-lives will take 6, 24, 40 and 60 hours respectively. This is why it takes warfarin to decrease the amount of vitamin K-dependent coagulation factor synthesized in the liver by up to 50%. This highlights the need for warfarin to be started in conjunction with heparin in order to initiate warfarin in the system before taking the patient off heparin.

Warfarin is measured as a ratio against a standard PTT. A standard level represents 25% of the normal rate, and this should be maintained for a longer-term therapy. Warfarin should be omitted if normal activity is less than 20% until activity rises to above 20%. The international normalized ratio (INR) represents the recommended target levels of between 2.5 and 3.5.

Blood tests need to be taken regularly to determine the maintenance dose prescribed. INR should be measured once monthly in long-term patients. Once a patient has suffered a PE, the risk of it recurring is high. Warfarin given after heparin therapy should continue for at least 6 months as recurrent multiple emboli may require life-long therapy.

Patients on warfarin need to be warned about bleeding disorders that may occur, especially with elderly patients. This is due to the reduced effect of platelets and coagulation factors. Occurrence of any of the above factors would mean a withdrawal from the drug, which restores normal clotting factors. For warfarin poisoning, vitamin K is given slowly intravenously as an antidote. This reverse may take several hours; therefore, in urgent cases, FFP is given.

The primary result of excessive usage of the drug is bleeding of the gums when brushing teeth, excessive or easy skin bruising and unexplained nose bleeds. The vital signs the nurse has to look for include when a patient appears to be in shock or having difficulty in breathing and pain.

Immunosuppressants

These are used to prevent tissue rejection after organ transplantation and to treat autoimmune diseases:

- Prednisolone is used in combination with azathioprine.
- Mycophenolate mofetil, ciclosporin and tacrolimus are potent immuno-suppressants that are used with prednisolone.

These drugs have serious adverse effects and, similar to cytotoxic drugs, increase a critical care patient's vulnerability to infection.

Ensure that strict hand washing is adopted when nursing immunosup-pressed patients.

Hyperglycaemic and Hypoglycaemic Agents

Hyperglycaemic Agents

Glucagon is used to treat drug-induced hypoglycaemic states where IV glucose cannot be administered. Nausea is a principal side effect, and the preparation needs to be protected from light.

Hypoglycaemic Agents

There are two different types, parenteral and oral:

1. Parenteral − insulin administered IV or subcutaneously − used in type I diabetes:
   a. The greater the concentration of zinc or the presence of protamine in the insulin preparation, the more prolonged the duration and delayed the action of the insulin itself.
   b. Types:
      i. Neutral insulin − clear, generally short acting
      ii. Lente or isophane − cloudy and intermediate acting
      iii. Mixed insulin suspensions of the above two to lengthen the action and reduce the number of daily injections required
      iv. Sources of insulin − bovine (ox), porcine (pig) and human (genetically modified for commercial use)
2. Oral hypoglycaemic agents − used in type II diabetes
   a. Sulphonylureas
      i. Stimulate the release of insulin from the pancreas
      ii. Inhibit the process of gluconeogenesis (forming glucose from amino acids and fatty acids) in the liver
      iii. Increase the number of insulin receptors on target cells
      iv. Adverse effects − hypoglycaemia overdose, allergy, depression of bone marrow and gastrointestinal disturbances

  v. Available − chlorpropamide, glibenclamide, gliclazide, glipizide, tolazamide and tolbutamide
b. Biguanide (metformin)
  i. Acts by promoting glucose uptake into cells through enhanced insulin-receptor binding
  ii. Slows absorption of glucose from the gut
  iii. Inhibits glucagon secretion and stimulates tissue glycolysis
  iv. Adverse effects − drug tolerance and acidosis

6.4 DRUG CALCULATIONS

In critical care, there are cardiac support and other drugs, which require careful and meticulous calculations to ensure that the correct dose is given to patients. Therefore, I have included some of the common drug formulas and useful information.

IV and oral therapy are common administration routes for drugs in critical care. It is in your interest to use some of your time to observe and learn some of the drugs that patients are prescribed. In addition to this, in your role as a critical care nurse, you will be expected to check and calculate the dosage and draw up the drugs.

The following are some of the drug calculation formulae that may help you in this role:

1. 1000 mg in 1 mg
   1000 mg in 1 g.
2. Ampicillin 500 mg diluted in 10 mL; you require 200 mg
   {What you want/What you have got} × What it is in.
   {200/500} × 10 = 4 mL
3. Adrenaline comes in strengths of 1:1000 (1 mg/mL) and 1:10,000 (1 mg/10 mL)
   a. If you require 1.6 mg of 1:1000 strength adrenaline, using the formula:
   {What you want/What you have got} × What it is in.
   {1.6/1} × 1 = 1.6 mL
   b. If you require 2.5 mg of 1:10,000 strength adrenaline, using the formula:
   {What you want/What you have got} × What it is in.
   {2.5/1} × 10 = 25 mL
4. Lidocaine comes in either a 1% solution or a 2% solution; this means that:
   a. A 1% solution is equal to 1 g in 100 mL
   1000 mg in 100 mL
   10 mg/mL

b. A 2% solution is equal to 2 g in 100 mL
2000 mg in 100 mL.
20 mg/mL

5. There are other drugs such as dopamine, adrenaline, dobutamine and noradrenaline, which require to be calculated in mg/kg/min
First, calculate micrograms/millilitre
Then use the formula: mg required 3 kg 3 min/concentration in micrograms.

Always check your calculations with someone more senior if you are unsure of your answer.

6.5 NURSE/NONMEDICAL PRESCRIBING

Any critical care nurse who is interested in the extension of nurse prescribing rights will appreciate the significance of the Crown Report. The Crown Report (Department of Health, 1999) made three main recommendations:

- The majority of patients continue to receive medicine on an individual patient basis.
- The current prescribing authority of doctors, dentists and certain nurses (in respect of a limited list of medicines) continues.
- New groups of professionals would be able to apply for authority to prescribe in specific clinical areas, where this would improve patient care, and patient safety could be assured.

Nonmedical Prescribing

Nursing is moving into the reality of nurse prescribing and allied health professionals (Beckwith and Franklin, 2011). Currently, this includes nurses, pharmacists, optometrists, physiotherapists, chiropodists, radiographers and community practitioners. Nonmedical prescribing includes responsibilities such as ensuring patient safety, better access to medications, patient involvement in choices of medications and decisions, improved use of skills and more flexible team working across the National Health Service (NHS). It involves trained healthcare professionals managing patients' medications with long-term conditions, undertake medication review and provide emergency care, mental health services and the homeless, and palliative care.

Independent Prescribing

Critical care nurses who are currently prescribing from the *Nurse Formulary* are able to prescribe any medication for any medical condition within their competence, including any controlled drug. However, these nurses and others not currently able to prescribe, who are in a position to undertake the assessment of patients with undiagnosed conditions, for example, hypo-kalaemia, and make a prescribing decision, for example, potassium added to fluids, can become a newly legally authorized independent prescriber. To undertake this role of nurse prescriber, a critical care nurse will have to undertake a relevant nurse prescribing course.

Dependent/Supplementary Prescribing

The dependent/supplementary prescriber is someone who may prescribe any medicine (including controlled drugs), within the nursing care plan of a patient, which has been agreed by the doctor. Supplementary prescribers do not have the diagnostic and assessment ability to make a decision about an initial prescription but will have sufficient knowledge to determine whether that prescription should be continued or whether to alter the dosage. Furthermore, a dependent/supplementary prescriber may still be able to prescribe a drug for the first time, but this would be within the parameters of clinical guidelines for a given condition and the care plan of a patient. This is about protocol arrangement.

Critical care nurse practitioners who consider themselves working at specialist level could, by undertaking a recognized accredited nurse prescriber course, become an independent or dependent prescriber.

References

ACAS, 2014. Bullying and Harassment at Work: A Guide for Employees. Available at: m.acas.org. uk/media/pdf/r//l/Bullying-and-harrassment-at-work-a-guide-for-employees.pdf [accessed 15/04/18].

Addington-Hall, Higginson, I., 2001. Palliative Care for Non-cancer Patients. Oxford University Press, Oxford.

Al-khalisy, H., et al., 2015. A widened pulse pressure: a potential valuable prognostic indicator of mortality in patients with sepsis. Journal of Community Hospital Internal Medicine Perspectives 5 (6), 29426. https://doi.org/10.3402/jchimp.v5.29426.

Allen, D.M., et al., 2011. ECG Interpretation Made Incredibly Easy. Lippincott Williams & Wilkins, London.

Arbour, R.B., Wiegand, D.L., 2014. Self-described nursing roles experienced during care of dying patients and their families: a phenomenological study. Intensive and Critical Care Nursing 30 (4), 211–218.

Baird, M.S., 2016. Manual of Critical Care Nursing - Nursing Interventions and Collaborative Management, seventh ed. Elsevier, Georgia.

BAPEN, 2016. Available at: https://www.bapen.org.uk/screening-and-must/must/introducing-must [accessed: 27/10/18]

BAPEN, 2018. Available at: https://www.bapen.org.uk/malnutrition-undernutrition/introduction-to-malnutrition [accessed: 27/10/18].

Beckwith, S., Franklin, P., 2011. Oxford Handbook of Prescribing for Nurses and Allied Health Professionals, second ed. Oxford University Press, Oxford.

Birati, E.Y., Jessop, M., 2015. Left ventricular assisted devices in the management of heart failure. Cardiac Failure Review 1 (1), 25–30.

Bogert, M.J., Goosens, A., Dongelmans, A., 2015. What are effective strategies for the implementation of care bundles in ICUs: a systematic review. Implementation Science 10 (119), 1–11. https://doi.org/10.1186/s13012-015-0306-1.

Boud, D., Keogh, R., Walker, D., 1985. Reflection: Turning Experience into Learning. Kogan Page, London.

British National Formulary, 2018. BNF 75 March-September. Royal Pharmaceutical Society, London.

Butler, V., 2005. Non-invasive ventilation NIV an adult audit across the north central London critical care network NCLCCN. Intensive and Critical Care Nursing 214, 243–256.

Carper, B.A., 1978. Fundamental patterns of knowing in nursing. Advances in Nursing Science 11, 13–23.

Cartwright, M.M., 2004. The metabolic response to stress: a case of complex nutrition support management. Critical Care Nursing Clinics of North America 16, 467–487. https://doi.org/10.1016/j.ccell.2004.07.001.

Chioncel, O., Collins, S.P., Ambrosy, A.P., Gheorghiade, M., Filippatos, G., 2015. Pulmonary odema - therapeutic targets. Cardiac Failure Review 1 (1), 38–45.

Chochinov, H.M., 2006. Dying, dignity, and new horizons in palliative end-of-life care. CA: A Cancer Journal for Clinicians 56 (2), 84–103.

Clarke, D.J., Holt, J., 2001. Philosophy: a key to open the door to critical thinking. Nurse Education Today 21, 71–78.

Comisso, I., Lucchini, A., 2018. Cardiovascular assessment. In: Comisso, et al. (Eds.), Nursing in Critical Care Setting: An Overview from Basic to Sensitive Outcomes. Available at: http://ebookcentral.proquest.com/lib/rcn/ (downloaded 30 November 2018).

Cook, L., 2014. Wound assessment. British Journal of Nursing 21 (Suppl. 20a), 4–6.

Coombs, M.A., Addington-Hall, J., Long-Sutehall, T., 2012. Challenges in transition from intervention to end of life care in intensive care: a qualitative study. International Journal of Nursing Studies 49 (5), 519–527.

Darzi, A., 2008. High Quality Care for All: NHS Next Stage Review Final Report. Department of Health, London.

Davidson, A.C., Banham, S., Elliott, M., et al., 2016. BTS/ICS guideline for the ventilatory management of acute hypercapnic respiratory failure in adults. Thorax 71 (Suppl. 2), ii1–35. https://doi.org/10.1136/thoraxjnl-2015-208209.

Davies, C.H., Ormerod, J.M., 1998. Failed coronary thrombolysis. The Lancet 351, 1191–1196.

Department of Health, 1999. Review of Prescribing: Supply and Administration of Medicines. Final Report. DoH, London.

Dewar, B., 2011. Caring about Caring: An Appreciative Inquiry about Compassionate Relationship Centred Care. Unpublished PhD thesis. Edinburgh Napier University, Edinburgh.

Dewey, J., 1933. How We Think: A Restatement of the Relation of Reflective Thinking to the Educative Process. Heath, Boston.

Edwards, S., Axe, S., 2015. The ten 'R's of safe multidisciplinary drug administration. Nurse Prescribing 13 (8), 352–360.

Edwards, S.L., Axe, S., 2018. Medication management: reducing drug errors, striving for safer practice. Nurse Prescribing 16 (8), 380–389.

Edwards, S.L., O'Connell, C.F., 2007. Exploring bullying: implications for nurse educators. Nurse Education in Practice 7, 26–35.

Edwards, S.L., 2001. Shock: types, classifications and exploration of their physiological effects. Emergency Nurse 9 (2), 29–38.

Edwards, S.L., 2002. Nursing knowledge: defining new boundaries. Nursing Standard 17 (2), 40–44.

Edwards, S.L., 2003a. Cellular pathophysiology Part 1: changes following tissue injury. Professional Nurse 18 (10), 562–565.

Edwards, S.L., 2003b. Cellular pathophysiology Part 2: responses following hypoxia. Professional Nurse 18 (11), 636–639.

Edwards, S.L., 2004. Compartment syndrome. Emergency Nurse 123, 32–38.

Edwards, S.L., 2007. Critical thinking: a two phase framework. Nurse Education in Practice 7, 303–314.

Edwards, S.L., 2014. Finding a place for story: looking beyond reflective practice. International Practice Development Journal 4 (2), 1–14.

Edwards, S.L., 2017. Reflecting differently: new dimensions – reflection-before and –beyond action. International Practice Development Journal 16 (2), 1–14.

Elliot, R., et al., 2016. Posttraumatic stress symptoms in intensive care patients: an exploration of associated factors. American Psychological Association 16 (2), 141–150.

Ferns, T., 2006. Violence, aggression and physical assault in healthcare settings. Nursing Standard 21 (13), 42–46.

Frazier, S.K., et al., 2012. 'Critical care nurses' assessment of patients' anxiety: reliance on physiological and behavioural parameters. American Journal of Critical Care 11 (1), 57—64.

Galbraith, A., Bullock, S., Manias, E., Hunt, B., Richards, A., 2007. Fundamentals of Pharmacology: An Applied Approach for Nursing and Health. Pearson Prentice Hall, Harlow.

Gao, F., Melody, T., Daniels, D.F., Giles, S., Fox, S., 2005. The impact of compliance with 6 hour sepsis bundle on hospital mortality in patients with severe sepsis: a prospective observational study. Critical Care 9, 764—770.

Garretson, S., Malberti, S., 2007. Understanding hypovolaemic, cardiogenic and septic shock. Nursing Standard 21 (50), 46—55.

Giuliani, E., 2018. The burden of not-weighted factors — nursing workload in a medical Intensive Care Unit. Intensive and Critical Care Nursing 47, 98—101.

Griffiths, R.D., Bongers, T., 2005. Nutrition support for patients in the intensive care unit. Post Graduate Medical Journal 81, 629—636.

Guyton, A.C., Hall, J., 2016. Pocket Companion to Guyton and Hall Textbook of Medical Physiology, thirteenth ed. Elsevier, Philadelphia.

Harrington, L., 2004. Nutrition in critically ill adults: key processes and outcomes. Critical Care Nursing Clinics of North America 16, 459—465.

Harrison, D., et al., 2014. External validation of the intensive care national audit & research centre (ICNARC) risk prediction model in critical care units in Scotland. BioMed Centre Anaesthesiology 14 (116). http://www.biomedcentral.com/1471-2253/14/116.

Higgins, C., 2013. Understanding Laboratory Investigations, for Nurses, Midwives and Health Professionals, third ed. Wiley and Sons, Chichester.

Hill, B.T., 2018. Role of central venous pressure monitoring in critical care settings. Nursing Standard 32 (23), 41—48.

Intravenous Nurses Society INS, 2016. Standards for Infusion Therapy. Becton Dickinson, Cambridge, MA.

Kiekkas, P., et al., 2008. Association between nursing workload and mortality of intensive care unit patients. Journal of Nursing Scholarship fourth quarter, 385—390.

Kisorio, L.C., Langley, 2016. End-of-live care in intensive care unit: family experiences. Intensive and Critical Care Nursing 35, 57—65.

Kiwanuka, F., Imanipour, M., Akhavan Rad, S., Masaba, R., Hagos Alemayehu, Y.H., 2019. Family members' experiences in adult intensive care units: a systematic review. Scandinavian Journal of Caring Sciences. https://doi.org/10.1111/scs.12675 [accessed: 4/4/19].

Knaus, W.A., et al., 1991. The APACHE III prognostic system risk prediction of hospital mortality for critically III hospitalized adults. Chest 100 (6), 1619—1636.

Lavallee, J.F., Gray, T.A., Dumville, J., Russell, W., Cullum, N., 2017. The effects of care bundles on patient outcomes: a systematic review and meta-analysis. Implementation Science 12 (1), 142.

Lecky, F., et al., 2014. Trauma scoring systems and databases. British Journal of Anaesthesia 113 (2), 286—294.

Logan, G., 2015. Clinical judgment and decision- making in wound assessment and management: is experience enough? British Journal of Community Nursing S21-2—S24-8.

Maher, A.B., 2016. Neurological assessment. International Journal of Orthopaedic and Trauma Nursing 22, 44—53.

Marieb, E.N., Keller, S., 2017. Essentials of Human Anatomy and Physiology, twelfth ed. Pearson, Harlow.

McCance, K.L., Huether, S.E., 2018. Pathophysiology: The Biologic Basis for Disease in Adults and Children, eighth ed. Mosby, St. Louis.

McInroy, A., Edwards, S.L., 2002. Preventing sensory alteration: a preventative approach. Nursing in Critical Care 75, 247−254.

McLernon, S., 2014. The Glasgow Coma Scale 40 years on: a review of its practical use. British Journal of Neuroscience Nursing 10 (4), 179−184.

Milovanovic, Z., Adeleye, A., 2017. Making Sense of Fluids and Electrolytes. Taylor and Francis, London.

Mitchell, M., Dwan, T., Takashima, M., Beard, K., Birgan, S., Wetzig, K., Tonge, A., 2019. The needs of families of trauma intensive care patients: a mixed methods study. Intensive and Critical Care Nursing 50, 11−20.

Molter, N.C., 1979. Needs of relatives of critically ill patients: a descriptive study. Heart Lung 8, 332−339.

National Institute for Health Care Excellence, 2013. Acute Kidney Injury: Prevention, Detection and Management. https://www.nice.org.uk/guidance/cg169.

National Institute for Health Care Excellence, 2014. Acute Coronary Syndromes in Adults. https://www.nice.org.uk/guidance/qs68.

National Institute for Health Care Excellence, 2017. Intravenous Fluid Therapy in Adults in Hospital. From: www.nice.org.uk.

National Institute for Health Care Excellence, 2018a. Non-invasive Ventilation − Improving Patient Experience and Outcomes through Understanding (INTU). From: https://www.nic.org.uk/sharedlearning/non-invasive-ventilation-improving-patient-experience-and-outcomes-through-understanding-intu.

National Institute for Health Care Excellence, 2018b. Heart Failure. http://www.nice.org.uk/guidance/conditions-and-diseases/cardiovascular-conditions/heart-failure.

Neal, M.J., 2005. Medical Pharmacology at a Glance, fifth ed. Blackwell Science, Oxford.

NICE, 2012. Venous Thromboembolic Disease: Diagnosis, Management and Thrombophilia Testing (updated 2015).

Noome, M., Dijkstra, B.M., van Leeuwen, E., Vloet, L.C., 2016. Exploring family experiences of nursing aspects of end-of-life care in the ICU: a qualitative study. Intensive and Critical Care Nursing 33, 56−64.

Nursing and Midwifery Council, 2015. The Code: Professional Standards of Practice and Behaviour for Nurses and Midwives. NMC, London.

Nursing and Midwifery Council, 2018. The Code - Professional Standards of Practice and Behaviour for Nurses, Midwives and Nursing Associates. NMC, London.

Nursing and Midwifery Council, 2018. Council Minutes 28th March Item 7b Standards for Prescribing and Medicines Management. NMC, London. https://www.nmc.org.uk/globalassets/sitedocuments/councilpapersanddocuments/council-2018/council-papers-march-2018.pdf.

Ochieng, B., Ward, K., 2018. Safeguarding of vulnerable adults training: assessing the effect of continuing professional development. Nursing Management 25 (4), 30−35.

Ojo, O., 2017. Enteral feeding for nutritional support in critically ill patients. British Journal of Nursing 26 (12), 666−669.

Orban, J.C., Walrave, Y., Mongardon, N., Allaouchiche, B., Argaud, L., Aubrun, F., et al., 2017. Causes and characteristics of death in intensive care units: a prospective multicentre study. Anesthesiology 126 (5), 882−889.

O'Tuathail, C., Taqi, R., 2011. Evaluation of three commonly used pressure ulcer risk assessment scale'. British Journal of Nursing 20 (6), s27−s34 (Tissue Viability Supplement).

Pritchard, M., 2010. Measuring Anxiety in surgical patients using a visual analogue scale. Nursing Standard 25 (11), 4−44.

Raghubir, A.G., 2018. Emotional intelligence in professional nursing practice: a concept review using Rodgers's evolutionary analysis approach. International Journal of Nursing Science. From: http://www.elsevier.com/journals/international-journal-of-nursing-sciences/2352-0132.

Reid, M.B., Allard-Gould, P., 2004. Malnutrition and the critically ill elderly patient. Critical Care Nursing Clinics of North America 16, 531–536.

Richards, A., Edwards, S.L., 2014. Essential Pathophysiology for Nursing and Healthcare Students. McGraw-Hill Education, Maidenhead.

Richards, A., Edwards, S.L., 2018. A Nurse's Survival Guide to the Ward, third ed. updated. Elsevier, Edinburgh.

Richards, A., 2009. A Nurse's Survival Guide to Drugs in Practice. Elsevier, Edinburgh.

Roberts, D., Ousey, K., 2004. Problem based learning: developing the triggers Experiences from a first wave site. Nurse Education in Practice 4 (3), 154–158.

Rodriguez, L., 2004. Nutritional status: assessing and understanding its value in the critical care setting. Critical Care Nursing Clinics of North America 16, 509–514.

Rogers, K.M.A., McCutcheon, K., 2013. Understanding arterial blood gases. The Journal of Perioperative Practice 23 (9), 191–197.

Rolfe, G., 2000. Research, Truth Authority: Post Modern Perspectives on Nursing. Macmillan, London.

Rowan, C.M., et al., 2015. Implementation of continuous capnography is associated with a decreased utilization of blood gases. Journal of Clinical Medicine Research 7 (2), 71–75.

Royal College of Nursing, 2015. Safeguarding Adults – Everyone's Responsibility: RCN Guidance for Nursing Staff. RCN, London.

Royal College of Nursing, 2016. Standards for Infusion Therapy. RCN, London.

Royal College of Physicians, 2017. National Early Warning Score (NEWS2) Standardising and the Assessment of Acute-Illness Severity in the NHS London. Royal College of Physicians.

Schantz, M.L., 2007. Compassion: a concept analysis. Nursing Forum 42 (2), 48–55.

Schell-Chaple, H.M., et al., 2018. Rectal and bladder temperature vs forehead core temperatures measured with SpotOn monitoring system. American Journal of Critical Care 27 (1), 43–50.

Schneiderbanger, D., Johannsen, S., Roewer, N., Schuster, F., 2014. Management of malignant hyperthermia: diagnosis and treatment. Therapeutics and Clinical Risk Management 10, 355–362.

Schon, D., 1983. The Reflective Practitioner. Basic Books, New York.

Shuvy, M., Atar, D., Steg, P.G., Halvorsen, S., Jolly, S., Yusuf, S., Lotan, C., 2013. Oxygen therapy in acute coronary syndrome: are the benefits worth the risk? European Heart Journal 34, 1630–1635.

Singer, P., Cohen, C., 2016. Severe undernutrition. In: Preiser, J. (Ed.), The Stress Response to Critical Illness. Springer International Publishing, Cham, pp. 187–195.

Smith, G.B., Osgood, V.M., Crane, S., 2002. ALERT – a multiprofessional training course in the care of the acutely ill adult patient. Resuscitation 52, 281–286.

Sving, E., et al., 2014. Factors contributing to evidence-based pressure ulcer prevention. A cross-sectional study. International Journal of Nursing Studies 51, 717–725.

Talbot, L.S., McGlinchey, E.L., Kaplan, K.A., Dahl, R.E., Harvey, A.G., 2010. Sleep deprivation in adolescents and adults: changes in affect. Emotion 10 (6), 831–841.

Tito, A., et al., 2018. Comparison of Revised Trauma Score Based on Intracranial Haemorrhage Volume among Head Injury Patients. Prague Medical Report 119 (1), 52–60.

Uleberg, O., et al., 2015. Temperature measurements in trauma patients: is the ear the key to the core? Scandinavian Journal of Trauma, Resuscitation and Emergency Medicine 23 (101). https://doi.org/10.1186/s13049-015-0178-z.

Venkataraman, R., 2018. Mortality prediction using acute physiology and chronic health evaluation II and acute physiology and chronic health evaluation IV scoring systems: is there a difference? Indian Journal of Critical Care Medicine 22 (5), 23–25.

Vincent, J.-L., Moreno, R., 2010. Clinical review: scoring systems in the critically ill. Critical Care 14 (207). http://ccforum.com/content/14/2/207.

Weijs, P.J.M., et al., 2014. Proteins and amino acids are fundamental to optimal nutrition support in critically ill patients. Critical Care 18 (591). http://ccforum.com/content/18/6/591.

WHO, 1996. Cancer Pain Relief, second ed. WHO, Geneva.

Wilson, J., 2012. Infection Control in Clinical Practice, fourth ed. Baillière Tindall, London.

Woodrow, P., 2004. Arterial blood gas analysis. Nursing Standard 18 (21), 45–52.

Woodrow, P., 2015. Neurological deficits. In: Woodrow, P. (Ed.), Nursing Acutely Ill Adults Routledge, pp. 183–193. http://ebookcentral.proquest.com/lib/rcn/detail.action?docID=2166421.

Wounds, U.K., 2017. Meeting CQUIN Targets: 'Improving the Assessment of Wounds'. https://www.wounds-uk.com.

Wung, S.F., Malone, D.C., Szalacha, L., 2018. Sensory overload and technology in critical care. Critical Care Nursing Clinics of North America 30 (2), 179–190.

Yogarajah, M., 2015. Disturbances of consciousness. In: Yogarajah, M., et al. (Eds.), Crash Course Neurology, Updated Edition. Elsevier, China, pp. 39–45. http://ebookcentral.proquest.com/lib/rcn/detail.action?docID=4336294.

Yucha, C., 2004. Renal regulation of acid-base balance. Nephrology Nursing Journal 31 (2), 201–206.

Relevant websites

www.afpp.org.uk

www.answers.com/topic/apache-ii

www.apache-msi.com/solutions/pspm.html

www.brit-thoracic.org.uk

www.brit-thoracic.org.uk/guide/guidelines.html

www.health.adelaide.edu.au/icu/qeh/files/icu_notes/outcome_icu.pdf

www.hpc-uk.org

www.nice.uk.org

www.nmc-uk.org

Further reading

Adam, S., Osborne, S., 2017. Critical Care Nursing: Science and Practice, third ed. Oxford University Press, Oxford.

Benner, P., 1984. From Novice to Expert: Excellence and Power in Clinical Nursing Practice. Addison-Wesley, London.

Bersten, A.D., Handy, J., 2018. Oh's Intensive Care Manual, eighth ed. Elsevier, Edinburgh.

Chioncel, O., Collins, S.P., Ambrosy, A.P., Gheorghiade, M., Filippatos, G., 2013. Pulmonary oedema — therapeutic targets. Cardiac Failure Review 1 (1), 38—45.

Cole-King, A., Gilbert, P., 2011. Compassionate care: the theory and the reality. Journal of Holistic Healthcare 8, 29—37.

Department of Health, 2000. Comprehensive Critical Care: A Review of Adult Critical Care Services. HMSO, London.

Edwards, S.L., O'Connell, C., 2007. Exploring bullying: implications for nurse educators. Nurse Education in Practice 7, 26—35.

Edwards, S.L., 2006. Tissue viability: understanding the mechanisms of injury and repair. Nursing Standard 21 (3), 48—57.

Edwards, S.L., 2007. Critical thinking: a two phase framework. Nurse Education in Practice 7, 303—314.

Edwards, S.L., 2008. Pathophysiology of acid base balance: the theory practice relationship. Intensive and Critical Care Nursing 24 (1), 28—40.

Gibbs, G., 1988. Learning by Doing: A Guide to Teaching and Learning Methods. Oxford Polytechnic Education Unit, Oxford.

Hall, J., Schmidt, G., Kress, J.P., 2015. Principles of Critical Care, fourth ed. McGraw-Hill Education, London.

Hall, J., 2015. Guyton and Hall Textbook of Medical Physiology, thirteenth ed. WB Saunders, Philadelphia PA.

Hillman, K., Bishop, G., 2009. Clinical Intensive Care and Acute Medicine, second ed. Cambridge University Press, Cambridge, UK.

Hughes, M., Grant, I. (Eds.), 2011. Advanced Respiratory Critical Care. Oxford University Press, Oxford.

Irwin, R.S., Rippe, J.M., Lisbon, A., Heard, S.O., 2012. Procedures, Techniques and Minimally Invasive Monitoring in Intensive Care Medicine, fifth ed. Lippincott Williams & Wilkins, Philadelphia.

Johns, C., 1995. Framing learning through reflection within Carper's fundamental ways of knowing in nursing. Journal of Advanced Nursing 22 (2), 226—234.

Khandelwal, N., Kross, E.K., Engelberg, R.A., Coe, N.B., Long, A.C., Curtis, J.R., 2015. Estimating the effect of palliative care interventions and advance care planning in ICU utilisation: a systematic review. Critical Care Medicine 43 (5), 1102—1111.

Langley, K.L.C., 2016. Intensive care nurses' experiences of end-of-life care. Intensive and Critical Care Nursing 30 (8), 30—38, 33.

Lansberg, J., 2017. Clinical Practice Manual for Pulmonary and Critical Care Medicine. Elsevier, Philadelphia.

Marmo, L., 2013. In: D'Arcy, Y.M. (Ed.), Compact Clinical Guide to Critical Care, Trauma, and Emergency Pain Management: An Evidence-Based Approach for Nurses. Springer Publishing, New York.

Martin, N.D., Kaplan, L.J., 2018. Principles of Adult Surgical Critical Care. Springer, Switzerland.

McCance, K.L., Huether, S.E., 2017. Pathophysiology: A Biological Basis for Practice, eighth ed. Mosby, St Louis.

McGloin, S., McLeod, A., 2010. Advanced Practice in Critical Care: A Case Study Approach. Blackwell Publishing Limited, Chichester.

Moore, T., Woodrow, P., Couling, S., 2009. High-dependency Nursing Care: Observation, Intervention and Support for Level 2 Patients, second ed. Routledge, London.

National Institute for Health Care Excellence, 2016. Extracorporeal Carbon Dioxide Remove for Acute Respiratory Failure. From: https://www.nice.org.uk/guidance/ipg564/chapter/3-the-procedure.

Padilha, K.G., et al., 2007. Nursing workload in intensive care units: a study using the Therapeutic Intervention Scoring System-28 (TISS-28). Intensive and Critical Care Nursing 23, 162—169.

Paw, H., Shulman, R., 2014. Handbook of Drugs in Intensive Care: An A—Z Guide, fifth ed. Cambridge University Press, Cambridge.

Peck, T.E., Hill, S.A., 2014. Pharmacology for Anaesthesia and Intensive Care. Cambridge University Press, Cambridge.

Rang, H.P., Ritter, J.M., Flower, R.J., Henderson, G., 2015. Pharmacology, eighth ed. Elsevier, Churchill Livingstone, Edinburgh.

Rehn, M., 2011. Prognostic models for the early care of trauma patients: a systematic review. Scandinavian Journal of Trauma, Resuscitation and Emergency Medicine 19 (17), 1—8. http://www.sjtrem.com/content/19/1/17.

Ridley, S., Smith, G., Batchelor, A. (Eds.), 2008. Core Cases in Critical Care. Greenwich Medical Media, London.

Seymour, J., 2001. Critical Moments: Death and Dying in Intensive Care. Open University Press, Buckingham.

Shailer, T.L., Harvey, C.J., Guyer, F., 1992. Principles of oxygen transport in the critically ill obstetric patient. NAACOGS: Clinical Issues in Perinatal & Womens Health Nursing 3, 392—398.

Skillbeck, J., Mott, L., Page, H., et al., 1998. Palliative care in chronic obstructive airways disease: a needs assessment. Palliative Medicine 12, 245—254.

Taylor, B.E., et al., 2016. Guidelines for the provision and assessment of nutrition support therapy in the adult critically ill patient: society of critical care medicine (SCCM) and American society for parenteral and enteral nutrition (A.S.P.E.N.). The Society of Critical Care Medicine and American Society for Parental and Enteral Nutrition 44 (2), 309—438.

Toth, P.P., Cannon, C.P., 2018. Comprehensive Cardiovascular Medicine in the Primary Care Setting.

VanBlarcom, A., McCoy, M.A., 2018. New nutrition guidelines; promoting enteral nutrition via a nutrition bundle. Critical Care Nurse 38 (3), 46—52.

Venkataraman, R., 2018. Mortality prediction using acute physiology and chronic health evaluation II and acute physiology and chronic health evaluation IV scoring systems: is there a difference? Indian Journal of Critical Care Medicine 22 (5), 23–25.

Wiseley, D., 2018. Advanced Mechanical Ventilation Made Easy: A Bedside Reference for RRTs, RNs, and Medical Residents.

Woodrow, P., 2011. Intensive Care Nursing: a Framework for Practice. Routledge, London.

Zuo, X.-L., Meng, F.-J., 2015. A care bundle for pressure ulcer treatment in intensive care units. International Journal of Nursing Science 2, 340–347.

Appendix 1

Units of measurement

UNITS (INTERNATIONAL SYSTEM OF UNITS), THE METRIC SYSTEM AND CONVERSIONS

The International System of Units (SI) or Système International d'Unités is the measurement system used for scientific, medical and technical purposes in most countries. In the United Kingdom, SI units have replaced those of the Imperial System, for example, the kilogram is used for mass instead of the pound (in everyday situations, both mass and weight are measured in kilograms although weight, which varies with gravity, is really a measure of force).

The SI comprises seven base units with several derived units. Each unit has its own symbol and is expressed as a decimal multiple or submultiple of the base unit by using the appropriate prefix, for example, millimetre is one-thousandth of a metre.

Base units

Quantity	Base unit and symbol
Length	Metre (m)
Mass	Kilogram (kg)
Time	Second (s)
Amount of substance	Mole (mol)
Electric current	Ampere (A)
Thermodynamic temperature	Kelvin ($°K$)
Luminous intensity	Candela (cd)

Derived units

Derived units for measuring different quantities are reached by multiplying or dividing two or more base units.

Quantity	Derived unit and symbol
Work, energy, quantity of heat	Joule (J)
Pressure	Pascal (Pa)
Force	Newton (N)
Frequency	Hertz (Hz)
Power	Watt (W)
Electrical potential, electromotive force, potential difference	Volt (V)
Absorbed dose of radiation	Grey (Gy)
Radioactivity	Becquerel (Bq)
Dose equivalent	Sievert (Sv)

Factors, decimal multiples and submultiples of SI units

Multiplication factor	Prefix	Symbol
10^{12}	Tera	T
10^{9}	Giga	G
10^{6}	Mega	M
10^{3}	Kilo	k
10^{2}	Hecto	h
10^{1}	Deca	da
10^{21}	Deci	d
10^{22}	Centi	C
10^{23}	Milli	M
10^{26}	Micro	μ
10^{29}	Nano	N
10^{212}	Pico	P
10^{215}	Femto	F
10^{218}	Atto	A

Rules for using units and writing large numbers and decimals

- The symbol for a unit is unaltered in the plural and should not be followed by a full stop except at the end of a sentence: 5 cm not 5 cm. or 5 cms.
- Large numbers are written in three-digit groups (working from right to left) with spaces not commas (in some countries, the comma is used to indicate a decimal point): fifty thousand is written as 50,000; five hundred thousand is written as 500,000.
- Numbers with four digits are written without space, for example, four thousand is written as 4000.
- The decimal sign between digits is indicated by a full stop positioned near the line, for example, 50.25. If the numerical value of the decimal is <1, a zero should appear before the decimal sign: 0.125 not .125.

- Decimals with more than four digits are also written in three-digit groups, but this time working from left to right, for example, 0.00025.
- 'Squared' and 'cubed' are expressed as numerical powers and not by abbreviation: square centimetre is cm^2 not sq. cm.

Commonly used measurements requiring further explanation

- Temperature – although the SI base unit for temperature is the Kelvin, by international convention, temperature is measured in degrees Celsius (°C).
- Energy – the energy of food or individual requirements for energy are measured in kilojoules (kJ); the SI unit is the joule (J). In practice, many people still use the kilocalorie (kcal), a non-SI unit, for these purposes.
- 1 calorie = 4.2 J.
- 1 kilocalorie (large calorie) = 4.2 kJ.
- Volume – volume is calculated by multiplying length, width and depth. Using the SI unit for length, the metre (m), means ending up with a cubic metre (m^3), which is a huge volume and is certainly not appropriate for most purposes. In clinical practice, the litre (l or L) is used. A litre is based on the volume of a cube measuring 10 cm × 10 cm × 10 cm. Smaller units still, for example, millilitre (mL) or one-thousandth of a litre, are commonly used in clinical practice.
- Time – the SI base unit for time is the second (s), but it is acceptable to use minute (min), hour (h) or day (d). In clinical practice, it is preferable to use 'per 24 hours' for the excretion of substances in urine and faeces: g/24 h.
- Amount of substance – the SI base unit for amount of substance is the mole (mol). The concentration of many substances is expressed in moles per litre (mol/L) or millimoles per litre (mmol/L), which replaces milli-equivalents per litre (mEq/L). Some exceptions exist and include haemo-globin and plasma proteins in grams per litre (g/L); and enzyme activity in International Units (IU, U or iu).
- Pressure – the SI unit of pressure is the pascal (Pa), and the kilopascal (kPa) replaces the old non-SI unit of millimetres of mercury pressure (mm Hg) for blood pressure and blood gases. However, mm Hg is still widely used for measuring blood pressure. Other anomalies include cerebrospinal fluid, which is measured in millimetres of water (mm H_2O), and central venous pressure, which is measured in centimetres of water (cm H_2O).
- To convert mm Hg to kPa, divide by 7.5 or multiply to do the opposite.
- To convert g/L to g/dL (decilitres), multiply by 10 or divide to do the opposite.

MEASUREMENTS, EQUIVALENTS AND CONVERSIONS (SI OR METRIC AND IMPERIAL)

Length

1 kilometre (km)	= 1000 metres (m)
1 metre (m)	= 100 centimetres (cm) or 1000 millimetres (mm)
1 centimetre (cm)	= 10 millimetres (mm)
1 millimetre (mm)	= 1000 micrometres (µm)
1 micrometre (µm)	= 1000 nanometres (nm)

Conversions

1 metre (m)	= 39.370 inches (in)
1 centimetre (cm)	= 0.3937 inches (in)
30.48 centimetres (cm)	= 1 foot (ft)
2.54 centimetres (cm)	= 1 inch (in)

Volume

1 litre (L)	= 1000 millilitres (mL)
1 millilitre (mL)	= 1000 microlitres (µL)

The millilitre (mL) and the cubic centimetre (cm^3) are usually treated as being the same.

Conversions

1 litre (L)	= 1.76 pints (pt)
568.25 millilitres (mL)	= 1 pint (pt)
28.4 millilitres (mL)	= 1 fluid ounce (fl oz)

Weight or mass

1 kilogram (kg)	= 1000 grams (g)
1 gram (g)	= 1000 milligrams (mg)
1 milligram (mg)	= 1000 micrograms (µg)
1 microgram (µg)	= 1000 nanograms (ng)

To avoid any confusion with milligram (mg), the word microgram (µg) should be written in full on prescriptions.

Conversions

1 kilogram (kg)	= 2.204 pounds (lb)
1 gram (g)	= 0.0353 ounce (oz)
453.59 grams (g)	= 1 pound (lb)
28.34 grams (g)	= 1 ounce (oz)

Temperature conversions

To convert Celsius to Fahrenheit, multiply by 9, divide by 5, and add 32 to the result:
For example, 36°C to Fahrenheit:

$$36 \times 9 = 324 \div 5 = 64.8 + 32 = 96.8°F$$

Therefore, 36°C = 96.8°F.

To convert Fahrenheit to Celsius, subtract 32, multiply by 5, and divide by 9:
For example, 104°F to Celsius:

$$104 - 32 = 72 \times 5 = 360 \div 9 = 40°C$$

Therefore, 104°F = 40°C.

Temperature comparison

Degree Celsius	Degree Fahrenheit
100	212
95	203
90	194
85	185
80	176
75	167
70	158
65	149
60	140
55	131
50	122
45	113
44	112.2
43	109.4
42	107.6
41	105.8
40	104
39.5	103.1
39	102.2
38.5	101.3
38	100.4
37.5	99.5
37	98.6
36.5	97.7
36	96.8
35.5	95.9
35	95
34	93.2
33	91.4

32	89.6
31	87.8
30	86
25	77
20	68
15	59
10	50
5	41
0	32
25	23
210	14

Boiling point = 100°C = 212°F.
Freezing point = 0°C = 32°F.

Appendix 2

Normal values

The values below represent an 'average' reference range, in adults, for blood, cerebrospinal fluid, urine and faeces. These ranges should be used as a guide only. Reference ranges vary between individual laboratories, and readers should consult their own laboratory for those used locally. This is especially important where reference values depend upon the analytical equipment and temperatures used.

BLOOD (HAEMATOLOGY)

Test	Reference range
Activated partial thromboplastin time	30–40 s
C-reactive protein	0–10 mg/L
Erythrocyte sedimentation rate	
Adult women	3–15 mm/h
Adult men	1–10 mm/h
Fibrinogen	1.5–4.0 g/L
Folate (serum)	4–18 µg/L
Haemoglobin	
Women	115–165 g/L (11.5–16.5 g/dL)
Men	130–180 g/L (13–18 g/dL)
Haptoglobins	0.3–2.0 g/L
International normalised ratio	0.9–1.1 s
Mean cell haemoglobin	27–32 pg
Mean cell haemoglobin concentration	30–35 g/dL
Mean cell volume	78–99 fL
Packed cell volume (haematocrit)	
Women	0.35–0.47 (35%–47%)
Men	0.4–0.54 (40%–54%)
Platelets (thrombocytes)	150–400 × 10^9/L
Prothrombin time	12–16 s
Red cells (erythrocytes)	
Women	3.8–5.3 × 10^{12}/L
Men	4.5–6.5 × 10^{12}/L
Reticulocytes (newly formed red cells in adults)	25–100 × 10^9/L
White cells total (leukocytes)	4.0–11.0 × 10^9/L

BLOOD VENOUS PLASMA (BIOCHEMISTRY)

Test	Reference range
Alanine aminotransferase (ALT)	10–40 U/L
Albumin	36–47 g/L
Alkaline phosphatase	40–125 U/L
Amylase	<200 U/L
Aspartate aminotransferase	10–35 U/L
Bicarbonate (arterial)	22–26 mmol/L
Bilirubin (total)	2–17 µmol/L
Caeruloplasmin	150–600 mg/L
Calcium	2.1–2.6 mmol/L
Chloride	95–105 mmol/L
Cholesterol (total)	Ideally below 5.2 mmol/L
HDL–cholesterol	>1.2 mmol/L
$PaCO_2$	4.4–6.1 kPa
Copper	13–24 µmol/L
Cortisol (at 08.00 h)	160–565 nmol/L
Creatine kinase (total)	
Women	30–135 U/L
Men	55–170 U/L
Creatinine	55–105 µmol/L
Gamma-glutamyl transferase	
Women	5–35 U/L
Men	10–55 U/L
Globulins	24–37 g/L
Glucose (venous blood, fasting)	3.6–5.8 mmol/L
Glycosylated haemoglobin (HbA_1)	4%–6%
Hydrogen ion concentration (arterial)	35–45 nmol/L
Iron	
Women	10–28 µmol/L
Men	14–32 µmol/L
Iron-binding capacity total	45–70 µmol/L
Lactate (arterial)	0.3–1.4 mmol/L
Lactate dehydrogenase (total)	230–460 U/L
Lead (adults, whole blood)	<0.5 µmol/L
Magnesium	0.7–1.0 mmol/L
Osmolality	275–290 mmol/kg
PaO_2	12–15 kPa
Oxygen saturation (arterial)	97%
pH	7.35–7.45
Phosphate (fasting)	0.8–1.4 mmol/L
Potassium (serum)	3.6–5.0 mmol/L
Protein (total)	60–80 g/L
Sodium	136–145 mmol/L
Transferrin	2–4 g/L
Triglycerides (fasting)	0.6–1.8 mmol/L
Urate	
Women	0.12–0.36 mmol/L
Men	0.12–0.42 mmol/L

Urea	2.5—6.5 mmol/L
Serum urate	
Women	0.09—0.36 mmol/L
Men	0.1—0.45 mmol/L
Venous oxygen saturation	65%—75%
Zinc	11—22 µmol/L

CEREBROSPINAL FLUID

Test	Reference range
Calcium	1.1—1.3 mmol/L
Chloride	120—170 mmol/L
Culture	Sterile
Glucose	2.5—4.0 mmol/L
Opening pressures (adult)	5—18 cm/H_2O
Protein	100—400 mg/L
Sodium	100—250 mmol/L
White cell count	0—5 white blood cell/µL
White cell type	Lymphocytes

URINE

Test	Reference range
Albumin/creatinine ratio	<3.5 mg albumin/mmol creatinine
Calcium (diet dependent)	<12 mmol/24 h (normal diet)
Copper	0.0—1.1 µmol/24 h
Cortisol	9—50 µmol/24 h
Creatinine	9—17 mmol/24 h
5-Hydroxyindole-3-acetic acid	10—45 µmol/24 h
Magnesium	2.4—6.5. mmol/24 h
Oxalate	
Women	0.04—0.31 mmol/24 h
Men	0.10—0.41 mmol/24 h
pH	4—8
Phosphate	600—1500 mg/24 h
Porphyrins (total)	90—370 µmol/24 h
Potassium (depends on intake)	25—100 mmol/24 h
Protein (total)	No more than 0.3 g/L
Sodium (depends on intake)	100—200 mmol/24 h
Urea	170—500 mmol/24 h
Zinc	300—600 µg/24 h

FAECES

Test	Reference range
Fat content (daily output on normal diet)	<7 g/24 h
Fat (as acid steatocrit)	<31%

Appendix 3

Drug measurement and calculations

The International System of Units is used for drug doses and concentrations and patient data (including weight and body surface area), drug levels in the body and other measurements (see Appendix 1 for more information).

WEIGHT

Grams (g) and milligrams (mg) are the units most often encountered in drug dosages. Doses of <1 g should be expressed in milligrams, for example, 250 mg rather than 0.25 g. Similarly, doses <1 mg should be expressed in micrograms, for example, 200 µg rather than 0.2 mg. Whenever drugs are prescribed in microgram dosages, the units should be written in full, for example, digoxin 250 micrograms, as the use of the contracted terms µg or mcg may in practice be mistaken for mg and, as this dose is 1000 times greater, disastrous consequences may follow.

Drug dosages are often described in terms of unit dose per kilogram of body weight, that is, mg/kg, µg/kg, etc. This method of dosage is frequently used for children and allows dosages to be tailored to the individual patient's size.

VOLUME

Litres (l or L) and millilitres (ml or mL) account for almost all measurements expressed in unit volume for the prescription and administration of drugs.

CONCENTRATION

When expressing concentration of dosages of a medicine in liquid form, several methods are available.

- Unit weight per unit volume — describes the unit of weight of a drug contained in unit volume, for example, 1 mg in 1 mL, 40 mg in 2 mL.

Examples of drugs in common use expressed in these terms: pethidine injection 100 mg in 2 mL; chloral hydrate mixture 1 g in 10 mL; phenoxymethylpenicillin oral solution 250 mg in 5 mL.

- Percentage (weight in volume) — describes the weight of a drug expressed in grams (g) which is contained in 100 mL of solution, for example, calcium gluconate injection 10%, which contains 10 g in each 100 mL of solution or 1 g in each 10 mL or 100 mg (0.1 g) in each 1 mL.
- Percentage (weight in weight) — describes the weight of a drug expressed in grams (g), which is contained in 100 g of a solid or semisolid medicament, such as ointments and creams, for example, fusidic acid ointment 2%, which contains 2 g of fusidic acid in each 100 g of ointment.
- Volume containing '1 part' — a few liquids and to a lesser extent gases, particularly those containing drugs in very low concentrations, are often described as containing one part per 'x' units of volume. For liquids, 'parts' are equivalent to grams and volume to millimetres, for example, adrenaline injection 1 in 1000 which contains 1 g in 1000 mL or expressed as a percentage (w/v) — 0.1%.
- Molar concentration — only very occasionally are drugs in liquid form expressed in molar concentration. The mole is the molecular weight of a drug expressed in grams, and a 1 molar (1 M) solution contains this weight dissolved in each litre. More often, the millimole (mmol) is used to describe a medicinal product, for example, potassium chloride solution 20 mmol in 10 mL indicates a solution containing the molecular weight of potassium chloride in milligrams ×20 dissolved in 10 mL of solution.

BODY HEIGHT AND SURFACE AREA

Drug doses may be expressed in terms of microgram, milligram or gram per unit of body surface area. This is frequently the case where precise dosages tailored to individual patients' needs are required. Typical examples may be seen in cytotoxic chemotherapy or drugs given to children. Body surface area is expressed as square metres or m^2 and drug dosages as units per square metre or units/m^2, for example, cytarabine injection 100 mg/m^2.

FORMULAE FOR CALCULATION OF DRUG DOSES AND DRIP RATES
Oral drugs (solids, liquids)

$$\text{Amount required} = \frac{\text{strength required} \times \text{volume of stock strength}}{\text{Stock strength}}$$

Parenteral drugs

1. Solutions (intramuscular, intravenous [IV] injections)

$$\text{Volume required} = \frac{\text{strength required} \times \text{volume of stock strength}}{\text{Stock strength}}$$

2. Powders
   It is essential to follow the manufacturer's directions for dilution, then use the appropriate formula.
3. IV infusions

$$\text{Rate(drops/min)} = \frac{\text{volume of solution} \times \text{number of drops per mL}}{\text{Time(min)}}$$

   a. Using standard giving sets (20 drops/mL) — clear fluids

   $$\text{Rate(drops/min)} = \frac{\text{volume of solution(mL)} \times 20}{\text{Time(min)}}$$

   b. Using filtered giving sets (15 drops/mL) — blood

   $$\text{Rate(drops/min)} = \frac{\text{volume of solution(mL)} \times 15}{\text{Time(min)}}$$

4. Infusion pumps

$$\text{Rate(mL/h)} = \text{Volume(mL)} \div \text{Time(h)}$$

5. IV infusions with drugs

$$\text{Rate(mL/h)} = \text{Amount of drug required(mg/h)} \times \frac{\text{volume of solution(mL)}}{\text{Total amount of drug(mg)}}$$

N.B. After selecting the appropriate formula, ensure that all strengths are in the same units, otherwise convert.

One percent solution contains 1 g of solute dissolved in 100 mL of solution.

1:1000 means 1 g in 1000 mL of solution; therefore, 1 g in 1000 mL is equivalent to 1 mg in 1 mL.

Other useful formulae

Children's dose (Clarke's body weight rule)

$$\text{Child's dose} = \frac{\text{Adult dose} \times \text{weight of child(kg)}}{\text{Average adult weight(70 kg)}}$$

Children's dose (Clarke's body surface area rule)

$$\text{Child's dose} = \frac{\text{Adult dose} \times \text{surface area of child(m}^2)}{\text{Surface area of adult(1.7 m}^2)}$$

Glossary

ABCDE of resuscitation Airway, breathing, circulation, disability, exposure

Activated partial thromboplastin time (APTT) A blood test which measures the intrinsic pathway

Acute Short and severe, not long drawn out or chronic

Airway Entry to the larynx from the pharynx

Allergy An altered or exaggerated susceptibility to various foreign substances or physical agents

Alveolar-capillary membrane The membrane between the alveolus and the capillary. Gas diffuses across the membrane from the alveolus to the capillary and vice versa

Alveolar pressure The pressure within the alveolus

Ambient pressure Surrounding air pressure

Apyrexia Absence of fever

Atrial fibrillation (AF) Atrial rate is fast, but few impulses reach the AV node; ventricular response is irregular — can be fast or slow AF

Benign A disorder or condition which does not produce harmful effects

BGL Blood glucose level

Bi-level positive airway pressure Continuous positive airway pressure is delivered at two levels (bi-level). The inspiratory airway pressure (IPAP) provides positive ventilation support on inspiration. The expiratory airway pressure (EPAP) provides the peep to aid gaseous exchange and to keep the alveoli expanded. Usually used in patients with type two respiratory failure

Biopsy Removal of some tissue or organ of the body for examination to establish a diagnosis

Blood viscosity The thickness of the blood

Boyle's law When temperature is constant, the pressure of gas varies inversely with its volume

Bronchospasm Narrowing of the bronchi by muscular contraction in response to a stimulus. The patient can usually inhale air into the lungs but requires visible muscular effort to exhale. A wheeze will be present

Cannula A hollow tube for the introduction or withdrawal of fluid from the body

Central venous pressure (CVP) The pressure of the blood within the right atrium. An individual catheter and a pressure manometer measure it

Coagulation activation The activation of the blood clotting process

Colitis Inflammation of the colon

Continuous positive airways pressure (CPAP) The use of a positive end expiratory pressure (PEEP) valve in the circuit provides the positive pressure and a resistance thus allowing the alveoli to remain slightly expanded creating a greater surface area for gaseous exchange to take place

Convulsion Involuntary contraction of muscle resulting from abnormal cerebral stimulation

Dalton's law The total pressure exerted by a mixture of gases is the sum of the pressures exerted independently by each gas in the mixture. The pressure exerted by each gas is directly proportional to its percentage in the total gas mixture

D-dimer levels Fibrinolysis is the process whereby the body responds to clot formations by removing the thrombus. Fibrin degradation fragments in the blood is the result of plasmin activation. D-dimers are the by product of this process. Therefore, if D-dimer levels are raised, then the person is likely to have had a thrombus

Deep vein thrombosis An obstruction of a deep vein by a blood clot, generally in the calf of the leg

Defibrillation Any agent, e.g., electric shock, which arrests ventricular fibrillation and restores normal rhythm

Dorsiflexion Flexing the foot up and down, flexing at the ankle

Duplex Doppler A method of measuring blood flow, using ultrasound. It is useful for estimating venous blood flow and so diagnosing thrombosis

Electrocardiogram (ECG) Reading of the electrical impulses in the heart

Embolism The condition in which there is obstruction of an artery by the impact of a solid body, thrombi, fat globules or air

Extrinsic pathway Fast method of blood clotting. Tissue cell trauma causes the release of tissue factor, which activates the clotting process. The extrinsic pathway is the pathway used when blood clots in the tissues

Fibrinolytic activity The action of fibrin within the body. Fibrin is the final product of blood coagulation. It joins with other molecules in a mesh-like structure to form a clot

Gas exchange The movement of oxygen and carbon dioxide between the alveolus and the capillaries

Gastric Pertaining to the stomach

Haematemesis Vomiting of blood

Haematocrit The percentage of red blood cells to total blood volume

Haematuria Blood in urine

Haemoconcentration An increase in the proportion of red blood cells relative to the plasma brought about by a decrease in the volume of plasma. It may occur in any condition when the body is dehydrated

Henry's law The amount of gas dissolvable in liquid is proportional to its pressure and solubility

Hepatitis Inflammation of the liver

Hydrostatic Pressure exerted by fluid

Hypercalcaemia High blood levels of calcium

Hyperglycaemia Excessive glucose in the blood

Hyperkalaemia High blood concentrations of potassium

Hypernatraemia High blood concentrations of sodium

Hypertension Increased blood pressure

Hypobaric At a pressure lower than that of atmospheric pressure

Hypotension Low blood pressure relative to the patient's age

Hypoxaemia Reduction of the oxygen concentration in the arterial blood recognized by cyanosis

Hypoxic When a person has a deficiency of oxygen in the tissues

Interstitial fluid Fluid contained between the cells and the capillaries

Intravascular fluid Fluid contained within the blood vessels, sometimes called extracellular fluid

Intrinsic pathway A slow method of blood clotting. Factor 12 (FXII) is activated by being triggered by a negatively charged platelet. They cling to the surface and activate the clotting process. The process produces FIXa, FVIIIa and calcium ions to ultimately produce fibrin. The intrinsic pathway is the pathway which initiates blood clotting within the circulatory system

Ischaemia An inadequate flow of blood to a part of the body, caused by constriction or blockage of the blood vessels supplying it

Ischaemic heart disease Deficient blood supply to cardiac muscle

Malaise Feeling of illness and discomfort

Malignant A disorder that becomes progressively worse if untreated

Meningitis Inflammation of the meninges

Metastasis Transfer of a disease from one part of a body to another

Myocardial infarction (MI) Blockage/occlusion of a coronary artery

Nausea Feeling of impending vomiting

Necrosis Localized death of tissue

Oxygen disassociation curve The S-shaped curve produced when haemoglobin saturation is plotted against the partial pressure of oxygen

Oxyhaemoglobin concentration The amount of haemoglobin combined with oxygen in the bloodstream

Parenteral nutrition (PN) Feeding of a patient intravenously via a CVP or long line

Partial pressure The pressure exerted by a single component of a mixture of gases

Prothrombin time (PT) A blood test which measures the extrinsic pathway

Pulmonary Relating to the lungs

Pulmonary embolism (PE) Obstruction of the pulmonary artery, or one of its branches, by an embolus, such as a blood clot

Pyrexia Fever or high temperature

Respiratory pressures The partial pressures of carbon dioxide and oxygen in various parts of the respiratory system

Sublingual Beneath the tongue

Tachycardia Increased rapid heart rate, generally above 100 beats per minute

Tachypnoea Abnormally fast respiration − greater than 20 breaths per minute

Thrombophlebitis Inflammation of the wall of a vein with secondary thrombosis occurring within the affected segment of vein

Tracheostomy Direct access to the trachea through the anterior opening of the neck. This can be performed surgically or percutaneously to provide an artificial and often temporary airway. The latter approach is common in the intensive care unit usually to support weaning from ventilator support.

Tracheotomy Fenestration in the anterior wall of the trachea by removal of a circular piece of cartilage from the third and fourth rings for establishment of a safe airway

Transfusion Introduction of fluid into the body

Vasodilatation An increase in the diameter of blood vessels

Venous stasis Sluggish circulation in which the metabolic demands of the cells are barely met. It can result in cell death and necrotic tissue developing

Index